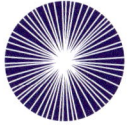

AMERICAN ACADEMY
OF OPHTHALMOLOGY®
Protecting Sight. Empowering Lives.

7 | Oculofacial Plastic and Orbital Surgery

Last major revision 2019–2020

2020–2021
BCSC
**Basic and Clinical
Science Course™**

EB○ Published after collaborative
review with the European Board
of Ophthalmology subcommittee

The American Academy of Ophthalmology is accredited by the Accreditation Council for Continuing Medical Education (ACCME) to provide continuing medical education for physicians.

The American Academy of Ophthalmology designates this enduring material for a maximum of 10 *AMA PRA Category 1 Credits*™. Physicians should claim only the credit commensurate with the extent of their participation in the activity.

CME expiration date: June 1, 2022. *AMA PRA Category 1 Credits*™ may be claimed only once between June 1, 2019, and the expiration date.

BCSC® volumes are designed to increase the physician's ophthalmic knowledge through study and review. Users of this activity are encouraged to read the text and then answer the study questions provided at the back of the book.

To claim *AMA PRA Category 1 Credits*™ upon completion of this activity, learners must demonstrate appropriate knowledge and participation in the activity by taking the posttest for Section 7 and achieving a score of 80% or higher. For further details, please see the instructions for requesting CME credit at the back of the book.

The Academy provides this material for educational purposes only. It is not intended to represent the only or best method or procedure in every case, nor to replace a physician's own judgment or give specific advice for case management. Including all indications, contraindications, side effects, and alternative agents for each drug or treatment is beyond the scope of this material. All information and recommendations should be verified, prior to use, with current information included in the manufacturers' package inserts or other independent sources, and considered in light of the patient's condition and history. Reference to certain drugs, instruments, and other products in this course is made for illustrative purposes only and is not intended to constitute an endorsement of such. Some material may include information on applications that are not considered community standard, that reflect indications not included in approved FDA labeling, or that are approved for use only in restricted research settings. **The FDA has stated that it is the responsibility of the physician to determine the FDA status of each drug or device he or she wishes to use, and to use them with appropriate, informed patient consent in compliance with applicable law.** The Academy specifically disclaims any and all liability for injury or other damages of any kind, from negligence or otherwise, for any and all claims that may arise from the use of any recommendations or other information contained herein.

All trademarks, trade names, logos, brand names, and service marks of the American Academy of Ophthalmology (AAO), whether registered or unregistered, are the property of AAO and are protected by US and international trademark laws. These trademarks include AAO; AAOE; AMERICAN ACADEMY OF OPHTHALMOLOGY; BASIC AND CLINICAL SCIENCE COURSE; BCSC; EYENET; EYEWIKI; FOCAL POINTS; FOCUS DESIGN (logo shown on cover); IRIS; ISRS; OKAP; ONE NETWORK; OPHTHALMOLOGY; OPHTHALMOLOGY GLAUCOMA; OPHTHALMOLOGY RETINA; PREFERRED PRACTICE PATTERN; PROTECTING SIGHT. EMPOWERING LIVES; and THE OPHTHALMIC NEWS & EDUCATION NETWORK.

Cover image: From BCSC Section 4, *Ophthalmic Pathology and Intraocular Tumors*. Photomicrograph depicting adenoid cystic carcinoma of the lacrimal gland. *(Courtesy of Vivian Lee, MD.)*

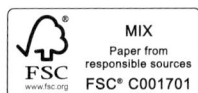

FSC® MIX Paper from responsible sources FSC® C001701 www.fsc.org

Printed in China.

Basic and Clinical Science Course

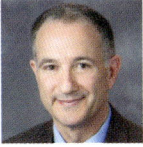

Christopher J. Rapuano, MD, Philadelphia, Pennsylvania
Senior Secretary for Clinical Education

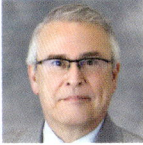

J. Timothy Stout, MD, PhD, MBA, Houston, Texas
Secretary for Lifelong Learning and Assessment

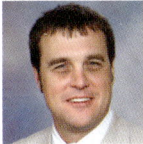

Colin A. McCannel, MD, Los Angeles, California
BCSC Course Chair

Section 7

Faculty for the Major Revision

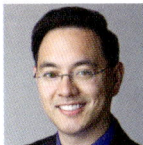

Bobby S. Korn, MD, PhD
Chair
La Jolla, California

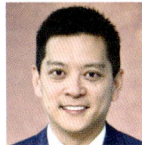

Pete Setabutr, MD
Chicago, Illinois

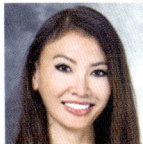

Cat N. Burkat, MD
Madison, Wisconsin

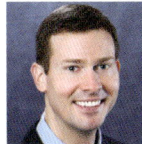

Eric A. Steele, MD
Portland, Oregon

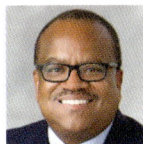

Keith D. Carter, MD
Iowa City, Iowa

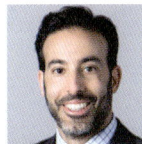

M. Reza Vagefi, MD
San Francisco, California

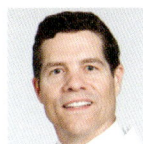

Julian D. Perry, MD
Cleveland, Ohio

The Academy wishes to acknowledge the *American Society of Ophthalmic Plastic and Reconstructive Surgery (ASOPRS)* for recommending faculty members to the BCSC Section 7 committee.

The Academy also wishes to acknowledge the following committees for review of this edition:

Committee on Aging: Claudia M. Prospero Ponce, MD, Houston, Texas

Vision Rehabilitation Committee: Terry L. Schwartz, MD, Cincinnati, Ohio

Practicing Ophthalmologists Advisory Committee for Education: Stephen R. Klapper, MD, *Primary Reviewer,* Carmel, Indiana; Bradley D. Fouraker, MD, *Chair,* Tampa, Florida; Alice Bashinsky, MD, Asheville, North Carolina; David J. Browning, MD, PhD, Charlotte, North Carolina; Cynthia S. Chiu, MD, Oakland, California; Steven J. Grosser, MD, Golden Valley, Minnesota; Troy M. Tanji, MD, Waipahu, Hawaii; Michelle S. Ying, MD, MSPH, Ladson, South Carolina

The Academy also wishes to acknowledge the following committee for assistance in developing Study Questions and Answers for this BCSC Section:

Self-Assessment Committee: Jurij R. Bilyk, MD, Philadelphia, Pennsylvania; Todd A. Goodglick, MD, Chevy Chase, Maryland; Renzo A. Zaldivar, MD, Morrisville, North Carolina

EB

European Board of Ophthalmology: Peter J. Ringens, MD, PhD, *EBO-BCSC Program Liaison,* Maastricht, Netherlands; Peter P. M. Raus, MD, *EBO Chair for BCSC Section 7,* Geel, Belgium; Lelio Baldeschi MD, PhD, Bruxelles, Belgium; Maria Borrelli, MD, Naples, Italy; Paul M. Jonckheere, MD, Antwerp, Belgium; Ilse Mombaerts, Prof. Dr, Leuven, Belgium

Financial Disclosures

Academy staff members who contributed to the development of this product state that within the 12 months prior to their contributions to this CME activity and for the duration of development, they have had no financial interest in or other relationship with any entity discussed in this course that produces, markets, resells, or distributes ophthalmic health care goods or services consumed by or used in patients, or with any competing commercial product or service.

The authors and reviewers state that within the 12 months prior to their contributions to this CME activity and for the duration of development, they have had the following financial relationships:*

Dr Burkat: Horizon Pharma (C)

Dr Browning: Aerpio Therapeutics (S), Alcon Laboratories (S), Alimera Sciences (C), Emmes (S), Genentech (S), Novartis Pharmaceuticals (S), Ohr Pharmaceutical (S), Pfizer (S), Regeneron Pharmaceuticals (S), Springer (P), ZEISS (O)

Dr Fouraker: Addition Technology (C, L), Alcon Laboratories (C, L), OASIS Medical (C, L)

Dr Grosser: InjectSense (O), Ivantis (O)

Dr Klapper: AdOM Advanced Optical Technologies (O)

Dr Korn: Elsevier (P), Horizon Pharma (C), Kaneka Pharma (C), Mallinckrodt Pharmaceuticals (C)

Dr Perry: Elsevier (P), US FDA Ophthalmic Devices Panel (C), Lacrimal Drainage Manometer Patent (P)

The other authors and reviewers state that within the past 12 months prior to their contributions to this CME activity and for the duration of development, they have had no financial interest in or other relationship with any entity discussed in this course that produces, markets, resells, or distributes ophthalmic health care goods or services consumed by or used in patients, or with any competing commercial product or service.

*C = consultant fee, paid advisory boards, or fees for attending a meeting; E = employed by or received a W2 from a commercial company; L = lecture fees or honoraria, travel fees or reimbursements when speaking at the invitation of a commercial company; O = equity ownership/stock options in publicly or privately traded firms, excluding mutual funds; P = patents and/or royalties for intellectual property; S = grant support or other financial support to the investigator from all sources, including research support from government agencies, foundations, device manufacturers, and/or pharmaceutical companies

Recent Past Faculty

Vikram D. Durairaj, MD
Jill Annette Foster, MD
Morris E. Hartstein, MD
Marsha C. Kavanagh, MD
Christine C. Nelson, MD

In addition, the Academy gratefully acknowledges the contributions of numerous past faculty and advisory committee members who have played an important role in the development of previous editions of the Basic and Clinical Science Course.

American Academy of Ophthalmology Staff

Dale E. Fajardo, EdD, MBA, *Vice President, Education*
Beth Wilson, *Director, Continuing Professional Development*
Ann McGuire, *Acquisitions and Development Manager*
Stephanie Tanaka, *Publications Manager*
Teri Bell, *Production Manager*
Susan Malloy, *Acquisitions Editor and Program Manager*
Jasmine Chen, *Manager of E-Learning*
Beth Collins, *Medical Editor*
Eric Gerdes, *Interactive Designer*
Naomi Ruiz, *Publications Specialist*
Debra Marchi, *Permissions Assistant*

American Academy of Ophthalmology
655 Beach Street
Box 7424
San Francisco, CA 94120-7424

Contents

PART III   Lacrimal System

14 Anatomy, Development, and Physiology of the Lacrimal Secretory and Drainage Systems

15 Abnormalities of the Lacrimal Secretory and Drainage Systems

General Introduction

The Basic and Clinical Science Course (BCSC) is designed to meet the needs of residents and practitioners for a comprehensive yet concise curriculum of the field of ophthalmology. The BCSC has developed from its original brief outline format, which relied heavily on outside readings, to a more convenient and educationally useful self-contained text. The Academy updates and revises the course annually, with the goals of integrating the basic science and clinical practice of ophthalmology and of keeping ophthalmologists current with new developments in the various subspecialties.

The BCSC incorporates the effort and expertise of more than 90 ophthalmologists, organized into 13 Section faculties, working with Academy editorial staff. In addition, the course continues to benefit from many lasting contributions made by the faculties of previous editions. Members of the Academy Practicing Ophthalmologists Advisory Committee for Education, Committee on Aging, and Vision Rehabilitation Committee review every volume before major revisions. Members of the European Board of Ophthalmology, organized into Section faculties, also review each volume before major revisions, focusing primarily on differences between American and European ophthalmology practice.

Organization of the Course

The Basic and Clinical Science Course comprises 13 volumes, incorporating fundamental ophthalmic knowledge, subspecialty areas, and special topics:

1 Update on General Medicine
2 Fundamentals and Principles of Ophthalmology
3 Clinical Optics
4 Ophthalmic Pathology and Intraocular Tumors
5 Neuro-Ophthalmology
6 Pediatric Ophthalmology and Strabismus
7 Oculofacial Plastic and Orbital Surgery
8 External Disease and Cornea
9 Uveitis and Ocular Inflammation
10 Glaucoma
11 Lens and Cataract
12 Retina and Vitreous
13 Refractive Surgery

References

Readers who wish to explore specific topics in greater detail may consult the references cited within each chapter and listed in the Basic Texts section at the back of the book. These references are intended to be selective rather than exhaustive, chosen by the BCSC faculty as being important, current, and readily available to residents and practitioners.

Multimedia

This edition of Section 7, *Oculofacial Plastic and Orbital Surgery,* includes videos related to topics covered in the book. The videos were selected by members of the BCSC faculty to present important topics that are best delivered visually. This edition also includes interactive features, or "activities," developed by members of the BCSC faculty. Both the videos and the activities are available to readers of the print and electronic versions of Section 7 (www.aao.org/bcscvideo_section07 and www.aao.org/bcscactivity_section07). Mobile-device users can scan the QR codes below (a QR-code reader must already be installed on the device) to access the videos and activities.

Videos

Activities

Self-Assessment and CME Credit

Each volume of the BCSC is designed as an independent study activity for ophthalmology residents and practitioners. The learning objectives for this volume are given on page 1. The text, illustrations, and references provide the information necessary to achieve the objectives; the study questions allow readers to test their understanding of the material and their mastery of the objectives. Physicians who wish to claim CME credit for this educational activity may do so by following the instructions given at the end of the book.

This Section of the BCSC has been approved as a Maintenance of Certification Part II self-assessment CME activity.

Conclusion

The Basic and Clinical Science Course has expanded greatly over the years, with the addition of much new text, numerous illustrations, and video content. Recent editions have sought to place greater emphasis on clinical applicability while maintaining a solid foundation in basic science. As with any educational program, it reflects the experience of its authors. As its faculties change and medicine progresses, new viewpoints emerge on controversial subjects and techniques. Not all alternate approaches can be included in this series; as with any educational endeavor, the learner should seek additional sources, including Academy Preferred Practice Pattern Guidelines.

The BCSC faculty and staff continually strive to improve the educational usefulness of the course; you, the reader, can contribute to this ongoing process. If you have any suggestions or questions about the series, please do not hesitate to contact the faculty or the editors.

The authors, editors, and reviewers hope that your study of the BCSC will be of lasting value and that each Section will serve as a practical resource for quality patient care.

Introduction to Section 7

With each major revision of a volume of the BCSC, the various contents *inside* the book undergo extensive review to modernize the information presented. Outdated material is eliminated, text is condensed and revised, figures are updated, and new treatments and features are introduced.

For approximately 4 decades, BCSC Section 7 has remained the same on the *outside,* carrying the title *Orbit, Eyelids, and Lacrimal System.* As of the 2019–2020 edition, the reader will note that the title changed to *Oculofacial Plastic and Orbital Surgery.* This change was a long time coming and reflects the continuing evolution of the subspecialty.

Sound knowledge of anatomy remains the bedrock of *Oculofacial Plastic and Orbital Surgery.* With this major revision, anatomy has been expanded beyond traditional drawings to include detailed anatomic sections to reflect more practical applications. Numerous clinical photos and diagrams have also been updated throughout, and 2 interactive online activity tools were added to enhance the learning of oculofacial anatomy and highlight the arterial danger zones of the face. In addition, several new videos highlighting clinical exam pearls and surgical techniques have been included.

This book is not meant as a thorough review of the field but rather serves as what a group of experts considers the most important highlights of the specialty. Readers interested in more comprehensive information can obtain additional detail from the selected references as well as from the sources listed on the Basic Texts page at the end of the book.

Objectives

Upon completion of BCSC Section 7, *Oculofacial Plastic and Orbital Surgery,* the reader should be able to

- describe the normal anatomy and function of orbital and oculofacial tissues

- identify general and specific pathophysiologic processes (including congenital, infectious, inflammatory, traumatic, neoplastic, and involutional) that affect the structure and function of these tissues

- select appropriate examination techniques and protocols for diagnosing disorders of the oculofacial and orbital systems

- select from among the various imaging and ancillary studies available those that are most useful for the particular patient

- describe appropriate differential diagnoses for disorders of the oculofacial and orbital tissues

- list the indications, advantages, and disadvantages for enucleation, evisceration, and exenteration

- describe functional and cosmetic indications in the medical and surgical management of oculofacial conditions

- state the principles of medical and surgical management of conditions affecting the oculofacial and orbital system

- describe the management of orbital compartment syndrome

- identify the major postoperative complications of oculofacial plastic and orbital surgery

PART I
Orbit

CHAPTER **1**

Orbital Anatomy

Highlights

- Sound knowledge of orbital anatomy is the foundation for diagnosis and management of orbital diseases.
- The orbit is composed of 7 bones that create a quadrilateral pyramid, which condenses to 3 walls at the orbital apex.
- Each of the orbital walls contains important landmarks and can be involved in disease processes.
- The optic canal and superior and inferior orbital fissures transmit the critical neurovascular structures of the orbit and can be anatomically subdivided by the annulus of Zinn.
- The vasculature of the orbit arises from the ophthalmic artery by way of the internal carotid artery. Branches of the ophthalmic artery subsequently form anastomoses with branches of the external carotid in the eyelid and periorbital region.
- The 4 paranasal sinuses are immediately adjacent to the orbit; they are rudimentary or very small at birth, developing and enlarging during childhood and adolescence.
- Pathologic processes in the paranasal sinuses can contribute to numerous diseases of the orbit.

BCSC Section 2, *Fundamentals and Principles of Ophthalmology*, also discusses ocular anatomy and includes many illustrations.

Dimensions

The orbits are bony cavities that contain the globes, extraocular muscles, nerves, fat, and blood vessels. Each bony orbit is pear shaped, tapering posteriorly to the apex and the optic canal. The medial orbital walls are approximately parallel and are separated by 25 mm in the average adult. The widest dimension of the orbit is approximately 1 cm behind the anterior orbital rim. Average measurements of the adult orbit are shown in Table 1-1. The intraorbital segment of the optic nerve has an S-shaped curve, allowing the eye to rotate and move forward with some freedom, without placing excessive tension on the posterior globe insertion (globe tenting).

Table 1-1 **Average Dimensions of the Adult Orbit**

Volume	30 cm³
Entrance height	35 mm
Entrance width	40–45 mm
Medial wall length	40–45 mm
Distance from posterior globe to optic foramen	18 mm
Length of orbital segment of optic nerve	25–30 mm

Topographic Relationships

The orbital septum arises anteriorly from the orbital rim. The paranasal sinuses are either rudimentary or very small at birth, and they increase in size through adolescence. They lie adjacent to the floor, medial wall, and anterior portion of the orbital roof. The orbital walls are composed of 7 bones: ethmoid, frontal, lacrimal, maxillary (maxilla), palatine, sphenoid, and zygomatic. The composition of each of the 4 walls and their location in relation to adjacent extraorbital structures are shown in Figures 1-1, 1-2, and 1-3 and summarized in the following sections.

Roof of the Orbit

The roof of the orbit is composed of the orbital plate of the frontal bone and the lesser wing of the sphenoid bone. It is located adjacent to the anterior cranial fossa and frontal sinus and includes the following important landmarks:

- the *fossa of the lacrimal gland,* which contains the orbital lobe of the lacrimal gland
- the *fossa for the trochlea of the superior oblique tendon,* located 5 mm behind the superonasal orbital rim
- the *supraorbital notch,* or *foramen,* which transmits the supraorbital vessels and the supraorbital branch of the frontal nerve

Lateral Wall of the Orbit

The lateral wall of the orbit is the thickest and strongest of the orbital walls. It is composed of the zygomatic bone and the greater wing of the sphenoid bone and is separated from the lesser wing (portion of the orbital roof) by the superior orbital fissure. It is located adjacent to the middle cranial fossa and the temporal fossa and commonly extends anteriorly to the equator of the globe, helping to protect the posterior half of the eye while still allowing wide peripheral vision. Important landmarks include the following:

- the *lateral orbital tubercle of Whitnall,* with multiple attachments, including the lateral canthal tendon, the lateral horn of the levator aponeurosis, the check ligament of the lateral rectus, and the Lockwood ligament (the suspensory ligament of the globe)
- the *Whitnall ligament,* which inserts onto the lateral orbital wall several millimeters (mm) above the lateral orbital tubercle via attachments to the lacrimal gland fascia
- the *frontozygomatic suture,* located 1 cm above the tubercle

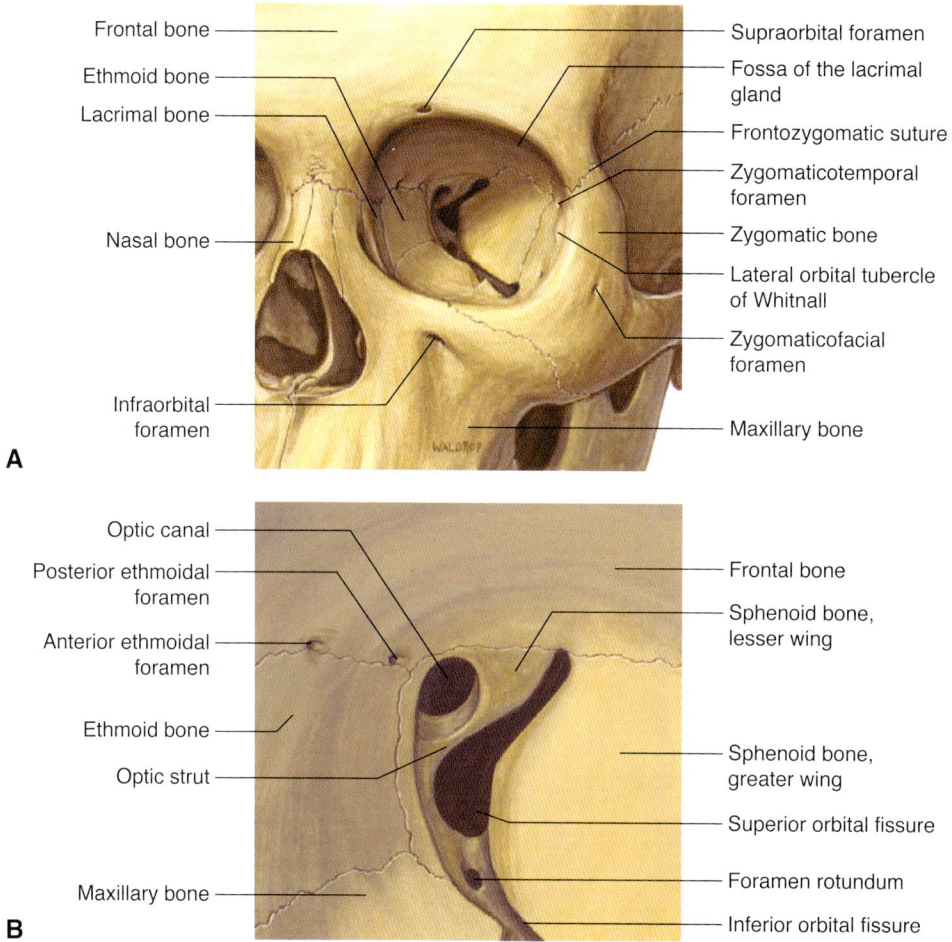

Frontal bone	Supraorbital foramen
Ethmoid bone	Fossa of the lacrimal gland
Lacrimal bone	Frontozygomatic suture
	Zygomaticotemporal foramen
Nasal bone	Zygomatic bone
	Lateral orbital tubercle of Whitnall
	Zygomaticofacial foramen
Infraorbital foramen	Maxillary bone

A

Optic canal	
Posterior ethmoidal foramen	Frontal bone
Anterior ethmoidal foramen	Sphenoid bone, lesser wing
Ethmoid bone	
Optic strut	Sphenoid bone, greater wing
	Superior orbital fissure
Maxillary bone	Foramen rotundum
	Inferior orbital fissure

B

Figure 1-1   Orbital bones. **A,** Frontal view. **B,** Apex. *(Reproduced with permission from Dutton JJ. Atlas of Clinical and Surgical Orbital Anatomy. Philadelphia: Saunders; 1994:8.)*

Medial Wall of the Orbit

The medial wall of the orbit is composed of the orbital plate of the ethmoid bone, the lacrimal bone, the frontal process of the maxillary bone, and the lesser wing of the sphenoid bone. Of these, only the lacrimal bone is wholly within the orbital confines. The medial wall of the orbit is located adjacent to the ethmoid and sphenoid sinuses and nasal cavity. The medial wall of the optic canal is formed by the lesser wing of the sphenoid, which is also the lateral wall of the sphenoid sinus.

An important landmark is the *frontoethmoidal suture,* which marks the approximate level of the cribriform plate, the roof of the ethmoids, the floor of the anterior cranial fossa, and the exit of the anterior and posterior ethmoidal arteries from the orbit.

The thinnest walls of the orbit are the *lamina papyracea,* between the orbit and the ethmoid sinuses along the medial wall, and the *maxillary bone,* particularly in its postero-medial portion. These are the bones most frequently fractured as a result of indirect, or

Sphenoid bone, greater wing
Superior orbital fissure
Anterior clinoid process
Optic canal
Sphenoid sinus
Pterygopalatine fossa

Frontal bone
Frontal sinus
Zygomaticotemporal foramen
Lateral orbital tubercle of Whitnall
Zygomatic bone
Zygomaticofacial foramen
Inferior orbital fissure
Maxillary bone
Maxillary sinus

A

Anterior cranial fossa
Frontal bone
Ethmoid bone
Lacrimal bone

Anterior ethmoidal foramen
Posterior ethmoidal foramen
Optic canal
Pituitary fossa
Sphenoid bone
Palatine bone

Maxillary bone
Maxillary sinus

Pterygopalatine fossa

WALDROP

B

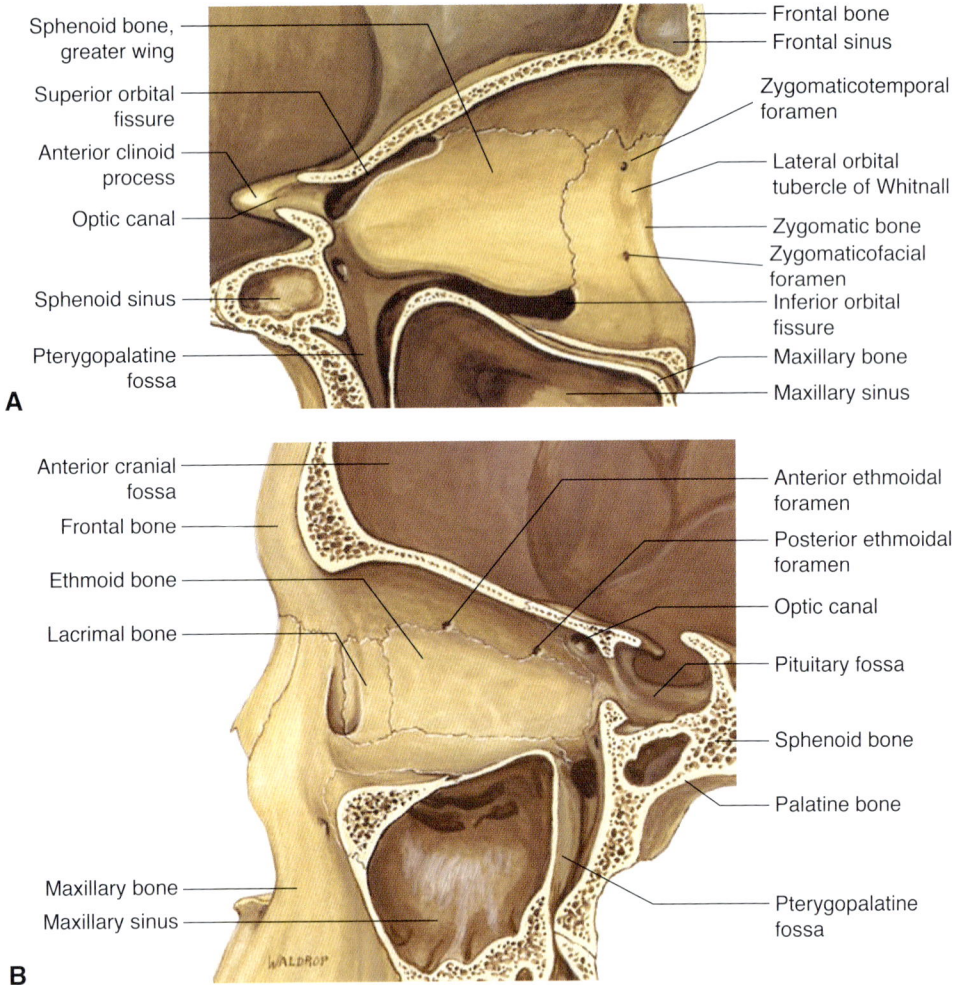

Figure 1-2 Orbital bones, internal views. **A,** Lateral wall. **B,** Medial wall. *(Modified with permission from Dutton JJ.* Atlas of Clinical and Surgical Orbital Anatomy. *Philadelphia: Saunders; 1994:9–10.)*

blowout, fractures (see Chapter 6 in this volume). Acute bacterial infections of the ethmoid sinuses may extend through the lamina papyracea or neurovascular perforations to form a subperiosteal abscess and extend into the orbital soft tissues.

Floor of the Orbit

The orbital floor is made up of the maxillary bone, the palatine bone, and the orbital plate of the zygomatic bone. The floor of the orbit forms the roof of the maxillary sinus. It does not extend to the orbital apex but instead ends at the pterygopalatine fossa; hence, it is the shortest of the orbital walls.

Important landmarks include the *infraorbital groove* and *infraorbital canal,* which transmit the infraorbital artery and the maxillary division of the trigeminal nerve.

Dutton JJ. *Atlas of Clinical and Surgical Orbital Anatomy.* 2nd ed. Philadelphia: Saunders; 2011.

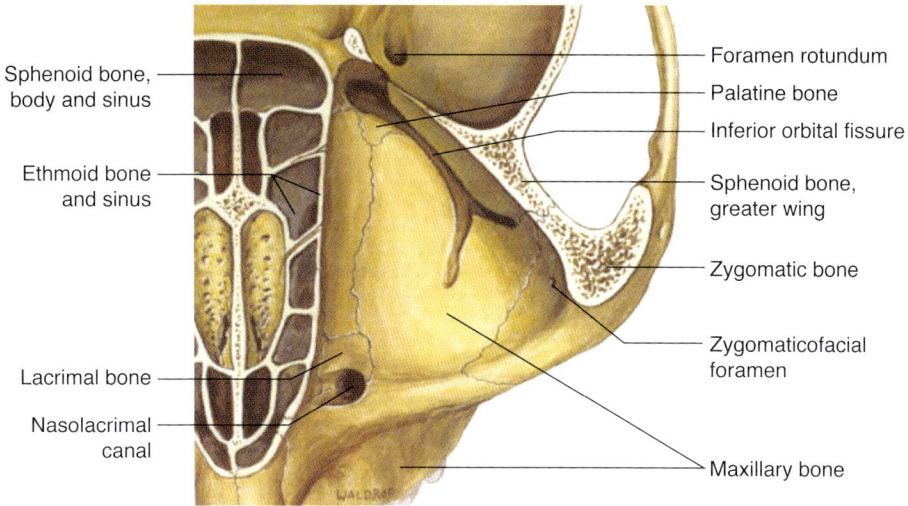

Figure 1-3 Orbital bones, orbital floor, internal view. *(Modified with permission from Dutton JJ.* Atlas of Clinical and Surgical Orbital Anatomy. *Philadelphia: Saunders; 1994:11.)*

Apertures

The orbital walls are perforated by several important apertures (see Figs 1-1 through 1-3).

Ethmoidal Foramina

The anterior and posterior ethmoidal arteries pass through the corresponding ethmoidal foramina in the medial orbital wall along the frontoethmoidal suture. These foramina provide a potential route of entry into the orbit for pathogens and neoplasms from the sinuses, and they also serve as a surgical landmark for the superior extent of medial wall surgery. Limiting manipulation of the medial orbital wall to the area below the level of the foramina helps prevent inadvertent entry into the cranial vault. Damage to the medial wall above the level of the foramina may disrupt a plane superior to the cribriform plate.

Superior Orbital Fissure

The superior orbital fissure separates the greater and lesser wings of the sphenoid bone and transmits cranial nerves (CNs) III, IV, and VI; the first (*ophthalmic*) division of CN V; and sympathetic nerve fibers. Most of the venous drainage from the orbit passes through this fissure via the superior ophthalmic vein to the cavernous sinus (Fig 1-4; see also Fig 1-1).

Inferior Orbital Fissure

The inferior orbital fissure is bounded by the sphenoid, maxillary, and palatine bones and lies between the lateral orbital wall and the orbital floor. It transmits the second

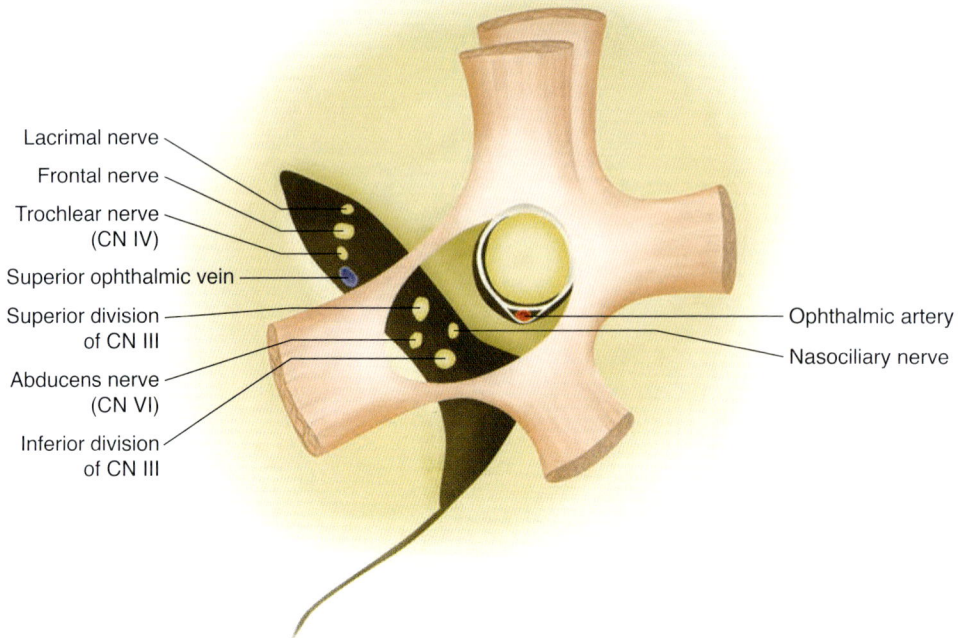

Lacrimal nerve
Frontal nerve
Trochlear nerve
(CN IV)
Superior ophthalmic vein
Superior division
of CN III
Abducens nerve
(CN VI)
Inferior division
of CN III

Ophthalmic artery
Nasociliary nerve

Figure 1-4 View of orbital apex, right orbit. The ophthalmic artery enters the orbit through the optic canal, whereas the superior and inferior divisions of cranial nerve (CN) III, CN VI, and the nasociliary nerve enter the muscle cone through the oculomotor foramen. CN IV, the frontal and lacrimal nerves, and the ophthalmic vein enter through the superior orbital fissure and thus lie within the periorbita but outside the muscle cone. Note that the presence of many nerves and arteries along the lateral side of the optic nerve mandates a superonasal surgical approach to the optic nerve in the orbital apex. *(Illustration by Cyndie C. H. Wooley.)*

(*maxillary*) division of CN V, including the zygomatic nerve, and branches of the inferior ophthalmic vein leading to the pterygoid plexus. The maxillary nerve (V_2) exits the skull through the foramen rotundum and travels through the pterygopalatine fossa to enter the orbit at the infraorbital groove. After giving off the zygomatic branch, the nerve becomes the infraorbital nerve and travels anteriorly in the floor of the orbit through the infraorbital canal, emerging on the face of the maxillary bone 1 cm below the inferior orbital rim. The infraorbital nerve carries sensation from the lower eyelid, cheek, upper lip, upper teeth, and gingiva.

Zygomaticofacial and Zygomaticotemporal Canals

The zygomaticofacial canal and zygomaticotemporal canal transmit vessels and branches of the zygomatic nerve through the lateral orbital wall to the cheek and the temporal fossa, respectively.

Nasolacrimal Canal

The nasolacrimal canal extends from the lacrimal sac fossa to the inferior meatus beneath the inferior turbinate in the nose. This canal transmits the nasolacrimal duct, which is continuous from the lacrimal sac to the nasal mucosa (see Part III, Lacrimal System).

Optic Canal

The optic canal is 8–10 mm long and is located within the lesser wing of the sphenoid bone. This canal is separated from the superior orbital fissure by the bony optic strut. The optic nerve, ophthalmic artery, and sympathetic nerves pass through this canal. The orbital end of the canal is the *optic foramen*, which normally measures less than 6.5 mm in diameter in adults. Optic canal enlargement accompanies the expansion of the nerve, as seen with optic nerve gliomas. Narrowing of the canal occurs in disorders such as fibrous dysplasia. Blunt trauma may cause an optic canal fracture or shearing of the pial vessels in the foramen, resulting in optic nerve damage.

Soft Tissues

Periorbita

The periorbita is the periosteal lining of the orbital bones. At the orbital apex, it fuses with the dura mater covering the optic nerve. Anteriorly, the periorbita is continuous with the orbital septum and the periosteum of the facial bones. The line of fusion of these layers at the orbital rim is called the *arcus marginalis*. The periorbita adheres loosely to the bone except at the orbital margin, sutures, fissures, foramina, tubercles, and canals. In an exenteration, the periorbita can be easily separated except where these firm attachments are present. Subperiosteal fluid, such as pus or blood, is usually loculated within these boundaries. The periorbita is richly innervated by sensory nerves.

Intraorbital Optic Nerve

The intraorbital portion of the optic nerve is approximately 30 mm long, which allows for eye movement without traction on the insertion of the nerve onto the globe. The optic nerve is 4 mm in diameter and is surrounded by the internal sheath, the arachnoid sheath, and the dural sheath, which are continuous with the pia mater, arachnoid mater, and dural mater covering the brain. The dura mater covering the posterior portion of the intraorbital optic nerve fuses with the annulus of Zinn at the orbital apex and is continuous with the periosteum of the optic canal.

Extraocular Muscles and Orbital Fat

The extraocular muscles are responsible for the movement of the eye and for synchronous movements of the eyelids. All of the extraocular muscles, except the inferior oblique muscle, originate at the orbital apex and travel anteriorly to insert onto the eye or eyelid. The 4 *rectus muscles* (superior, medial, lateral, and inferior) originate at the annulus of Zinn. The *levator palpebrae superioris muscle* arises above the annulus on the lesser wing of the sphenoid bone. The *superior oblique muscle* originates slightly medial to the levator muscle origin and travels anteriorly through the trochlea on the superomedial orbital rim, where it turns posterolaterally and inserts on the globe beneath the superior rectus muscle. The *inferior oblique muscle* originates in the anterior orbital floor lateral to the lacrimal sac and travels posterolaterally within the lower eyelid retractors to insert inferolateral to the macula.

In the anterior portion of the orbit, the rectus muscles are connected by a membrane known as the *intermuscular septum*. When viewed in the coronal plane, this membrane forms a ring that divides the orbital fat into the *intraconal fat (central surgical space)* and the *extraconal fat (peripheral surgical space)*. These anatomic designations are helpful for describing the location of a mass on magnetic resonance imaging (MRI) or a computed tomography (CT) scan. A knowledge of these spaces helps direct the surgical dissection to the mass.

The orbit is further divided by many fine fibrous septa that unite and support the globe, optic nerve, and extraocular muscles (Fig 1-5). Accidental or surgical orbital trauma can disrupt this supporting system and contribute to globe displacement and restriction. In some cases of diplopia after a fracture, restriction of eye movement is caused by the entrapment of the orbital connective tissue rather than by the muscles themselves.

The motor innervation of the extraocular muscles arises from cranial nerves III, IV, and VI. The superior rectus and levator muscles are supplied by the superior division of CN III *(oculomotor nerve)*. The inferior rectus, medial rectus, and inferior oblique muscles are supplied by the inferior division of CN III. The lateral rectus is supplied by CN VI *(abducens nerve)*. The cranial nerves to the rectus muscles enter the orbit posteriorly through the superior orbital fissure and travel through the intraconal fat to enter the intraconal surface of the muscles at the junction of the posterior third and anterior two-thirds.

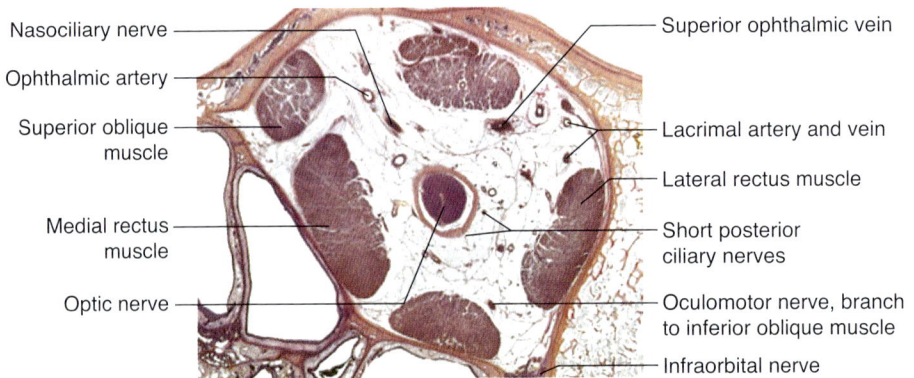

Figure 1-5 Cross section of the orbit at mid-orbit and at the widest extent of the extraocular muscles. Note the pink-stained fibrous tissue septa in the intraconal space. *(Modified with permission from Dutton JJ. Atlas of Clinical and Surgical Orbital Anatomy. Philadelphia: Saunders; 1994:151.)*

Cranial nerve IV (*trochlear nerve*) crosses over the levator muscle and innervates the superior oblique on the superior surface at its posterior third. The nerve to the inferior oblique muscle travels anteriorly on the lateral aspect of the inferior rectus to enter the muscle on its posterior surface.

Annulus of Zinn

The annulus of Zinn is the fibrous ring formed by the common origin of the 4 rectus muscles (Fig 1-6). The ring encircles the optic foramen and the central portion of the superior orbital fissure. The superior origin of the lateral rectus muscle separates the superior orbital fissure into 2 compartments. The portion of the orbital apex enclosed by the annulus is called the *oculomotor foramen.* This opening transmits CN III (upper and lower divisions), CN VI, and the nasociliary branch of the ophthalmic division of CN V (*trigeminal*). The superior and lateral aspect of the superior orbital fissure external to the muscle cone transmits CN IV as well as the frontal and lacrimal branches of the ophthalmic division of CN V. Cranial nerve IV is the only nerve that innervates an extraocular muscle and does not pass directly into the muscle cone when entering the orbit. A retrobulbar block therefore spares this muscle's action. Cranial nerves III and VI pass directly into the muscle cone through the oculomotor foramen. The superior ophthalmic vein passes through the superior and lateral portion of the superior orbital fissure outside the oculomotor foramen.

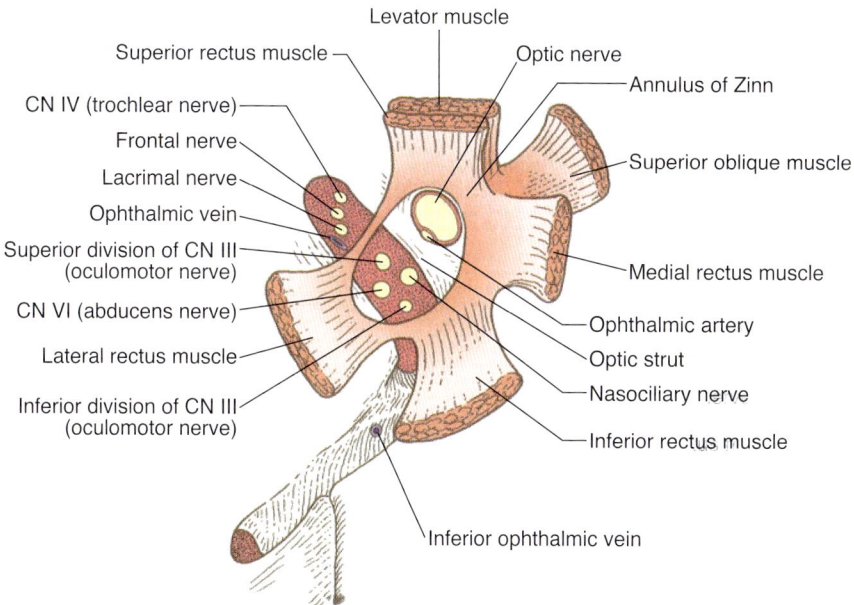

Figure 1-6 Anterior view of the right orbital apex showing the distribution of nerves as they enter through the superior orbital fissure and optic canal. This view also shows the annulus of Zinn, the fibrous ring formed by the common origin of the 4 rectus muscles. *(Modified with permission from Nerad JA.* Techniques in Ophthalmic Plastic Surgery. *Philadelphia: Saunders; 2010.)*

Vasculature of the Orbit

The blood supply to the orbit arises primarily from the *ophthalmic artery* (Figs 1-7, 1-8), which is a branch of the internal carotid artery. Smaller contributions come from the external carotid artery by way of the internal maxillary and facial arteries. The ophthalmic artery travels underneath the intracranial optic nerve through the dura mater along the optic canal to enter the orbit. The major branches of the ophthalmic artery are the

- branches to the extraocular muscles
- central retinal artery (to the optic nerve and retina)
- posterior ciliary arteries (long to the anterior segment and short to the choroid)

Terminal branches of the ophthalmic artery travel anteriorly and form rich anastomoses with branches of the external carotid in the face and periorbital region (Fig 1-9).

The *superior ophthalmic vein* provides the main venous drainage of the orbit (see Figs 1-7, 1-8). This vein originates in the superonasal quadrant of the orbit and extends posteriorly through the superior orbital fissure into the cavernous sinus. Frequently, the superior ophthalmic vein appears on axial orbital CT scans as the only structure coursing diagonally through the superior orbit. Many anastomoses occur anteriorly with the veins of the face as well as posteriorly with the pterygoid plexus.

Lymphatic System of the Orbit

The presence of a human orbital lymphatic system has not been established. However, experimental studies in monkeys have identified orbital lymphatic vessels by means of enzyme histochemistry and electron microscopy in the conjunctiva, lacrimal glands, and dura and arachnoid of the optic nerve. Despite the controversy, it is likely that human orbital lymphatics exist and may clinically explain the drainage of orbital edema fluid and the existence of orbital lymphatic malformations (*lymphangiomas*).

Dickinson AJ, Gausas RE. Orbital lymphatics: do they exist? *Eye (Lond).* 2006; 20(10):1145–1148.

Nerves

Sensory innervation to the periorbital area is provided by the ophthalmic and maxillary divisions of CN V (Fig 1-10). After branching off at the trigeminal ganglion, the ophthalmic division of CN V travels in the lateral wall of the cavernous sinus, where it divides into 3 main branches: frontal, lacrimal, and nasociliary. The *frontal nerve* and *lacrimal nerve* enter the orbit through the superior orbital fissure above the annulus of Zinn (see Fig 1-6) and travel anteriorly in the extraconal fat to innervate the medial canthus (*supratrochlear branch*), upper eyelid (*lacrimal* and *supratrochlear branches*), and forehead (*supraorbital branch*). The *nasociliary branch* enters the orbit through the superior orbital fissure within the annulus of Zinn, entering the intraconal space and traveling anteriorly to innervate the eye via the ciliary branches. The short ciliary nerves penetrate the sclera after passing through the ciliary ganglion without synapse. The long ciliary nerves pass by the ciliary ganglion and enter the sclera, where they extend anteriorly to supply the iris, cornea, and ciliary muscle.

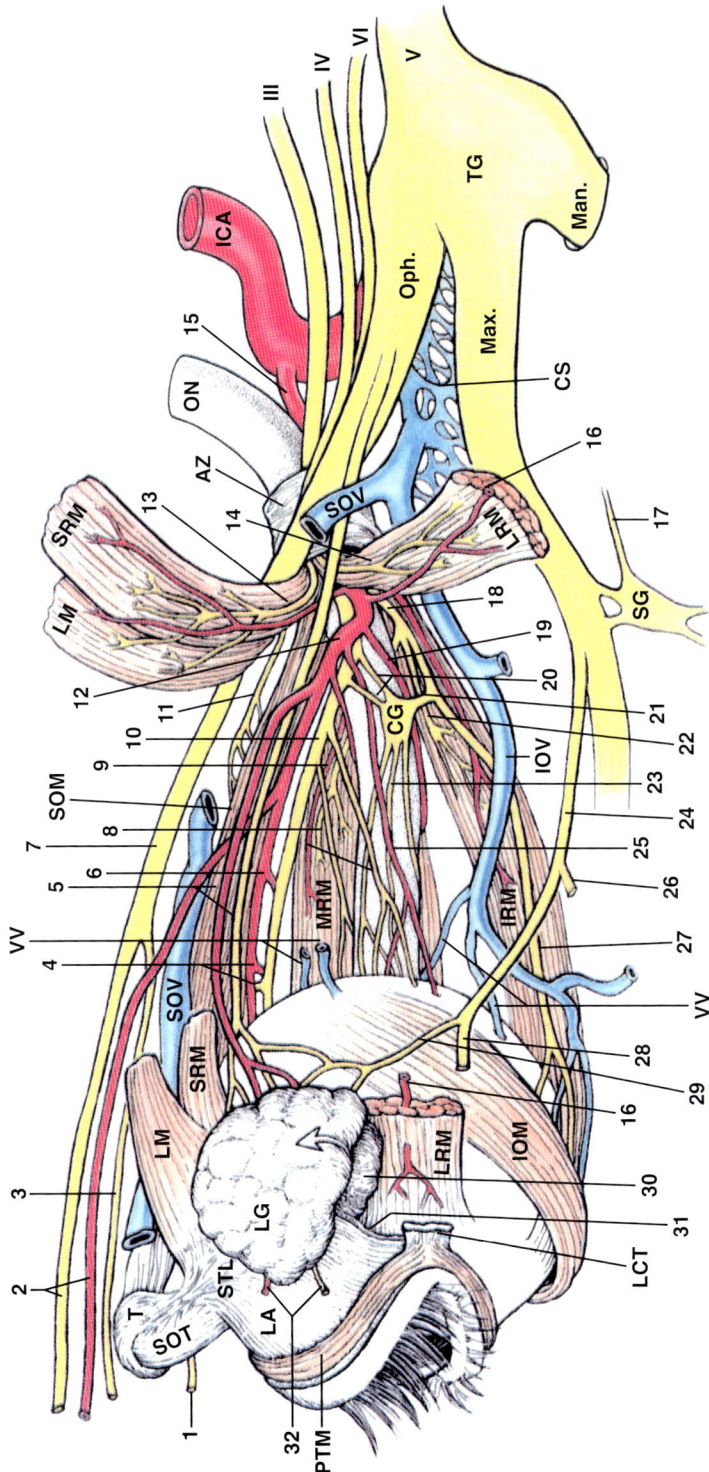

Figure 1-7 Side view of left orbit. AZ, annulus of Zinn; CG, ciliary ganglion; CS, cavernous sinus; ICA, internal carotid artery; IOM, inferior oblique muscle; IOV, inferior ophthalmic vein; IRM, inferior rectus muscle; LA, levator aponeurosis; LCT, lateral canthal tendon; LG, lacrimal gland; LM, levator muscle; LRM, lateral rectus muscle; Man., mandibular nerve; Max., maxillary nerve; MRM, medial rectus muscle; ON, optic nerve; Oph., ophthalmic nerve; PTM, pretarsal muscle; SG, sphenopalatine ganglion; SOM, superior oblique muscle; SOT, superior oblique tendon; SOV, superior ophthalmic vein; SRM, superior rectus muscle; STL, superior transverse ligament; T, trochlea; TG, trigeminal (Gasserian) ganglion; VV, vortex veins; 1, infratrochlear nerve; 2, supraorbital nerve and artery; 3, supratrochlear nerve; 4, anterior ethmoid nerve and artery; 5, lacrimal nerve and artery; 6, posterior ethmoid artery; 7, frontal nerve; 8, long ciliary nerves; 9, branch of CN III to medial rectus muscle; 10, nasociliary nerve; 11, CN IV; 12, ophthalmic (orbital) artery; 13, superior ramus of CN III; 14, CN VI; 15, ophthalmic artery, origin; 16, anterior ciliary artery; 17, vidian nerve; 18, inferior ramus of CN III; 19, central retinal artery; 20, sensory branches from ciliary ganglion to nasociliary nerve; 21, motor (parasympathetic) nerve to ciliary ganglion from nerve to inferior oblique muscle; 22, branch of CN III to inferior rectus muscle; 23, short ciliary nerves; 24, zygomatic nerve; 25, posterior ciliary arteries; 26, zygomaticofacial nerve; 27, nerve to inferior oblique muscle; 28, zygomaticotemporal nerve; 29, lacrimal secretory nerve; 30, lacrimal gland–palpebral lobe; 31, lateral horn of levator aponeurosis; 32, lacrimal artery and nerve terminal branches. *(Reproduced from Stewart WB, ed. Ophthalmic Plastic and Reconstructive Surgery. 4th ed. San Francisco: American Academy of Ophthalmology Manuals Program; 1984.)*

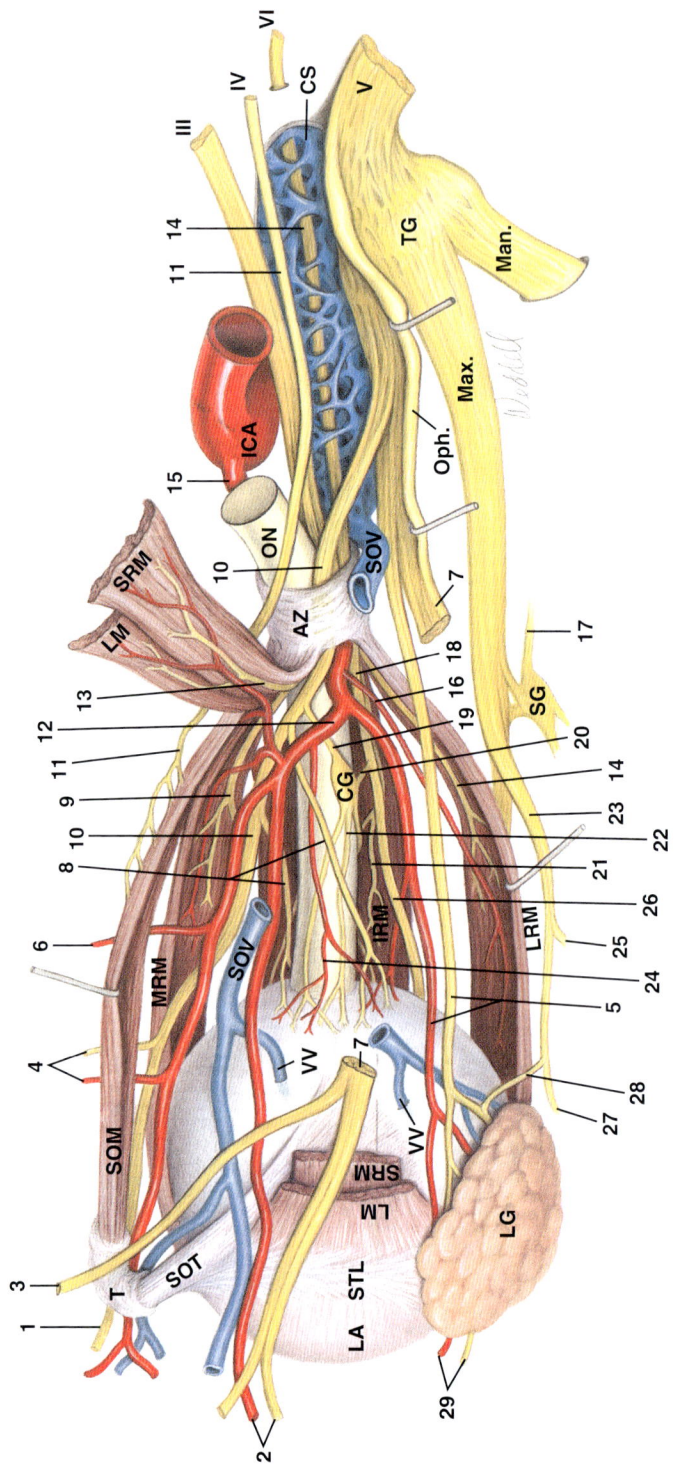

Figure 1-8 Top view of left orbit. AZ, annulus of Zinn; CG, ciliary ganglion; CS, cavernous sinus; ICA, internal carotid artery; IRM, inferior rectus muscle; LA, levator aponeurosis; LG, lacrimal gland; LM, levator muscle; LRM, lateral rectus muscle; Man., mandibular nerve; Max., maxillary nerve; MRM, medial rectus muscle; ON, optic nerve; Oph., ophthalmic nerve; SG, sphenopalatine ganglion; SOM, superior oblique muscle; SOT, superior oblique tendon; SOV, superior ophthalmic vein; SRM, superior rectus muscle; STL, superior transverse ligament; T, trochlea; TG, trigeminal (Gasserian) ganglion; VV, vortex veins; 1, infratrochlear nerve; 2, supraorbital nerve and artery; 3, supratrochlear nerve; 4, anterior ethmoid nerve and artery; 5, lacrimal nerve and artery; 6, posterior ethmoid artery; 7, frontal nerve; 8, long ciliary nerves; 9, branch of CN III to medial rectus muscle; 10, nasociliary nerve; 11, CN IV; 12, ophthalmic (orbital) artery; 13, superior ramus of CN III; 14, CN VI; 15, ophthalmic artery, origin; 16, anterior ciliary artery; 17, vidian nerve; 18, inferior ramus of CN III; 19, sensory branches from ciliary ganglion to nasociliary nerve; 20, motor (parasympathetic) nerve to ciliary ganglion from nerve to inferior oblique muscle; 21, branch of CN III to inferior rectus muscle; 22, short ciliary nerves; 23, zygomatic nerve; 24, posterior ciliary arteries; 25, zygomaticofacial nerve; 26, nerve to inferior oblique muscle; 27, zygomaticotemporal nerve; 28, lacrimal secretory nerve; 29, lacrimal artery and nerve terminal branches. *(Reproduced from Stewart WB, ed. Ophthalmic Plastic and Reconstructive Surgery. 4th ed. San Francisco: American Academy of Ophthalmology Manuals Program; 1984.)*

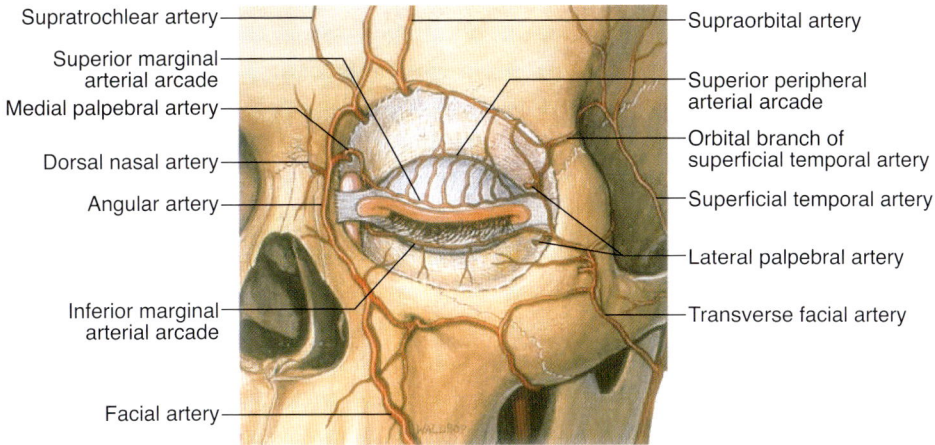

Figure 1-9 Periorbital and eyelid arteries, frontal view. *(Reproduced with permission from Dutton JJ.* Atlas of Clinical and Surgical Orbital Anatomy. *Philadelphia: Saunders; 1994.)*

The muscles of facial expression, including the orbicularis oculi, procerus, corrugator supercilii, and frontalis muscles, receive their motor supply by way of branches of CN VII (the facial nerve) that enter on the undersurface of each muscle.

The parasympathetic innervation, which controls accommodation, pupillary constriction, and lacrimal gland stimulation, follows a complicated course. Parasympathetic innervation enters the eye as the short posterior ciliary nerves after synapsing within the ciliary ganglion. Parasympathetic innervation to the lacrimal gland originates in the lacrimal nucleus of the pons and eventually joins the lacrimal nerve to enter the lacrimal gland.

Sympathetic activity originates in the hypothalamus, with sympathetic fibers descending through the brainstem to the spinal cord, where they continue. Fibers destined for the orbit synapse in the ciliospinal center of Budge-Waller and then travel with branches of the carotid artery to enter the orbit. The sympathetic nerves carry innervation for pupillary dilation, vasoconstriction, smooth muscle function of the eyelids and orbit, and hidrosis. The nerve fibers follow the arterial supply to the pupil, eyelids, and orbit and travel anteriorly in association with the long ciliary nerves. Interruption of this innervation results in the familiar signs of Horner syndrome: ptosis of the upper eyelid, elevation of the lower eyelid, miosis, anhidrosis, and vasodilation. See Chapter 1 in BCSC Section 5, *Neuro-Ophthalmology,* for detailed discussion of neuro-ophthalmic anatomy.

Lacrimal Gland

The lacrimal gland is composed of a larger *orbital lobe* and a smaller *palpebral lobe*. The gland is located within a fossa of the frontal bone in the superotemporal orbit. Ducts from both lobes pass through the palpebral lobe and empty into the upper conjunctival fornix. Frequently, a portion of the palpebral lobe is visible on slit-lamp examination with the upper eyelid everted. Biopsy is generally not performed on the palpebral lobe or temporal conjunctival fornix because it can interfere with lacrimal drainage. The orbital lobe of the lacrimal gland may prolapse inferiorly out of the fossa and present as a mass in the lateral upper eyelid.

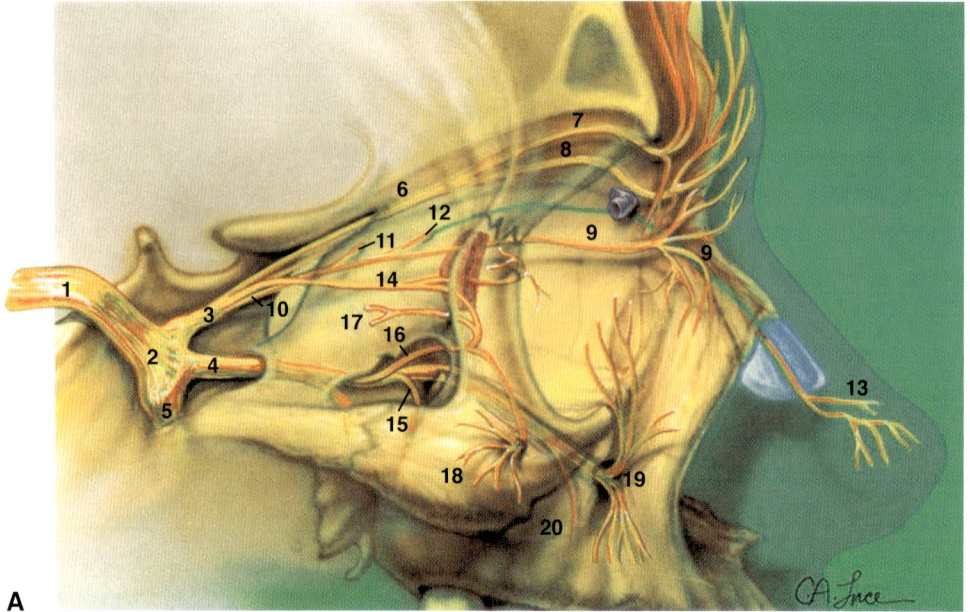

A

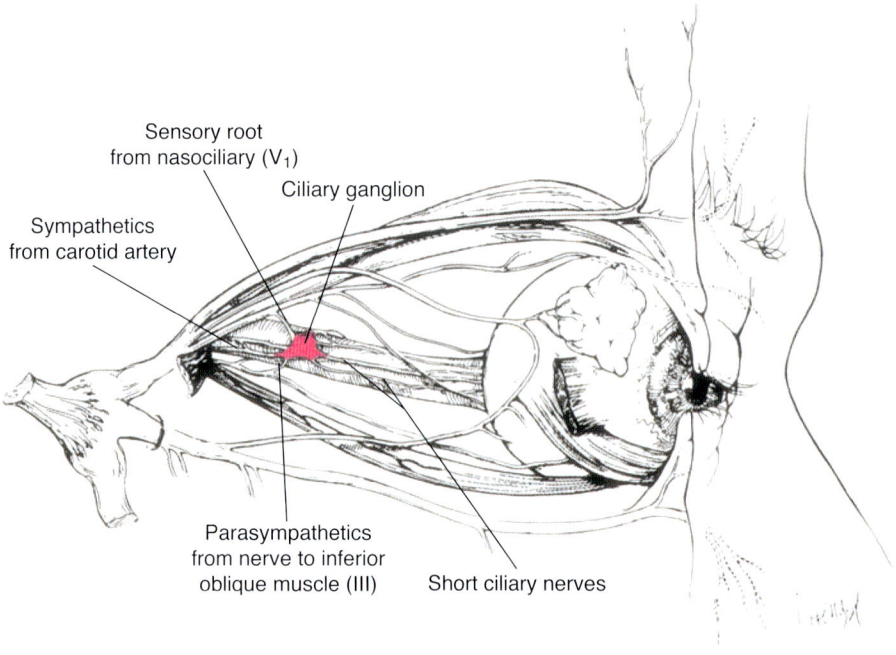

Sensory root
from nasociliary (V₁)

Ciliary ganglion

Sympathetics
from carotid artery

Parasympathetics
from nerve to inferior
oblique muscle (III)

Short ciliary nerves

B

Figure 1-10   Sensory innervation of the periorbital area. **A,** Sensory nerves. 1, CN V (trigemi-nal); 2, trigeminal ganglion; 3, ophthalmic division of CN V (V_1); 4, maxillary division of CN V (V_2); 5, mandibular division of CN V (V_3); 6, frontal nerve; 7, supraorbital nerve; 8, supratrochlear nerve (trochlea noted by purple); 9, infratrochlear nerve; 10, nasociliary nerve; 11, posterior ethmoidal nerve; 12, anterior ethmoidal nerve; 13, external or dorsal nasal nerve; 14, lacri-mal nerve; 15, posterior superior alveolar nerve; 16, zygomatic nerve; 17, zygomaticotemporal nerve; 18, zygomaticofacial nerve; 19, infraorbital nerve; 20, anterior superior alveolar nerve. **B,** Contributions to the ciliary ganglion. *(Part A reproduced with permission from Zide BM, Jelks GW, eds.* Sur-gical Anatomy of the Orbit. *New York: Raven; 1985:12. Part B reproduced with permission from Doxanas MT, Anderson RL.* Clinical Orbital Anatomy. *Baltimore: Williams & Wilkins; 1984.)*

Periorbital Structures

Nose and Paranasal Sinuses

The bones forming the medial, inferior, and superior orbital walls are close to the nasal cavity and are pneumatized by the paranasal sinuses, which arise from and drain into the nasal cavity. The sinuses decrease the weight of the skull and function as resonators for the voice. The sinuses also support the nasal passages by trapping irritants and by warming and humidifying inhaled air. Pathophysiologic processes in these spaces that secondarily affect the orbit include sinonasal carcinomas, inverted papillomas, zygomycoses, granulomatosis with polyangiitis (formerly, Wegener granulomatosis), and mucoceles, as well as sinusitis, which may cause orbital cellulitis or abscess.

The nasal cavity is divided into 2 nasal fossae by the nasal septum. The lateral wall of the nose has 3 bony projections: the superior, middle, and inferior conchae (*turbinates*). The turbinates are covered by nasal mucosa, and they overhang the corresponding meati. Just cephalad to the superior concha is the *sphenoethmoidal recess*, into which the sphenoid sinus drains. The frontal sinus, the maxillary sinus, and the anterior and middle ethmoid air cells drain into the middle meatus. The nasolacrimal duct opens into the inferior meatus. The nasal cavity is lined by a pseudostratified, ciliated columnar epithelium with copious goblet cells. The mucous membrane overlying the lateral alar cartilage is hair-bearing and, therefore, less suitable for use as a composite graft in eyelid reconstruction than the mucoperichondrium over the nasal septum.

The *frontal sinuses* develop from evaginations of the frontal recess and cannot be seen radiographically until the sixth year of life. Pneumatization of the frontal bone continues through childhood and is complete by early adulthood (Fig 1-11). The sinuses can develop asymmetrically and vary greatly in size and shape. Each frontal sinus drains through a separate frontonasal duct and empties into the anterior portion of the middle meatus.

The *ethmoid air cells* are thin-walled cavities that lie between the medial orbital wall and the lateral wall of the nose. They are present at birth and expand as the child grows.

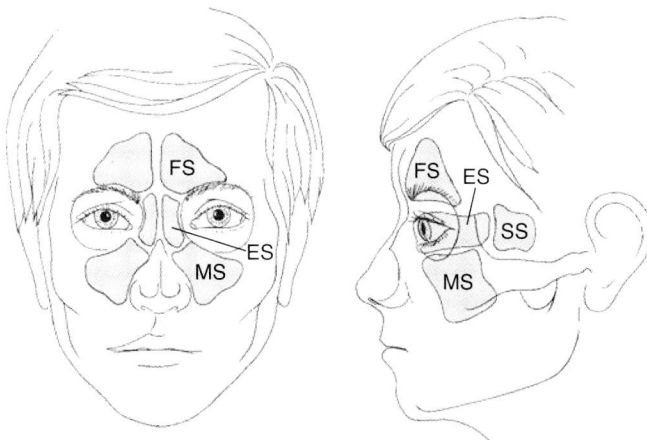

Figure 1-11 Relationship of the orbits to the paranasal sinuses. FS, frontal sinus; ES, ethmoid sinus; MS, maxillary sinus; SS, sphenoid sinus.

Ethmoid air cells can extend into the frontal, lacrimal, and maxillary bones and may extend into the orbital roof (*supraorbital ethmoids*). The numerous small, thin-walled air cells of the *ethmoid sinus* are divided into anterior, middle, and posterior. The anterior and middle air cells drain into the middle meatus; the posterior air cells, into the superior meatus. Sinusitis in the ethmoids is a common cause of orbital cellulitis and medial orbital subperiosteal abscess when the inflammation or infection spreads into the orbit.

The *sphenoid sinus* evaginates from the posterior nasal roof to pneumatize the sphenoid bone. It is rudimentary at birth and reaches full size after puberty. The sinus drains into the sphenoethmoidal recess of each nasal fossa. The optic canal is located immediately superolateral to the sinus wall. Pathologic processes involving the sphenoid sinus compress the optic nerve, leading to visual field abnormalities and vision loss.

The *maxillary sinuses* are the largest of the paranasal sinuses. The roof of the maxillary sinus forms the floor of the orbit. The maxillary sinuses extend posteriorly in the maxillary bone to the inferior orbital fissure. The infraorbital nerve and artery travel along the roof of the sinus from posterior to anterior. The bony nasolacrimal canal lies within the medial wall. The sinus drains into the middle meatus of the nose by way of the maxillary ostium. Orbital blowout fractures commonly disrupt the floor of the orbit medial to the infraorbital canal, where the bone is thinnest. The infraorbital nerve is often compromised, causing hypoesthesia of the cheek, upper lip, and maxillary teeth.

CHAPTER **2**

Evaluation of Orbital Disorders

Highlights

- Historical information guides the diagnosis of orbital disorders.
- The evaluation of an orbital disorder should distinguish orbital from periorbital and intraocular lesions.
- Orbital disorders often present with globe displacement, and careful physical examination of the pattern of change is necessary in the clinical workup.
- Select orbital disorders can present with characteristic periorbital changes that guide in diagnosis.
- Orbital disease can be categorized into 5 basic clinical patterns:
  - inflammatory (acute, subacute, and chronic)
  - mass effect (causing globe displacement with axial or nonaxial proptosis)
  - structural (congenital or acquired change in the bony orbital structure)
  - vascular (venous or arterial lesions with characteristic dynamic changes)
  - functional (sensory and/or motor dysfunction of neurovascular structures)
- Computed tomography and magnetic resonance imaging are the primary imaging modalities for orbital disorders.

History

The history establishes a probable diagnosis and guides the initial workup and therapy. It should include the following:

- onset, course, and duration of symptoms (pain, altered sensation, diplopia, changes in vision) and signs (erythema, palpable mass, globe displacement)
- prior disease (eg, thyroid eye disease, sinus disease) and therapy
- injury (head or facial trauma)
- systemic conditions (eg, cancer, inflammatory disease)
- family history
- old photographs for establishing a timeline of the process

Pain

Pain may be a symptom of inflammatory or infectious lesions, orbital hemorrhage, malignant lacrimal gland tumors, invasion from adjacent nasopharyngeal carcinoma, or metastatic lesions.

Progression

The rate of progression can be a helpful diagnostic indicator. Conditions with onset occurring over days to weeks include nonspecific orbital inflammation (NSOI), scleritis, myositis, dacryoadenitis, orbital cellulitis, hemorrhage, thrombophlebitis, fulminant neoplasia (rhabdomyosarcoma, neuroblastoma), and metastatic tumors. Conditions with onset occurring over months to years include dermoid cyst, benign mixed tumor, neurogenic tumor, cavernous hemangioma, lymphoma, fibrous histiocytoma, fibrous dysplasia, or osteoma.

Periorbital Changes

Periorbital changes may provide clues to the underlying disorders. For example, ecchymosis of the eyelid skin may be a sign of metastatic neuroblastoma (Fig 2-1), leukemia, or amyloidosis. Table 2-1 lists various periorbital signs and their common causes.

Physical Examination

Special attention should be given to visual acuity, pupillary responses, color vision and visual field testing, ocular motility, globe position, and ophthalmoscopy. Diagnostic and imaging studies are often required in addition to the basic workup.

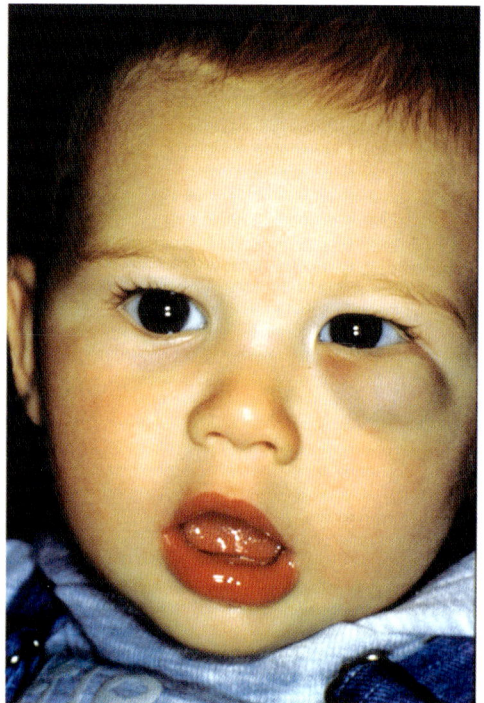

Figure 2-1 Left lower eyelid ecchymosis in child with metastatic neuroblastoma. *(Courtesy of Keith D. Carter, MD.)*

Table 2-1 Periorbital Changes Associated With Orbital Disease

Sign	Etiology
Salmon-colored mass in cul-de-sac	Lymphoma (see Fig 5-17)
Eyelid retraction and lid lag	Thyroid eye disease (see Fig 4-9)
Vascular congestion over the insertions of the rectus muscles (particularly the lateral rectus)	Thyroid eye disease (see Fig 4-8)
Corkscrew conjunctival vessels	Arteriovenous fistula (see Fig 5-5A)
Vascular anomaly of eyelid skin	Lymphatic malformation, varix, or hemangioma (see Fig 5-1)
S-shaped eyelid	Plexiform neurofibroma (see Fig 5-10 and Video 5-1) or lacrimal gland mass
Eczematous lesions of the eyelids	Mycosis fungoides (T-cell lymphoma)
Ecchymosis of eyelid skin	Metastatic neuroblastoma, leukemia, or amyloidosis (see Fig 2-1)
Prominent temple	Sphenoid wing meningioma (see Fig 5-11), metastatic neuroblastoma
Edematous swelling of lower eyelid	Meningioma, inflammatory tumor, metastases
Frozen globe	Metastases or zygomycosis
Black-crusted lesions in nasopharynx	Zygomycosis
Facial asymmetry	Fibrous dysplasia (see Fig 5-15A) or neurofibromatosis

Inspection

Globe displacement is the most common clinical manifestation of an orbital abnormality. It usually results from a tumor, a vascular abnormality, an inflammatory process, or a traumatic event.

Several terms are used to describe the position of the eye and orbit. *Proptosis* or *exophthalmos* denotes a forward displacement or protrusion of the globe. *Exorbitism* refers to an angle between the lateral orbital walls that is greater than 90°, which may also be associated with shallow orbital depth. This condition contrasts with *hypertelorism,* or *telorbitism,* which refers to a wider-than-normal separation between the medial orbital walls. Generally, exorbitism and hypertelorism are congenital or traumatic abnormalities. *Telecanthus* denotes an abnormal increased distance between the medial canthi. The eye may also be displaced vertically (*hyperglobus* or *hypoglobus*) or horizontally by an orbital mass. Retrodisplacement of the eye into the orbit, called *enophthalmos,* may occur as a result of volume expansion of the orbit (fracture, silent sinus syndrome), in association with orbital varix, or secondary to sclerosing orbital tumors (eg, metastatic breast carcinoma).

Because the globe is usually displaced away from the site of a mass, proptosis often indicates the location of that mass. Axial displacement is usually indicative of an intraconal mass behind the globe; such lesions include cavernous hemangioma, glioma, meningioma, metastases, and arteriovenous malformations. Nonaxial displacement is caused by lesions with a prominent component outside the muscle cone. Superior displacement is produced by maxillary sinus tumors invading the orbital floor and pushing the globe upward. Inferomedial displacement can result from orbital dermoid cysts and lacrimal gland tumors. Inferolateral displacement can result from frontoethmoidal mucoceles, abscesses, osteomas, and ethmoid sinus carcinomas.

In adults, bilateral proptosis is caused most often by thyroid eye disease (TED); however, other disorders can also produce bilateral proptosis, including lymphoma, vasculitis, NSOI, metastatic tumors, carotid-cavernous fistulas, cavernous sinus thrombosis, and leukemic infiltrates. TED is also the most common cause of unilateral proptosis in adults. In children with bilateral proptosis, the clinician should consider TED, NSOI, metastatic neuroblastoma, or leukemic infiltrates. Unilateral proptosis in children should raise concern for orbital cellulitis, vascular malformation, and malignancy.

Exophthalmometry is a measurement of the anterior-posterior position of the globe, generally from the lateral orbital rim to the anterior corneal surface (Hertel exophthalmometry, Fig 2-2A). The Naugle exophthalmometer uses the frontal and maxillary bones as its reference structures (Fig 2-2B); this exophthalmometer is useful in trauma patients when the lateral orbital rim has been displaced or in patients who have had the lateral orbital rim removed as part of decompressive surgery.

Globe position varies by gender and ethnicity. The mean normal values are 16.5 mm in white males, 18.5 mm in black males, 15.4 mm in white females, and 17.8 mm in black females. Asymmetry of greater than 2 mm between an individual patient's eyes suggests proptosis or enophthalmos. These conditions may best be appreciated clinically when the examiner looks up from below with the patient's head tilted back (the so-called *worm's-eye view*; Fig 2-3).

Pseudoproptosis is either the simulation of abnormal prominence of the eye or a true asymmetry that is not the result of increased orbital contents. Diagnosis should be postponed until a mass lesion has been ruled out. Causes of pseudoproptosis include the following:

- enlarged globe or irregular cornea (eg, axial myopia, staphyloma, keratoconus)
- contralateral enophthalmos (prior orbital trauma, surgery, silent sinus syndrome)

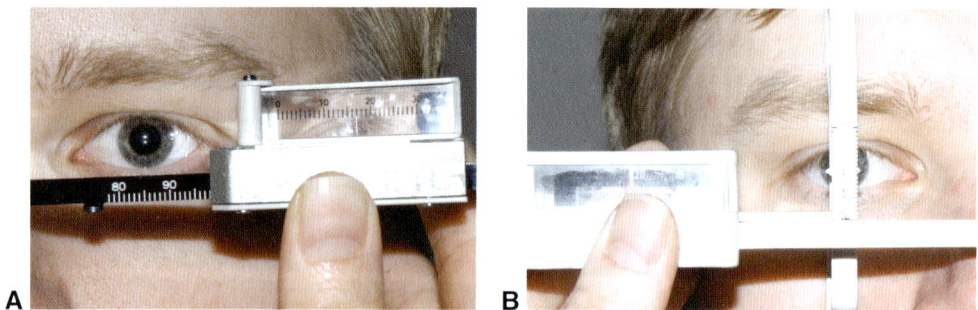

A **B**

Figure 2-2 Types of exophthalmometers. **A,** The Hertel exophthalmometer uses the lateral canthus as its reference point. **B,** The Naugle exophthalmometer uses the frontal and maxillary bones as reference points. It can measure both proptosis and hyperglobus or hypoglobus. *(Courtesy of University of Iowa.)*

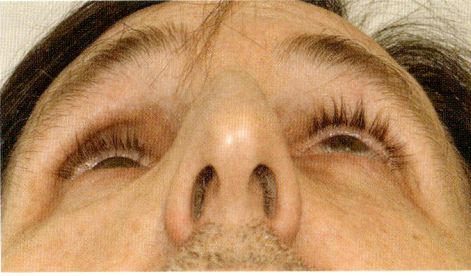

Figure 2-3 "Worm's-eye view" position. Note enophthalmos of the right eye. *(Courtesy of Bobby S. Korn, MD, PhD.)*

- asymmetric orbital size
- asymmetric palpebral fissures (usually caused by ipsilateral eyelid retraction, facial nerve paralysis, or contralateral ptosis)
- congenital deformity (microphthalmia)

Ocular movements may be restricted in a specific direction of gaze by neoplasm or inflammation. In TED, the inferior rectus is the muscle most commonly affected; this mechanically limits globe elevation and may cause hypotropia in primary gaze and restriction of upgaze. A large or rapidly enlarging orbital mass can also impede ocular movements, even in the absence of direct muscle invasion.

Eyelid abnormalities are common in TED. The *von Graefe sign* is a delay in the upper eyelid's descent ("lid lag") during downgaze and is highly suggestive of a diagnosis of TED. In fact, such lid lag and the retraction of the upper and lower eyelids are the most common physical signs of TED (see Chapter 4 in this volume).

Migliori ME, Gladstone GJ. Determination of the normal range of exophthalmometric values for black and white adults. *Am J Ophthalmol.* 1984;98(4):438–442.

Palpation

Palpation around the globe may disclose the presence of a mass in the anterior orbit, especially if the lacrimal gland is enlarged. Increased resistance to retrodisplacement of the globe is a nonspecific abnormality that may result either from a retrobulbar tumor or from diffuse inflammation such as that seen in TED. The physician should also palpate regional lymph nodes.

The differential diagnosis for a palpable mass in the superonasal quadrant may include mucocele, mucopyocele, encephalocele, neurofibroma, dermoid cyst, rhabdomyosarcoma, lymphoma, or amyloid. A palpable mass in the superotemporal quadrant may be a prolapsed lacrimal gland, a dermoid cyst, a lacrimal gland tumor, lymphoma, or NSOI. A lesion behind the equator of the globe is usually not palpable.

Pulsation of the eye is caused by transmission of the vascular pulse through the orbit. This may result from either abnormal vascular flow or transmission of normal intracranial pulsations through a bony defect in the orbital walls. Abnormal vascular flow may be caused by arteriovenous communications, such as carotid-cavernous fistulas. Defects in the bony orbital walls may result from sinus mucoceles, surgical removal of bone, trauma, or developmental abnormalities, including encephalocele, meningocele, or sphenoid wing dysplasia (associated with neurofibromatosis).

Primary Studies

Computed tomography (CT) and magnetic resonance imaging (MRI) are the primary studies for evaluation of orbital disorders. Ultrasonography (echography) may also be helpful for some disorders.

Computed Tomography

Computed tomography is essential in the management of orbital disorders. Tissues in a tomographic plane are assigned a density value proportional to their coefficient of absorption of x-rays. Either 2- or 3-dimensional images are digitally constructed from these density measurements.

CT is the most valuable technique for delineating the shape, location, extent, and character of lesions in the orbit (Fig 2-4). CT helps refine the differential diagnosis; and when orbitotomy is indicated, CT helps guide the selection of the surgical approach by showing the relationship of the lesion to the surgical space or spaces of the orbit. The resolution and soft-tissue contrast of CT are adequate for visualizing nearly all pathologic processes in the orbit, and the bony resolution is superior to that provided by any other modality, making CT the imaging technique of choice for orbital trauma and bony tumors. Orbital CT scans are usually obtained in 3-mm sections (as opposed to the thicker 5-mm sections typically utilized in head CT scans). For greater detail, fine cuts at 1.0-mm intervals may be requested.

The visualization of tumors that are highly vascularized (eg, meningioma) or that have altered vascular permeability is improved by the use of intravenous contrast-enhancing agents. Contrast is also helpful to identify an orbital abscess. If contrast is desired, it must be specifically ordered as part of the study. The resolution and tissue-contrast capabilities of CT allow imaging not only of bone but also of soft tissue and foreign bodies.

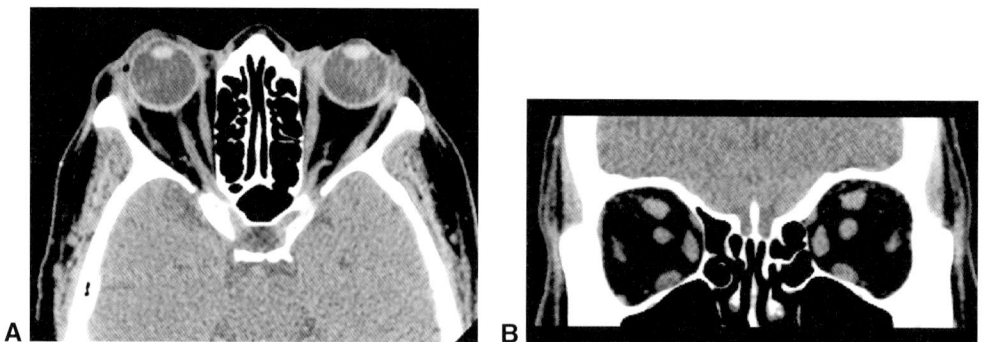

Figure 2-4 Computed tomography (CT) of the orbit demonstrating normal anatomy. **A,** Axial view. **B,** Coronal view. *(Courtesy of Bobby S. Korn, MD, PhD.)*

Orbital images can be obtained in the *axial plane,* parallel to the course of the optic nerve; in the *coronal plane,* showing the eye, optic nerve, and extraocular muscles in cross section; or in the *sagittal plane,* parallel to the nasal septum. CT scanners use software to reconstruct (reformat) any section in any direction (axial, coronal, or sagittal). Modern *spiral (helical) CT scanners* have multiple detector ports, and the scanner and the collecting tube move in a spiral fashion around the patient, generating a continuous data set. This results in rapid acquisition of a larger volume of data that allows highly detailed reconstructions in all imaging planes. *Direct coronal scans* are ideal for evaluation of the optic nerve and extraocular muscles as well as the bony roof and floor of the orbit. *Three-dimensional CT* allows reformatting of CT information into 3-dimensional projections of the bony orbital walls (Fig 2-5). Because this type of imaging requires thin sections and additional computer time, it is typically reserved for use in preparation for craniofacial surgery or repairs of complex orbital fractures.

Magnetic Resonance Imaging

MRI is a noninvasive imaging technique that does not employ ionizing radiation and has no known adverse biological effects (Fig 2-6). MRI is based on the interaction of 3 physical components: atomic nuclei possessing an electrical charge, radiofrequency (RF) waves, and a powerful magnetic field.

When tissue that contains hydrogen atoms is placed in the magnetic field, individual nuclei align themselves in the direction of the magnetic field. These aligned nuclei can be excited by an RF pulse emitted from a coil lying within the magnetic field. Excited nuclei align themselves against the static magnetic field; as the RF pulse is terminated, the nuclei flip

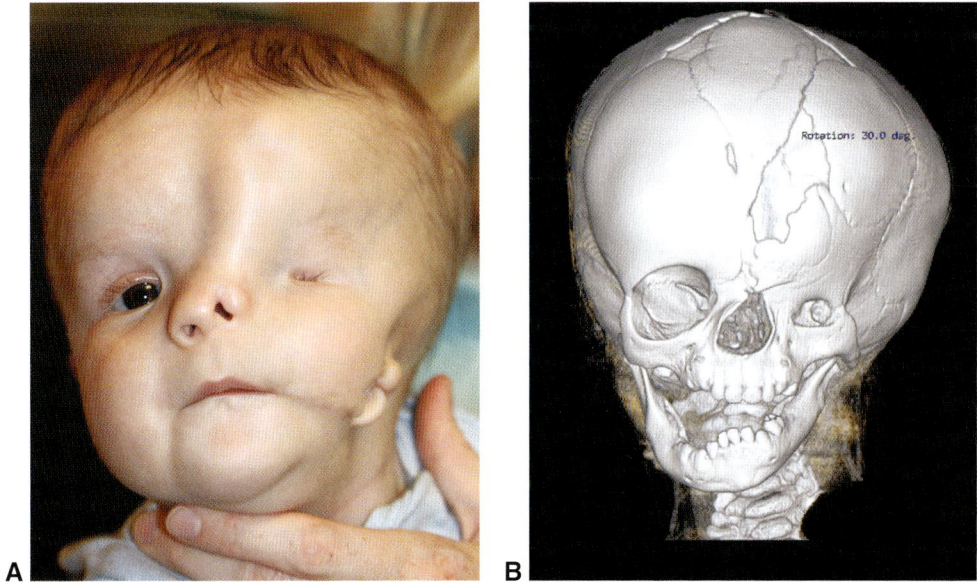

Figure 2-5 Hemifacial microsomia. **A,** Photograph of patient. **B,** Three-dimensional CT reconstruction of same patient. *(Courtesy of Jill Foster, MD.)*

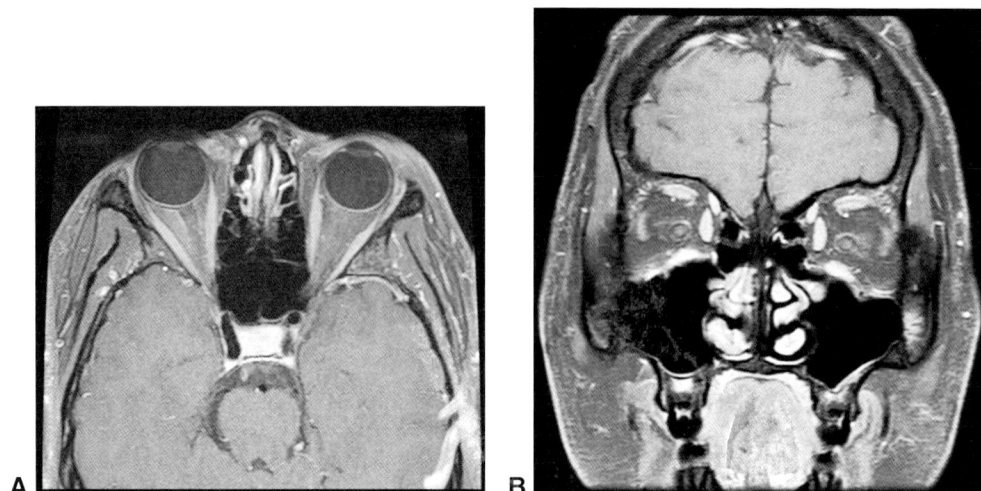

Figure 2-6 Gadolinium-enhanced T1-weighted magnetic resonance (MR) images of the orbit, with fat suppression. **A,** Axial view. **B,** Coronal view. *(Courtesy of Thomas Y. Hwang, MD, PhD, and Timothy J. McCulley, MD.)*

back to their original magnetized position. The time that this realignment takes (the relaxation time) can be measured.

Each orbital tissue has specific magnetic resonance (MR) parameters that provide the information used to generate an image. These parameters include tissue proton density and relaxation times. *Proton density* is determined by the number of protons per unit volume of tissue. Fat has greater proton density per unit volume than bone and, therefore, greater signal intensity. *T1,* or longitudinal relaxation time, is the time required for the net bulk magnetization to realign itself along the original axis. *T2,* or transverse relaxation time, is the mean relaxation time based on the interaction of hydrogen nuclei within a given tissue, an indirect measure of the effect the nuclei have on one another. Each tissue has different proton density and T1 and T2 characteristics, providing the image contrast necessary to differentiate tissues. Healthy tissue can have imaging characteristics different from those of diseased tissue, a good example being the bright signal associated with tissue edema seen on T2-weighted scans.

MRI is usually performed with images created from both T1 and T2 parameters. T1-weighted images generally offer the best anatomic detail of the orbit. T2-weighted images have the advantage of showing methemoglobin brighter than melanin, whereas these substances have the same signal intensity on T1-weighted images. The difference in brightness seen on T2-weighted images can be helpful in differentiating melanotic lesions from hemorrhagic processes. *Gadolinium,* a paramagnetic contrast agent given intravenously, allows enhancement of vascularized lesions so that they exhibit the same density as fat. It also enhances lesions that have abnormal vascular permeability. Special MR sequences have been developed to suppress the normal bright signal of fat on T1-weighted images (fat suppression; see Fig 2-6) and the bright signal of cerebrospinal fluid on T2-weighted images (fluid-attenuated inversion recovery, or FLAIR). *Gradient echo sequences* may reveal hemorrhage in vascular malformations that might be missed on T1- and T2-weighted images.

Comparison of CT and MRI

Although both CT and MRI are important modalities for the detection and characterization of orbital and ocular diseases, CT is currently the primary and most useful orbital imaging technique. Compared with MRI, it is faster, less expensive, and less sensitive to motion artifact. In general, CT provides better spatial resolution, allowing precise localization of a lesion. MRI generally provides better tissue contrast than CT; however, in most orbital disorders, the orbital fat provides sufficient natural tissue contrast to allow ready visualization of orbital tumors on CT. Each of the techniques has advantages in specific situations, some of which are discussed in the following text and in Table 2-2.

MRI offers advantages over CT in some situations. It allows the direct display of anatomic information in multiple planes (sagittal, axial, coronal, and any oblique plane). MRI provides better soft-tissue definition than does CT, a capability that is especially helpful in the evaluation of demyelination and in vascular and hemorrhagic lesions (Fig 2-7). As with CT, contrast agents are available to improve MRI detail.

Table 2-2 Comparison of CT and MRI in Orbital Disease

CT	MRI
Good technique for most orbital conditions, especially trauma and thyroid eye disease	Better technique for orbitocranial junction or intracranial imaging
Good view of bone and calcium	No view of bone or calcification
Limited definition of the orbital apex	Good view of orbital apex soft tissues unimpeded by bone
Better spatial resolution	More soft-tissue detail
Reformatting or rescanning required to image in multiple planes	Simultaneous imaging of multiple planes
Improved imaging with contrast in many cases	Improved imaging with contrast in many cases
Less motion artifact because of shorter scanning time	More motion artifact because of longer scanning time
Less claustrophobic environment in scanner	Tighter confines in scanner; "open scanners" now available but have lower resolution
Good technique for patients with metallic foreign bodies	More contraindications (eg, patients with ferromagnetic metallic foreign bodies, aneurysm clips, pacemakers)
Contraindicated in pregnancy; use should be limited in children	Can safely be used in pregnant women and children
Less expensive technique	More expensive technique
Contrast contraindicated in patients with allergy to iodine or with renal dysfunction	Use of gadolinium carries risk of nephrogenic systemic fibrosis in patients with severe renal failure (stage 4 or 5; GFR <30 mL/min/1.73 m^2)

CT = computed tomography; GFR = glomerular filtration rate; MRI = magnetic resonance imaging.

Compared with CT, MRI also provides better tissue contrast of structures in the orbital apex, intracanalicular portion of the optic nerve, structures in periorbital spaces, and orbitocranial tumors, because there is no artifact from the skull-base bones. Bone and calcification produce low signal on MRI. Bony structures may be evaluated by visualization of the signal void left by the bone. However, this is not possible when the bone is adjacent to structures that also create a signal void, such as air, rapidly flowing blood, calcification, and dura mater. Thus, CT is superior to MRI for the evaluation of fractures, bone destruction, and tissue calcification.

MRI is contraindicated in patients who have ferromagnetic metallic foreign bodies in the orbit or periorbital soft tissue, ferromagnetic vascular clips from previous surgery, magnetic intravascular filters, or electronic devices in the body such as cardiac pacemakers. If necessary, the presence of such foreign material can be ruled out with plain film x-ray or CT. Certain types of eye makeup can produce artifacts and should be removed prior to MRI. Dental amalgam is not a ferromagnetic substance and is not a contraindication to MRI, but this material produces artifacts and degrades the images on both MRI and CT.

Because CT and MRI yield different types of images, it is not unusual for both techniques to be employed in the evaluation of an orbital disorder. The use of these modalities

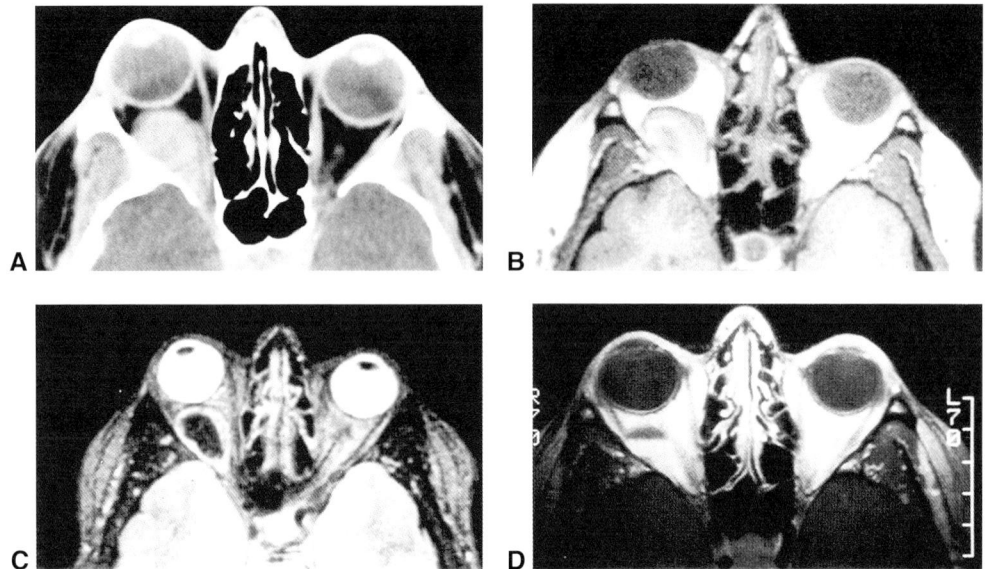

Figure 2-7 Acute proptosis. **A,** CT image of a patient with acute right proptosis resulting from spontaneous orbital hemorrhage. The hematoma exhibits discrete margins, homogeneous consistency, and a radiodensity similar to that of blood vessels and muscle. **B,** T1-weighted MR scan obtained 4 days after the hemorrhage demonstrates the transient bull's-eye pattern characteristic of a hematoma beginning to undergo physical changes and biochemical hemoglobin degradation. **C,** T2-weighted MR scan obtained the same day as the image in part B shows a characteristic ring pattern. **D,** T1-weighted MR scan performed 3 months later shows that the hematoma has decreased in size, and there is layering of the degraded blood components.

should be based on the specific patient's condition. In most cases, CT is the more effective and economical choice (see Table 2-2). MRI is the better primary technique for imaging the orbitocranial junction and brain, but CT scanning may enhance the assessment by providing better bone images. When the orbitocranial junction or brain is involved, CT scanning and MRI may be complementary; and in some cases, both may be required to evaluate complex lesions.

CT imaging should be obtained judiciously in children, as they are much more ra-diosensitive than adults. Extrapolation of lifetime risk of malignancy development from atomic bomb survivors led to a consensus statement that low-level radiation may have a small risk of causing cancer. When possible, MRI should be considered first for children, with CT reserved for select clinical scenarios.

Brody AS, Frush DP, Huda W, Brent RL; American Academy of Pediatrics Section on
Radiology. Radiation risk to children from computed tomography. *Pediatrics*. 2007;
120(3):677–682.

Ultrasonography

Orbital ultrasonography may be used to examine patients with orbital disorders. The size, shape, and position of normal and abnormal orbital tissues can be determined by means of contemporary ultrasound techniques. B-scan ultrasonography captures 2-dimensional im-ages of these tissues, while standardized A-scan ultrasonography provides 1-dimensional images rendered as a series of spikes of varying height and width that demonstrate the particular echogenic characteristics of each tissue. Areas of edema can sometimes be used to discern the degree of disease activity. Ultrasonography has high resolution in the area of the sclera and optic nerve insertion and is useful for evaluating scleritis and other types of anterior inflammation that produce fluid in the sub-Tenon space. Localization of foreign bodies is possible with ultrasonography. *Doppler ultrasonography* can provide specific in-formation regarding blood flow and can demonstrate arterialization, retrograde flow in the orbital veins in cases of dural cavernous fistula or arteriovenous malformation, or vas-cular abnormalities associated with increased blood flow. Vascular tumors can be identi-fied by active pulsation or, in the case of venous lesions, by compressibility and change in size with the Valsalva maneuver.

However, ultrasound analysis of orbital tissues and diseases requires specialized equip-ment and experienced personnel, and office-based equipment is generally not suitable for this purpose. Ultrasonography is of limited value in assessing lesions of the posterior orbit (because of sound attenuation) or the sinuses or intracranial space (because sound does not pass well through air or bone).

Secondary Studies

Secondary studies that are performed for specific indications include venography, arteri-ography, and stereotactic navigation. Although these studies are rarely used, they may be helpful in specific cases.

Venography

Before the advent of CT and MRI, orbital venography was used in the diagnosis and management of orbital varices and in the study of the cavernous sinus. Contrast material is injected into the frontal or the angular vein to reveal a venous abnormality. Subtraction and magnification techniques have been used to increase the resolution of venography. Because moving blood generates a signal void during MR imaging, larger venous abnormalities and structures can be visualized well on MR venography. Some orbitocranial vascular malformations or fistulas are best accessed directly via the superior ophthalmic vein, both for diagnosis and for possible treatment.

Arteriography

Arteriography is the gold standard for diagnosis of an arterial lesion such as an aneurysm or arteriovenous malformation. Retrograde catheterization of the cerebral vessels is performed through the femoral artery. However, there is a small risk of serious neurologic and vascular complications (1%–2%) because the technique requires installation of a catheter and injection of radiopaque dye into the arterial system; thus, the test is reserved for patients with a high probability of having a lesion.

Visualization can be maximized by the use of selective injection into the internal and external carotid arteries, magnification to allow viewing of the smaller-caliber vessels, and subtraction techniques to radiographically eliminate bone. An additional benefit of arteriography is the ability to simultaneously diagnose and embolize lesions using various glues and coils.

CT and MR Angiography

The development of better hardware and software has enabled precise CT and MR imaging for diagnosis of arteriovenous malformations, aneurysms, and arteriovenous fistulas without the expense, discomfort, and risks associated with intravascular catheterization use of contrast agents. MR angiography is useful for diagnosis of vertebrobasilar dolichoectasia seen in hemifacial spasm. However, MR angiography is less sensitive than direct catheter angiography for identifying carotid-cavernous fistulas. When determining which test to use, the ophthalmologist may consult with a radiologist to discuss the suspected lesion and to ensure selection of the imaging modality best suited to the patient.

Stereotactic Navigation

The use of computer-assisted 3-dimensional navigation (image guidance) is increasingly common in clinical practice (Fig 2-8). Stereotactic guidance can be useful when performing complex multidisciplinary surgeries in which orbital lesions are accessed through craniotomy and endoscopic skull-base approaches. However, in uncomplicated orbital surgery, while image guidance may have some utility for surgical training, it has a lesser role in procedures performed by experienced orbital surgeons.

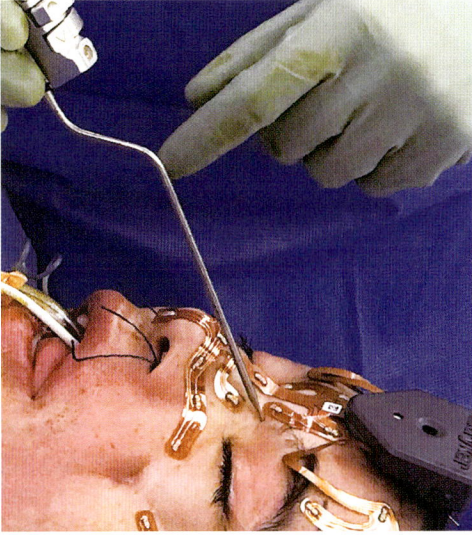

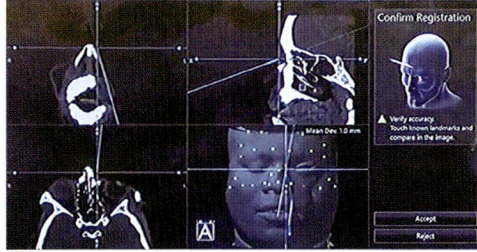

Figure 2-8 Computer-assisted 3-dimensional navigation (image guidance). *(Courtesy of M. Reza Vagefi, MD.)*

Ali MJ, Naik MN, Kaliki S, Dave TV. Interactive navigation-guided ophthalmic plastic surgery: the usefulness of computed tomography angiographic image guidance. *Ophthalmic Plast Reconstr Surg.* 2016;32(5):393–398.

Pathology

The diagnosis of an orbital lesion usually requires analysis of tissue obtained through an orbitotomy. Appropriate handling of the tissue specimen is necessary to ensure an accurate diagnosis. Most tissue samples are placed in formalin for permanent section analysis. If a lymphoproliferative lesion is suspected, some fresh tissue should be sent for flow cytometry analysis. Frozen section evaluation may be performed at the time of surgery, but it is generally not used for definitive diagnosis of an orbital tumor. However, when the area of proposed biopsy is not obvious, frozen sections are helpful to confirm that appropriate tissue has been obtained for permanent section analysis. Frozen section analysis is also used intraoperatively to determine tumor margins and ensure complete tumor removal. Tissue removed for frozen section analysis should be placed in a dampened saline gauze and sent promptly to the frozen section laboratory.

Because of the vast array of possible unusual tumor types in the orbit, preoperative consultation with a pathologist familiar with orbital disease may be helpful to maximize the information gained from any orbital biopsy. In many cases, fresh tissue should be obtained and frozen for cell-surface-marker studies. Cell-marker studies are required in the analysis of all orbital lymphoid lesions. These studies may allow differentiation between reactive lymphoid hyperplasia and lymphoma. Such studies may also indicate the presence of estrogen receptors in cases of metastatic prostate or breast carcinoma and thus provide useful information about sensitivity to hormonal therapy. Marker studies are also helpful in the diagnosis of poorly differentiated tumors when light microscopy alone is not definitive. Although cell-marker studies have largely replaced electron microscopy in the diagnosis of undifferentiated tumors, it may nevertheless be worthwhile in these cases to preserve fresh tissue in glutaraldehyde for possible electron microscopy. In noncohesive tumors (hematologic or lymphoid), a touch preparation may permit a diagnosis.

All biopsy specimens must be treated delicately to minimize crush and cautery artifacts, which can confuse interpretation. Permanent section tissue biopsy specimens should be placed in fixatives promptly. If fine-needle aspiration biopsy is planned, a cytologist or trained technician must be available to handle the aspirate. In special cases, the biopsy can be performed under either ultrasonographic or CT control. Although a fine-bore needle occasionally yields a sufficient cell block, the specimen is usually limited to cytologic study. Larger biopsy specimens, in which light and electron microscopy can be used to evaluate histologic patterns, may permit a more conclusive diagnosis.

As the technology improves and costs decrease, genomic analysis of tumors is increasingly being performed. This modality has implications for disease prognosis and the promise of precision therapy. Discussion with the pathologist prior to surgery is recommended so that tissues can be sent in the appropriate media for optimal genetic analysis.

See BCSC Section 4, *Ophthalmic Pathology and Intraocular Tumors,* for a more extensive discussion of pathology.

Laboratory Studies

Screening for abnormal thyroid function commonly includes T_4 and thyroid-stimulating hormone (TSH) tests. Results of these serum tests are abnormal in 90% of patients with TED. However, if the results are normal but thyroid disease is still strongly suspected, additional endocrine studies such as thyroid-stimulating immunoglobulins or TSH-receptor antibodies can be considered, as these tests have greater sensitivity for detecting thyroid disease.

Granulomatosis with polyangiitis (formerly called Wegener granulomatosis; see Chapter 4 in this volume) should be considered in patients with sclerokeratitis or coexisting sinus disease and orbital mass lesions. A useful test for this uncommon disease is the antineutrophil cytoplasmic autoantibody (ANCA) serum assay, which shows a cytoplasmic staining pattern (c-ANCA) in cases of granulomatosis with polyangiitis. However, the test results may initially be negative in cases of localized disease. Biopsy of affected tissues classically shows vasculitis, granulomatous inflammation, and tissue necrosis, although necrotizing vasculitis is not always present in orbital biopsies.

Testing for serum angiotensin-converting enzyme (ACE) and lysozyme may be helpful in the diagnosis of sarcoidosis. This multisystem granulomatous inflammatory condition may present with lacrimal gland enlargement, conjunctival granulomas, extraocular muscle or optic nerve infiltration, or solitary orbital granulomas. Diagnosis is confirmed through biopsy of one or more affected organs.

CHAPTER 3

Congenital Orbital Anomalies

Highlights

- Anophthalmia is rare and is usually associated with lethal mutations.
- Rehabilitation of the microphthalmic orbit is directed toward expansion of the hypoplastic orbit.
- Craniofacial clefts result from developmental arrest or mechanical disruption of development.
- Craniosynostosis occurs as an isolated abnormality or as part of a genetic syndrome.
- When symptomatic, dermoid cysts should be removed with the cyst wall intact.

Introduction

Developmental defects of the orbit can manifest clinically at any time from conception until late in life. Most significant congenital anomalies of the eye and orbit are apparent on ultrasonography, performed before birth. The more profound the abnormality, the earlier in development it occurred. Identifying the embryologic origin of the congenital malformation helps ophthalmologists understand and classify the physical changes in the patient.

If an anomaly is caused by a slowing or cessation of a normal stage of development, the resulting deformity can be considered a pure arrest.

In the examination of the child with an ocular or craniofacial malformation, the clinician should focus on carefully defining the severity of the defect and identifying associated changes. Some syndromes may have specific associated ocular changes or secondary ocular complications such as exposure keratitis or strabismus related to orbital maldevelopment.

See Section 6, *Pediatric Ophthalmology and Strabismus,* for detailed discussion, including illustrations, of many of the topics covered in this chapter.

Anophthalmia

True anophthalmia is defined as a total absence of tissues of the eye; it is classified into 3 types. *Primary anophthalmia,* which is rare and usually bilateral, occurs when the primary optic vesicle fails to grow out from the cerebral vesicle at the 2-mm stage of embryonic development. *Secondary anophthalmia* is rare and lethal and results from a gross abnormality in the anterior neural tube. *Consecutive anophthalmia* presumably results from a secondary degeneration of the optic vesicle.

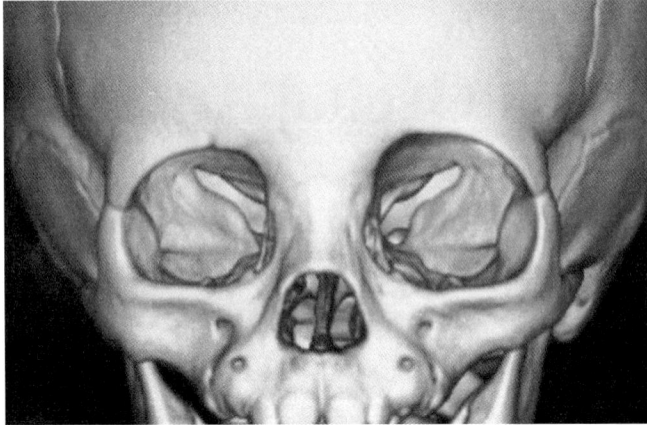

Figure 3-1 Right microphthalmic orbit. Three-dimensional computed tomography (CT) reconstruction shows a hypoplastic right orbit with microphthalmia. *(Courtesy of Bobby S. Korn, MD, PhD.)*

Because orbital development is partially dependent on the size and growth of the globe, the bones of the orbit, the eyelids, and also the adnexal structures fail to develop and remain hypoplastic in anophthalmia. Intervention requires measures that address all of these issues, not just the missing eye.

Microphthalmia

Microphthalmia is much more common than anophthalmia and is defined by the presence of a small eye with axial length that is at least 2 standard deviations below the mean axial length for age. Microphthalmic eyes vary in size depending on the severity of the defect. Most infants with a unilateral small orbit (Fig 3-1) and no visible eye actually have a microphthalmic globe. The defect may be isolated, or it may occur with a constellation of abnormalities as part of a well-defined syndrome. Because multiple genetic mutations have been reported in anophthalmia/microphthalmia, microphthalmia is considered a developmental phenotype that results from several different genetic rearrangements.

Treatment of Anophthalmia/Microphthalmia

All children with microphthalmia have hypoplastic orbits. Because most microphthalmic eyes have no potential for vision, treatment focuses on achieving a cosmetically acceptable appearance that is reasonably symmetrical. Treatment begins shortly after birth and consists of socket expansion with progressively larger conformers, which are used until the patient can be fitted with a prosthesis. Enucleation is usually not necessary for the fitting of a conformer or an ocular prosthesis and is ordinarily avoided because it may worsen the bony hypoplasia. Orbital volume may be augmented with autogenous materials, such as dermis-fat grafts (Fig 3-2), or with synthetic implants. When placed at an early age, dermis-fat grafts may grow with the child, resulting in progressive socket expansion. In cases of severe bony asymmetry, intraorbital tissue expanders can be progressively inflated to enlarge the hypoplastic orbit.

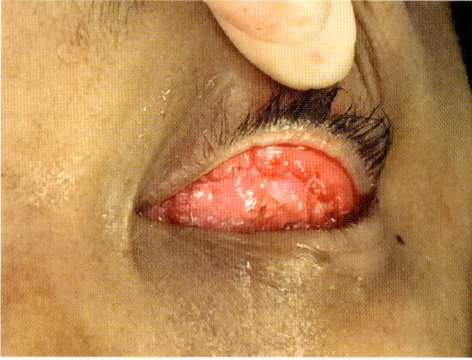

Figure 3-2 Dermis-fat graft in the left anophthalmic socket. *(Courtesy of Cat N. Burkat, MD.)*

Craniofacial techniques have been used to reposition and resize the orbit in patients with severe microphthalmia or anophthalmia or in older children with previously untreated microphthalmia. Such repairs are complex, as noted in the following discussion of craniofacial clefting.

Microphthalmia with orbital cyst results from failure of the choroidal fissure to close in the embryo (Fig 3-3). This condition is usually unilateral but may be bilateral. The

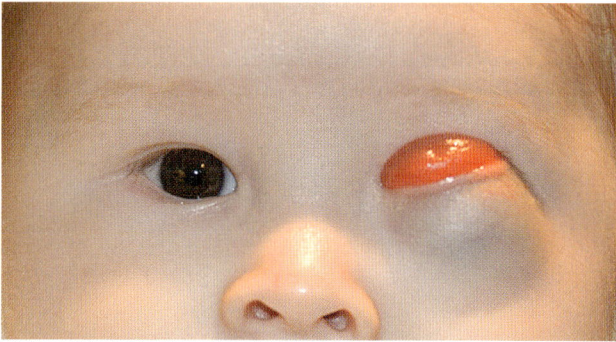

A

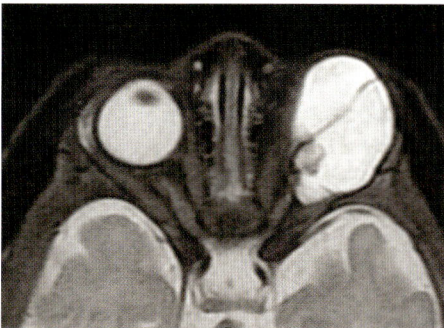

B

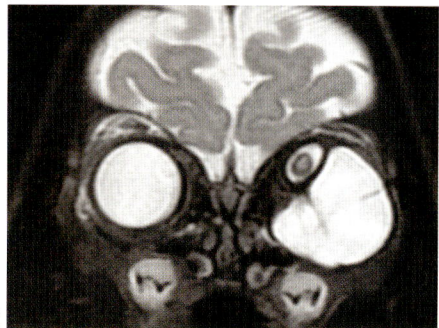

C

Figure 3-3 Microphthalmia with orbital cyst. **A,** Young child with left micropthalmia with orbital cyst. T2-weighted axial magnetic resonance imaging (MRI) **(B)** and coronal MRI **(C)** show the orbital cyst component. *(Courtesy of Don O. Kikkawa, MD.)*

presence of an orbital cyst may be beneficial for stimulating normal growth of the involved orbital bone and eyelids. In some cases, the orbital cyst may be removed to allow the fitting of an ocular prosthesis. When these conditions are bilateral, significant visual impairment can result. Prompt referral for low vision rehabilitation and early intervention should be initiated in infancy, as soon as vision impairment is suspected.

> American Academy of Ophthalmology Vision Rehabilitation Committee. Preferred
> Practice Pattern Guidelines. *Vision Rehabilitation.* San Francisco: American Academy of
> Ophthalmology; 2017. www.aao.org/ppp.

Craniofacial Clefting and Syndromic Congenital Craniofacial Anomalies

Craniofacial clefts occur as a result of a developmental arrest or mechanical disruption of development. Etiologic theories include a failure of neural crest cell migration and a failure of fusion or movement of facial processes. Facial clefts in the skeletal structures are distributed around the orbit and maxilla; clefts in the soft tissues are most apparent around the eyelids and lips. Examples of clefting syndromes affecting the orbit and eyelids include some forms of midline clefts with hypertelorism as well as the oculoauriculovertebral spectrum, which includes hemifacial microsomia, oculoauriculovertebral dysplasia (Goldenhar syndrome), and mandibulofacial dysostosis (Treacher Collins syndrome, Fig 3-4A).

The bones of the skull or orbit may also have congenital clefts through which the intracranial contents can herniate. These protruding contents can be the meninges *(meningocele),*

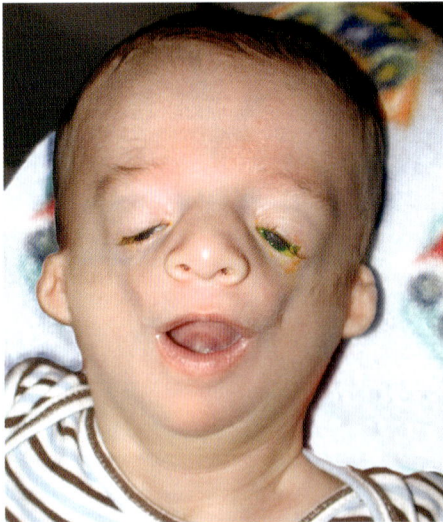

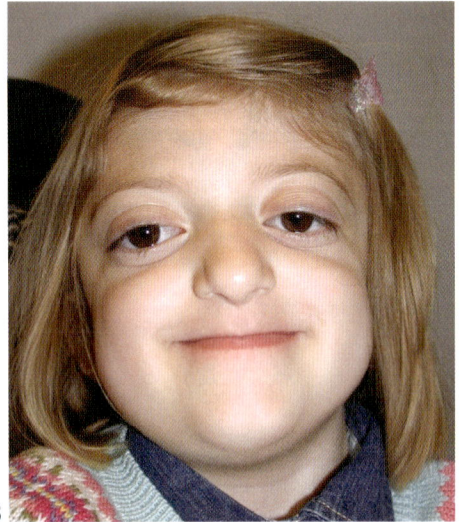

Figure 3-4 Craniofacial deformities. **A,** Mandibulofacial dysostosis (Treacher Collins syndrome). **B,** Craniofacial dysostosis (Crouzon syndrome). *(Courtesy of Jill Foster, MD.)*

brain tissue *(encephalocele),* or both meninges and brain tissue *(meningoencephalocele).* When these herniations involve the orbit, they most commonly present anteriorly with a protrusion subcutaneously near the medial canthus or over the bridge of the nose. Straining or crying may increase the size of the mass, and the globe may be displaced temporally and downward (inferolaterally). Such herniations less commonly move into the posterior orbit; these lesions may cause anterior displacement and pulsation of the globe. Intranasal extension may occur, causing life-threatening airway obstruction. Treatment is surgical and should be carried out in collaboration with a neurosurgeon. Meningoceles and encephaloceles adjacent to the orbit are frequently associated with anomalies of the optic nerve head, such as morning glory disc anomaly.

Craniosynostosis can occur as an isolated abnormality or in conjunction with other anomalies as part of a genetic syndrome. *Syndromic craniosynostosis* is the premature closure of 1 or more sutures in the bones of the skull and results in various skeletal deformities, including orbital defects. Associated ophthalmic problems include strabismus, astigmatism, ptosis, proptosis, nasolacrimal duct obstruction, and amblyopia. Secondary intracranial hypertension can be a complication. Hypertelorism and proptosis are frequently observed in craniosynostosis syndromes such as Crouzon syndrome (craniofacial dysostosis; Fig 3-4B) and Apert syndrome (acrocephalosyndactyly; Fig 3-5). Syndromic craniosynostosis is a genetically heterogeneous disorder, with mutations identified in several genes, predominantly the fibroblast growth factor receptor genes.

The severe orbital and facial defects associated with craniofacial disorders can sometimes be improved with surgery. Bony and soft tissue reconstruction is generally necessary. Such operations are often staged and usually require a team approach with multiple subspecialists.

Jadico SK, Huebner A, McDonald-McGinn DM, Zackai EH, Young TL. Ocular phenotype correlations in patients with TWIST versus FGFR3 genetic mutations. *J AAPOS.* 2006; 10(5):435–444.

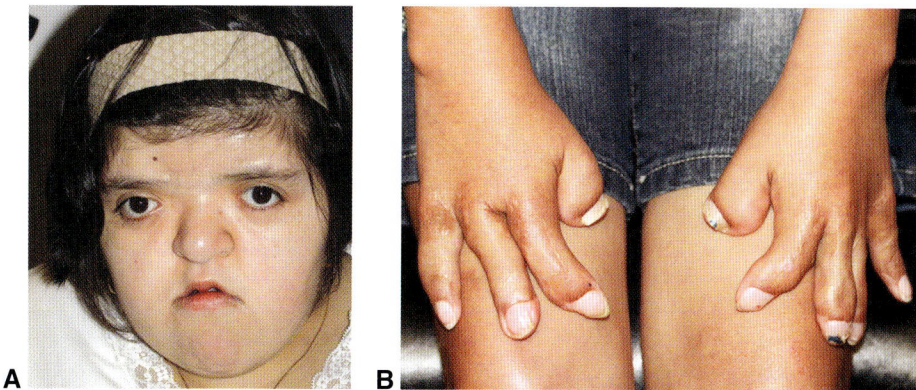

Figure 3-5 Apert syndrome (acrocephalosyndactyly). **A,** Hypertelorism and proptosis. **B,** Syndactyly. *(Courtesy of Jill Foster, MD.)*

Congenital Orbital Tumors

Hamartomas and Choristomas

Hamartomas are anomalous growths of tissue consisting only of mature cells normally found at the involved site. Classic examples are infantile (capillary) hemangiomas and the characteristic lesions of neurofibromatosis. *Choristomas* are tissue anomalies characterized by types of cells not normally found at the involved site. Classic examples are dermoid cysts, epidermoid cysts, dermolipomas, and teratomas. This chapter discusses only some of the choristomas; further discussion of these congenital and juvenile tumors can be found in BCSC Section 6, *Pediatric Ophthalmology and Strabismus*.

Dermoid cyst

Dermoid and epidermoid cysts are among the most common benign orbital tumors of childhood. These cysts are present congenitally and enlarge progressively. The more superficial cysts usually become symptomatic in childhood, but deeper orbital dermoids may not become clinically evident until adulthood. *Dermoid cysts* are lined by keratinizing epithelium and contain dermal appendages, such as hair follicles and sebaceous glands. They contain an admixture of oil and keratin. In contrast, *epidermoid cysts* are lined by epidermis only and are usually filled with keratin; they do not contain dermal appendages.

Orbital dermoid cysts occur most commonly in the area of the lateral brow adjacent to the frontozygomatic suture (Fig 3-6); less often they may be found in the medial upper

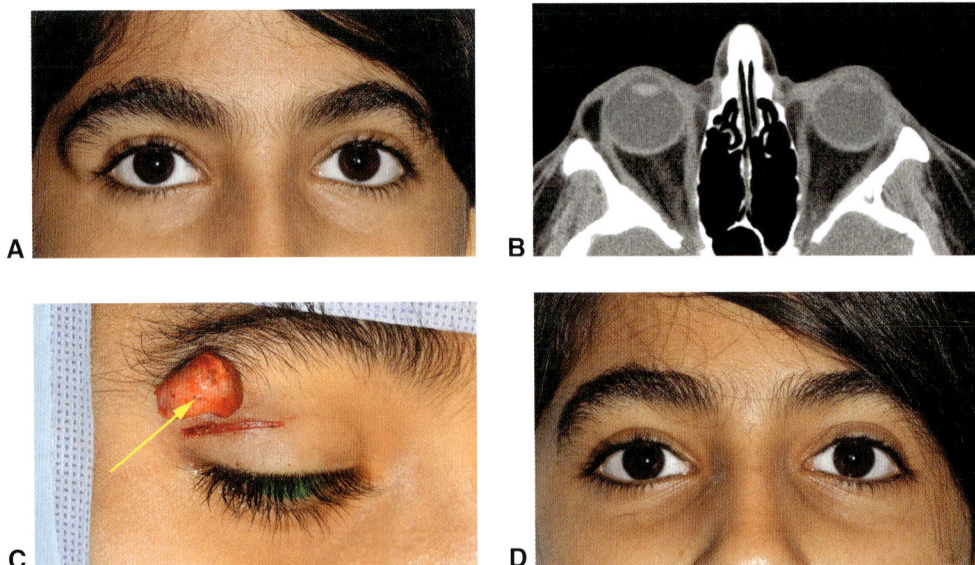

Figure 3-6   Orbital dermoid cyst. **A,** Young child with fullness of the right superolateral orbit. **B,** CT scan of the hypointense lesion in the axial plane is characteristic of a dermoid cyst (epithelial choristoma); note its location at the frontozygomatic suture line. **C,** Dermoid cyst removed through an upper eyelid crease incision shows dermal appendages (*arrow*). **D,** Postoperative photograph shows resolution of the eyelid fullness. *(Courtesy of Bobby S. Korn, MD, PhD.)*

eyelid adjacent to the frontoethmoidal suture. Dermoid cysts commonly present as palpable smooth, painless, oval masses that enlarge slowly. They may be freely mobile, or they may be fixed to periosteum at the underlying suture.

If the dermoid occurs in the temporal fossa, computed tomography (CT) is often indicated to rule out dumbbell expansion through the suture into the underlying orbit. A dumbbell dermoid cyst such as this can cause pulsating proptosis with mastication, a highly specific feature of this condition.

CT is also useful to evaluate medial lesions and to distinguish dermoids from congenital encephaloceles, dacryoceles, and vascular lesions that might also occur in this location. When viewed on a CT scan, an orbital dermoid cyst is typically well defined, and it has an enhancing wall and a nonenhancing lumen (see Fig 3-6B). A partially calcified margin or rim is visible in most cases. With magnetic resonance imaging, the lesion is best appreciated on fat-suppression sequences and appears as a well-defined round to ovoid structure of variable size. Most dermoids are relatively hypointense with respect to orbital fat on T1-weighted images and relatively hyperintense on T2-weighted images. Enhancement is minimal because of the lack of blood vessels in the cyst.

Dermoid cysts that do not present until adulthood often are not palpable because they are situated posteriorly in the orbit, usually in the superior and temporal portions adjacent to the bony sutures. The globe and adnexa may be displaced, causing progressive proptosis, and erosion or remodeling of bone can occur. Long-standing dermoid cysts may erode the orbital bones. In some cases, the clinical presentation of orbital dermoid cysts may be orbital inflammation, which is incited by leakage of oil and keratin from the cyst. Expansion of the dermoid cyst and inflammatory response to leakage may result in an orbitocutaneous fistula, which may also occur after incomplete surgical removal.

Management Dermoid cysts are usually removed surgically. Because dermoid cysts that present in childhood are often superficial, they can be excised through an incision placed in the upper eyelid crease or directly over the lesion. If possible, the cyst wall should be maintained during surgery. Rupture of the cyst can lead to an acute inflammatory process if part of the cyst wall or any of the contents remain within the eyelid or orbit. If the cyst wall is ruptured, the surgeon should remove the cyst contents. Complete surgical removal may be difficult if the cyst has leaked preoperatively and adhesions have developed.

Dermolipoma

Dermolipomas are solid tumors usually located in and beneath the conjunctiva over the globe's lateral surface. These benign lesions may have deep extensions that can extend to the levator aponeurosis and extraocular muscles. Superficially, dermolipomas may have fine hairs that can be irritating to patients (Fig 3-7). These tumors typically require no treatment unless the lesion is large and/or cosmetically objectionable. In these cases, only the anterior, visible portion should be excised; when possible, the overlying conjunctiva should be preserved. Care must be taken to avoid damage to the lacrimal gland ducts, extraocular muscles, and the levator aponeurosis. Lesions that may simulate dermolipomas include prolapsed orbital fat, prolapsed palpebral lobe of the lacrimal gland, and lymphomas (such processes are generally found only in adults).

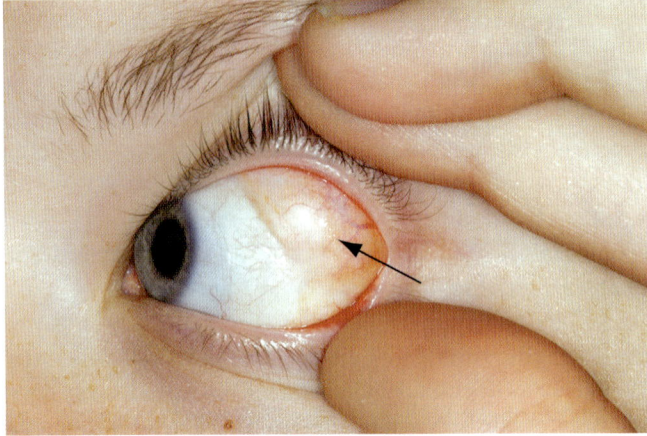

Figure 3-7 Dermolipoma of left lateral orbit. There are fine hairs on the surface of the tumor *(arrow). (Courtesy of Keith D. Carter, MD.)*

Teratoma

Teratomas are rare tumors that arise from all 3 germinal layers (ectoderm, mesoderm, and endoderm) and are usually cystic. On histologic examination, a teratoma is characterized by a complex arrangement of various tissues, including clear cysts lined by either epidermis or gastrointestinal or respiratory epithelium. Islands of hyaline cartilage, cerebral tissue, epidermal cysts, and choroid plexus are frequently found. A child with an orbital teratoma characteristically presents with severe unilateral proptosis at birth. As a consequence, the globe and optic nerve may be maldeveloped. The proptosis may increase over the first few days or weeks of life, and compression of the globe can result in corneal exposure and vision loss. When the lesion is smaller, the globe is often normal. Although teratomas in other parts of the body have been known to undergo malignant transformation, teratomas confined to the orbit are generally benign; for those that are malignant, exenteration may be necessary. However, some cystic teratomas can be removed and ocular function preserved.

CHAPTER 4

Orbital Inflammatory and Infectious Disorders

▶ *This chapter includes a related video, which can be accessed by scanning the QR code provided in the text or going to www.aao.org/bcscvideo_section07.*

Highlights

- Orbital inflammatory disease comprises a broad range of disorders that can be divided conceptually into those that have an identifiable cause (specific) and those that do not (nonspecific).
- All specific causes of orbital inflammation, such as infections or autoimmune diseases, must be eliminated before applying a diagnosis of nonspecific orbital inflammation.
- This chapter presents an overview of the major causes of orbital inflammation, with the goal of providing a working knowledge of the most common of these disorders (Table 4-1).

Infectious Inflammation

Cellulitis

Most cases of cellulitis stem from bacterial infection; however, cellulitis resulting from non-infectious (eg, autoimmune, malignant, foreign-body) etiologies may mimic bacterial cellulitis. Defining the etiology of the cellulitis allows prompt and effective treatment.

Bacterial infections of the orbit or periorbital soft tissues originate from 3 primary sources:

- direct spread from adjacent sinusitis, dacryocystitis, dacryoadenitis, or an odontogenic infection
- direct inoculation after trauma or skin infection
- hematologic spread from a distant focus (eg, otitis media, pneumonia, endocarditis)

Preseptal cellulitis

Preseptal cellulitis involves structures anterior to the orbital septum. Eyelid edema, erythema, and inflammation may be severe, but the globe and deep orbital tissues remain uninvolved

Table 4-1 Differential Diagnosis of Major Orbital Inflammations

Infectious (identify as preseptal or orbital cellulitis)
    Bacterial (identify the source)
        Direct inoculation (trauma, surgery)
        Spread from adjacent tissue (sinusitis, dacryocystitis, dacryoadenitis)
        Spread from distant focus (bacteremia, pneumonia)
        Opportunistic infection (necrotizing fasciitis, tuberculosis)
    Fungal
        Zygomycosis
        Aspergillosis
    Parasitic
        Echinococcosis
        Cysticercosis

Autoimmune
    Thyroid eye disease (TED)
    Immunoglobulin G4–related disease (IgG4-RD)

Vasculitic
    Giant cell arteritis
    Granulomatosis with polyangiitis
    Polyarteritis nodosa
    Vasculitis associated with connective tissue disorders

Granulomatous
    Sarcoidosis
    Foreign body

Nonspecific orbital inflammation (NSOI) (diagnosis of exclusion)

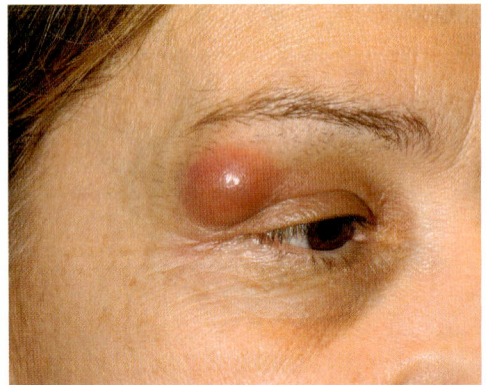

Figure 4-1 A patient with preseptal cellulitis of the right upper eyelid with formation of a localized abscess. The eye remains quiet with no chemosis or proptosis. *(Courtesy of Bobby S. Korn, MD, PhD.)*

(Fig 4-1). Therefore, pupillary reaction, vision, ocular motility, and globe position are not disturbed. Furthermore, pain on eye movement and chemosis are noticeably absent.

Although preseptal cellulitis in adults usually arises from penetrating cutaneous trauma or dacryocystitis, in children, it commonly arises from underlying sinusitis. Most pediatric cases are now caused by gram-positive cocci, but *Haemophilus influenzae* type B should still be considered, especially in nonimmunized children.

Treatment Antibiotic therapy and workup should begin as promptly as possible, particularly in children. If eyelid swelling precludes motility evaluation and, thus, the ability to exclude orbital cellulitis, workup should include computed tomography (CT) imaging of the orbit and sinuses. An optimal antibiotic regimen may be developed in collaboration with the patient's primary care physician or an infectious disease specialist.

In children with a reliable examination and follow-up plan, oral antibiotics (eg, cephalexin for an anterior etiology; amoxicillin clavulanate for a sinusitis-associated infection), frequent warm compresses, and nasal decongestants (eg, oxymetazoline nasal spray) for associated sinusitis typically improve the infection. For infants, children with an unreliable examination or follow-up plan, or for infections that progress on oral antibiotics, hospital admission and intravenous (IV) antibiotics (eg, ceftriaxone, vancomycin) may be considered.

In teenagers and adults, preseptal cellulitis usually arises from a superficial source and responds quickly to appropriate oral antibiotics (eg, ampicillin-sulbactam, trimethoprim-sulfamethoxazole [TMP-SMX], doxycycline, clindamycin) and warm compresses. Initial antibiotic selection depends on the history, clinical findings, and initial laboratory studies. Prompt culture and sensitivity studies allow for revising antibiotic therapy in unresponsive cases.

In older adults, infections behave differently and may not produce typical signs, such as erythema, calor, or fever. Response to antibiotics in patients in this age group may also be delayed, and surgical intervention to excise devitalized tissue may be necessary to clear an infection. Imaging studies and hospital admission for IV antibiotics should be considered to rule out underlying sinusitis if no direct inoculation site is identified, if the patient does not respond to oral antibiotics within 48 hours, or if orbital involvement becomes evident.

Preseptal cellulitis in any age group may require surgical drainage if it progresses to a localized abscess (see Fig 4-1). Incision and drainage directly over the abscess typically improve the infection, but dissection of the upper eyelid should preserve the orbital septum to avoid contaminating the orbital soft tissues and to prevent injury to the underlying levator aponeurosis.

In patients with preseptal cellulitis resulting from trauma, *Staphylococcus aureus* represents the most common pathogen. The infection usually responds rapidly to a penicillin used against penicillinase-resistant organisms, such as methicillin or ampicillin-sulbactam. However, *methicillin-resistant S aureus (MRSA)*, previously recognized as a cause of severe nosocomial infections, is now increasingly encountered in the community setting as well.

Community-acquired (CA)-MRSA infections tend to present as a fluctuant abscess with surrounding cellulitis. Eyebrow abscesses have a particularly high rate of CA-MRSA–positive cultures. The pain associated with the lesion is often out of proportion to its appearance. Classically, CA-MRSA has been susceptible to a wider range of antibiotics (including TMP-SMX, rifampin, or clindamycin), compared with susceptibility of hospital-associated (HA)-MRSA. Over the past decade, however, antibiotic-resistant CA-MRSA strains have migrated into the health care setting, and the genetic differences and outcomes between CA-MRSA and HA-MRSA infections have increasingly overlapped. Both types of MRSA may result in acute morbidity and long-term disability. MRSA has also been associated with necrotizing fasciitis, orbital cellulitis, endogenous endophthalmitis, panophthalmitis, and cavernous sinus thrombosis.

Carniciu AL, Chou J, Leskov I, Freitag SK. Clinical presentation and bacteriology of eyebrow infections: the Massachusetts Eye and Ear Infirmary experience (2008–2015). *Ophthalmic Plast Reconstr Surg.* 2017;33(5):372–375.

Mathias MT, Horsley MB, Mawn LA, et al. Atypical presentations of orbital cellulitis caused by methicillin-resistant Staphylococcus aureus. *Ophthalmology.* 2012;119(6):1238–1243.

Pelton RW, Klapper SR. Preseptal and orbital cellulitis. *Focal Points: Clinical Modules for Ophthalmologists.* San Francisco: American Academy of Ophthalmology; 2008, module 11.

Orbital cellulitis

Orbital cellulitis involves structures posterior to the orbital septum, and in the majority of cases it occurs as a secondary extension of acute or chronic bacterial sinusitis (Table 4-2). Clinical findings include fever, leukocytosis (75% of cases), erythema, proptosis, chemosis, ptosis, and restriction of and pain with ocular movement (Fig 4-2A, B). Decreased vision, impaired color vision, restricted visual fields, and pupillary abnormalities suggest optic neuropathy that demands immediate investigation and aggressive management. Delay in treatment may result in blindness, cavernous sinus thrombosis, cranial neuropathy, meningitis, or death. Treatment may require a multidisciplinary approach.

Orbital findings indicate that imaging is needed to identify sinusitis, which may require treatment from an otolaryngologist. Antibiotic therapy in adults should provide broad-spectrum coverage because such infections usually involve multiple organisms that may include gram-positive cocci, such as *H influenzae* and *Moraxella catarrhalis,* and anaerobes. Although nasal decongestants promote drainage of the infected sinus, sinus surgery is often required, especially if orbital findings progress during IV antibiotic therapy. In contrast, orbital cellulitis in children is more often caused by a single gram-positive organism and is less likely to require surgical sinus drainage.

Progressive proptosis, globe displacement, or lack of response to appropriate antibiotic therapy suggests abscess formation, which can be identified on orbital CT imaging with contrast. Abscesses usually localize in the subperiosteal space (Fig 4-2C, D), adjacent to the infected sinus, but may extend through the periosteum into the orbital soft tissues. When initial medical treatment fails, further imaging may identify an abscess and determine an approach for surgical intervention.

Table 4-2 Causes of Orbital Cellulitis

Extension from periorbital structures
Paranasal sinuses (sinusitis)
Face and eyelids, infection of
Lacrimal sac (dacryocystitis)
Dental (odontogenic infection)

Exogenous causes
Trauma (rule out foreign bodies)
Surgery (after any orbital or periorbital surgery)

Endogenous causes
Bacteremia with septic embolization

Intraorbital causes
Endophthalmitis
Dacryoadenitis

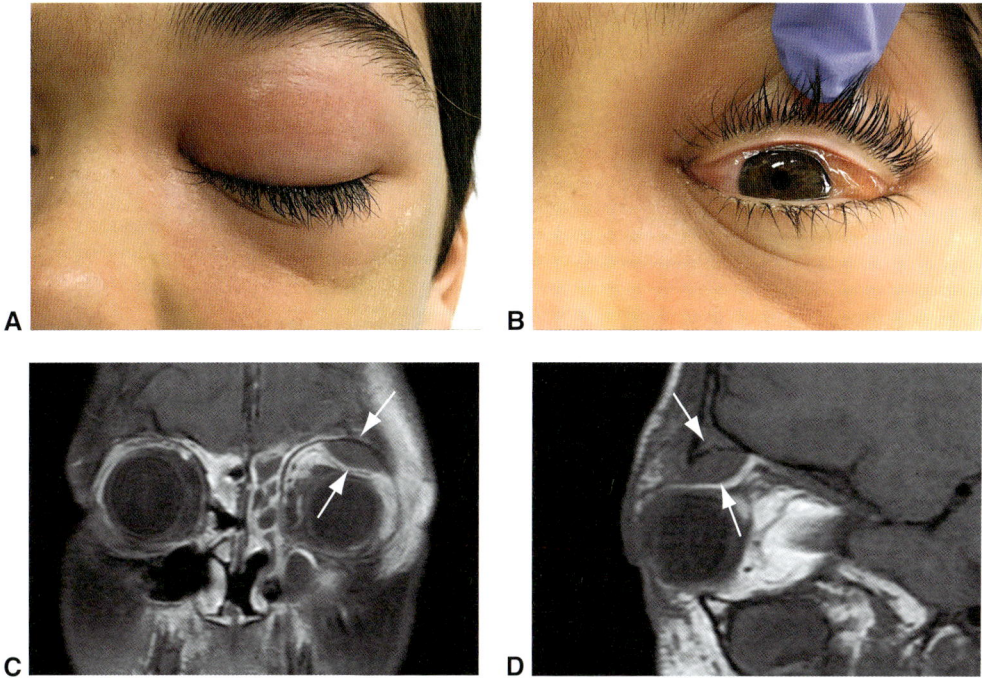

Figure 4-2 Left-sided orbital cellulitis. **A,** Marked periocular erythema is present, as well as upper eyelid ptosis. **B,** Chemosis is present with elevation of the eyelid. **C** and **D,** T-1 weighted magnetic resonance imaging (MRI) with gadolinium contrast reveals a superior subperiosteal abscess (*arrows*). *(Courtesy of Cat N. Burkat, MD.)*

However, not all subperiosteal abscesses (SPAs) require surgical drainage. Isolated medial or inferior SPAs in children younger than 9 years with underlying isolated ethmoid sinusitis, intact vision, and only moderate proptosis typically respond to medical therapy. Management may consist of careful observation *unless any of the following criteria are present:*

- patient aged 9 years or older
- presence of frontal sinusitis
- nonmedial SPA location
- large SPA
- suspicion of anaerobic infection (eg, presence of gas in abscess on CT)
- recurrence of SPA after prior drainage
- evidence of chronic sinusitis (eg, nasal polyps)
- acute optic nerve or retinal compromise
- infection of dental origin (anaerobic infection more likely)

In patients with these criteria or with infections refractory to medical therapy, surgical drainage coupled with appropriate antibiotic therapy typically leads to clinical improvement within 24–48 hours. Sinusitis may improve with concomitant sinus surgery. The refractory nature of orbital abscesses in adolescents and adults may relate to the frequent involvement of multiple and drug-resistant pathogens, particularly anaerobic organisms.

Treatment with corticosteroids may speed resolution of inflammation and decrease the length of hospital admission, although the timing and dose remain controversial. Their use should be balanced by the risk of masking infection progression.

Because orbital cellulitis and abscesses respond to therapy in most patients, orbital infections rarely spread posteriorly to the cavernous sinus. Cavernous sinus thrombosis is often heralded by the rapid progression of proptosis, the development of ipsilateral ophthalmoplegia, and the onset of anesthesia in both the first and second divisions of the trigeminal nerve. In rare instances, contralateral ophthalmoplegia, meningitis, or frank brain abscess may develop. Lumbar puncture may reveal acute inflammatory cells and the causative organism on stain and culture. Contrast-enhanced magnetic resonance imaging (MRI) confirms the diagnosis.

Orbital cellulitis caused by MRSA may occur without antecedent respiratory illness or trauma and without adjacent paranasal sinus disease on imaging. MRSA-caused orbital cellulitis may require surgical intervention more often than typical orbital cellulitis, and it may also lead to significant decrease in visual acuity more often, especially in cases in which referral for surgical intervention has been delayed. Because of the potentially aggressive nature of this pathogen, successful management demands a high degree of clinical suspicion and prompt medical and surgical intervention. In addition, consultation with specialists in infectious diseases may be warranted.

Orbital cellulitis following blowout fractures generally occurs in patients with underlying sinus disease or a medial wall fracture. Prophylactic antibiotics can be considered in these cases.

Odontogenic infections may spread through the sinuses to cause orbital cellulitis. These infections account for 2%–5% of all orbital cellulitis cases and can arise from any tooth, although most develop from maxillary premolar teeth. These infections are typically polymicrobial, often consisting of gram-positive aerobes and anaerobes.

Garcia GH, Harris GJ. Criteria for nonsurgical management of subperiosteal abscess of the orbit: analysis of outcomes 1988–1998. *Ophthalmology.* 2000;107(8):1454–1456, discussion 1458.

Pushker N, Tejwani LK, Bajaj MS, Khurana S, Velpandian T, Chandra M. Role of oral corticosteroids in orbital cellulitis. *Am J Ophthalmol.* 2013;156(1):178–183.

Necrotizing Fasciitis

Necrotizing fasciitis is a severe, potentially vision-threatening or life-threatening bacterial infection involving the subcutaneous soft tissues, particularly the superficial and deep fasciae. A variety of organisms may cause this disorder, including aerobic and anaerobic, gram-positive and gram-negative bacteria, but the organism most commonly responsible is group A β-hemolytic streptococcus.

This infection develops rapidly and requires immediate attention because it is potentially fatal. Although most patients are immunocompromised, it may occur in immunocompetent patients as well. The initial clinical presentation is similar to that of orbital or preseptal cellulitis, with swelling, erythema, and pain, but it may be accompanied by a shocklike syndrome. Because necrotizing fasciitis tends to track along avascular tissue planes, an early sign may be anesthesia over the affected area caused by involvement of deep cutaneous nerves. In addition, reports of disproportionate pain may suggest the presence of necrotizing fasciitis, as do skin color changes that progress from rose to blue-gray, with bullae formation and frank cutaneous necrosis. Usually, the course is rapid, and the patient requires treatment in an intensive care unit.

Treatment includes early surgical debridement along with IV antibiotics (Fig 4-3). If the involved pathogen is unknown, broad-spectrum coverage for gram-positive and gram-negative as well as anaerobic organisms is indicated. Clindamycin is effective in treating infections due to most causative organisms and acts against the toxins produced by group A streptococcus. To limit the inflammatory damage associated with the toxins, adjunctive corticosteroid therapy after the start of antibiotic therapy has been advocated. Some cases of necrotizing fasciitis can be cautiously followed with systemic antibiotic therapy and with little or no debridement, including cases that are limited to the eyelids, such those with clearly defined margins, and in which the patient shows no signs of toxic shock.

Patients may experience rapid deterioration, culminating in hypotension, renal failure, and adult respiratory distress syndrome. Although clinical series from all body sites

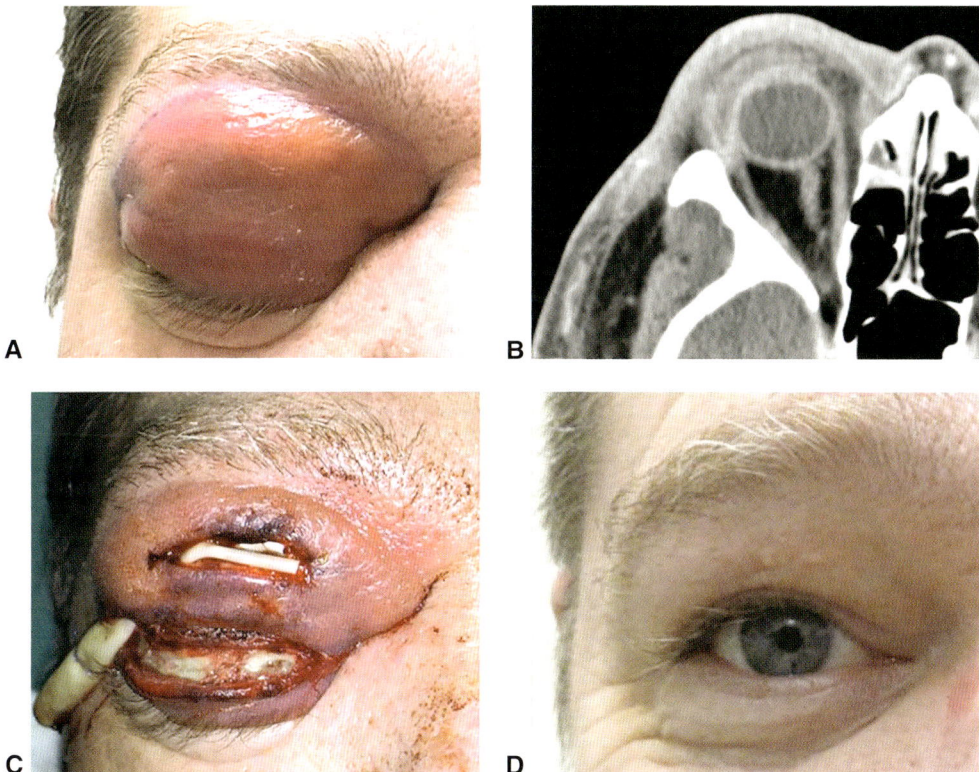

Figure 4-3 Necrotizing fasciitis. **A,** A patient with marked erythema and induration with early bullae formation. **B,** Axial computed tomography (CT) imaging study shows the spread of infection along preseptal fascial planes. **C,** Photograph taken immediately postoperatively demonstrates debrided tissues and drain. **D,** Photograph of patient after extensive debridement and systemic antibiotic therapy. *(Courtesy of Julian D. Perry, MD, and Catherine J. Hwang, MD.)*

report up to a 30% mortality rate, usually due to toxic shock syndrome, this occurs less commonly in patients who have infection in the periocular region.

Lazzeri D, Lazzeri S, Figus M, et al. Periorbital necrotising fasciitis. *Br J Ophthalmol.* 2010;94(12):1577–1585.

Mycobacterial Infection

Although it most commonly occurs in endemic areas of the developing world, tuberculosis may occur in the developed world as well, most often in individuals with HIV infection or in association with inner-city poverty. Orbital tuberculosis usually results after hematogenous spread from an often-subclinical pulmonary focus, but it may also arise from adjacent tuberculous sinusitis. Patients may present with proptosis, motility dysfunction, bone destruction, and chronic draining fistulas. Most orbital cases are unilateral and occur in children, in whom the infection may masquerade as an orbital malignancy. Pathologic specimens may not reveal acid-fast bacilli, but usually show caseating necrosis, epithelioid cells, and Langerhans giant cells. Skin testing and fine-needle aspiration biopsy with culture performed early in the course of the disease may help establish the diagnosis. Antituberculous therapy is usually curative.

Nontuberculous (atypical) mycobacteria may also infect the periocular tissues. Predisposing factors include immunosuppression, nasolacrimal duct obstruction, trauma, and a history of recent periocular surgery. Postoperative infections occur most commonly after lacrimal surgery but can occur after blepharoplasty as well (Fig 4-4). The causative organisms, which are identified in less than one-third of reported cases, are typically *Mycobacterium chelonae* or *Mycobacterium fortuitum.* Treatment consists of periocular debridement and systemic antituberculous antibiotics.

Klapper SR, Patrinely JR, Kaplan SL, Font RL. Atypical mycobacterial infection of the orbit. *Ophthalmology.* 1995;102(10):1536–1541.
Mauriello JA Jr; Atypical Mycobacterial Study Group. Atypical mycobacterial infection of the periocular region after periocular and facial surgery. *Ophthalmic Plast Reconstr Surg.* 2003;19(3):182–188.
Moorthy RS, Valluri S, Rao NA. Nontuberculous mycobacterial ocular and adnexal infections. *Surv Ophthalmol.* 2012;57(3):202–235.

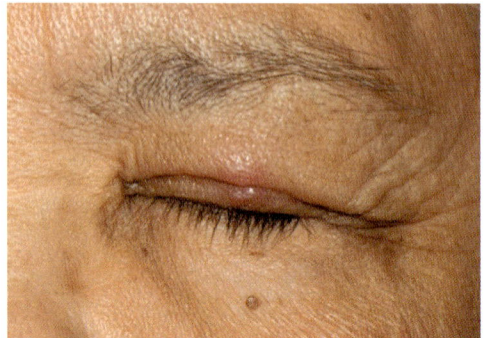

Figure 4-4 A patient presents with delayed infection of the left upper eyelid by nontuberculous (atypical) mycobacteria after blepharoplasty. *(Courtesy of Bobby S. Korn, MD, PhD.)*

Zygomycosis

Zygomycosis (also known as *phycomycosis* or *mucormycosis*) is the most common and the most virulent fungal disease involving the orbit. The specific fungal genus involved is usually *Mucor* or *Rhizopus*. These fungi, belonging to the class Zygomycetes, almost always extend into the orbit from an adjacent sinus or the nasal cavity. The fungi invade blood vessel walls, producing thrombosing vasculitis. The resultant tissue necrosis promotes further fungal invasion.

Patients commonly present with proptosis and an orbital apex syndrome (internal and external ophthalmoplegia, ptosis, decreased corneal sensation, and decreased vision). Ascending infection may result in cavernous sinus thrombosis (Fig 4-5). Because of the thrombosing vasculitis, the infection may not produce significant orbital inflammation and an unusually white and quiet eye should prompt concern for orbital ischemia.

Predisposing factors include systemic disease with associated metabolic acidosis, diabetes mellitus, malignancies, and treatment with antimetabolites or steroids. Biopsy of the necrotic-appearing tissues in the nasopharynx, involved sinus, or orbit confirms the diagnosis and shows nonseptate, large branching hyphae that stain with hematoxylin-eosin, unlike most fungi (see the discussion of zygomycosis in BCSC Section 5, *Neuro-Ophthalmology*).

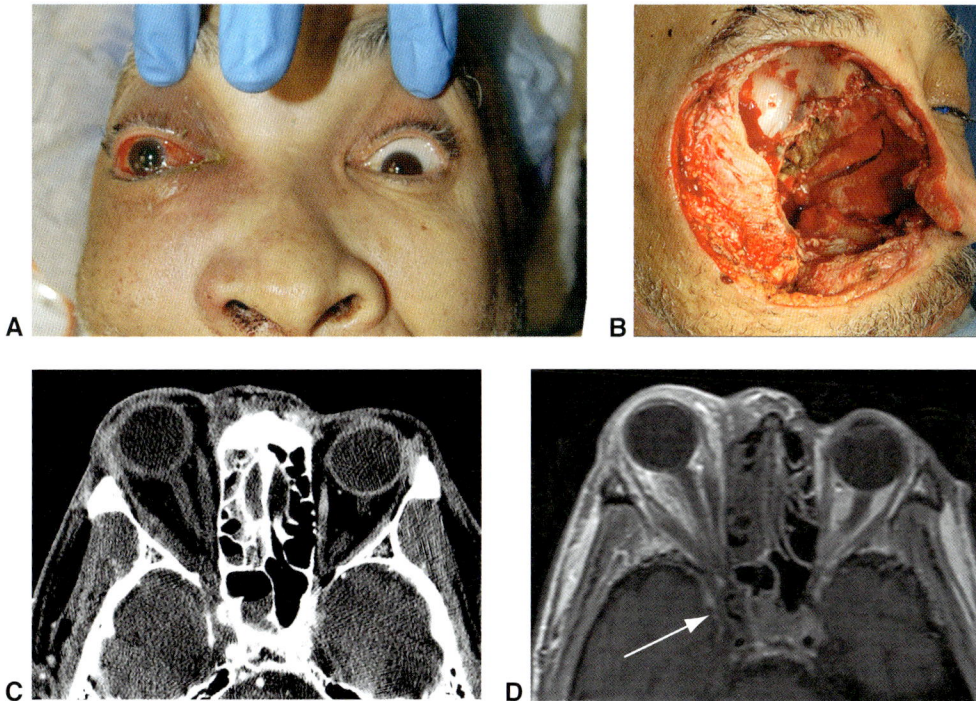

Figure 4-5 Right-sided sino-orbital zygomycosis in a patient with diabetic ketoacidosis. **A,** In this photograph, complete right upper eyelid ptosis and ophthalmoplegia are present in the patient. **B,** Wide surgical debridement consisting of orbital exenteration and sinus surgery was life-saving. CT **(C)** and MRI **(D)** axial scans show orbital and sinus involvement as well as cavernous sinus thrombosis *(arrow)*. *(Courtesy of Bobby S. Korn, MD, PhD.)*

Treatment should include a multidisciplinary team to address any underlying predisposing disease, perform wide surgical debridement, and administer antifungal therapy. Diabetic ketoacidosis, in particular, requires prompt correction; this condition produces more free serum iron, thought to be central for fungal pathogenesis. Antifungal therapy may consist of IV or liposomal amphotericin B; posaconazole or voriconazole may be used in patients who cannot tolerate the adverse effects of amphotericin. In addition, retrobulbar injection of amphotericin B may be considered. Adjunctive treatments include hyperbaric oxygen therapy. Despite aggressive surgical debridement, including exenteration, the prognosis for survival remains poor and often depends on whether the underlying systemic predisposing disease is immediately treatable.

Warwar RE, Bullock JD. Rhino-orbital-cerebral mucormycosis: a review. *Orbit.* 1998;17(4):237–245.

Aspergillosis

Fungi in the *Aspergillus* genus can affect the orbit in several distinct clinical entities. *Invasive aspergillosis* is a fungal disease characterized by fulminant sinus infection with secondary orbital invasion. Patients present with severe periorbital pain, decreased vision, and proptosis. Diagnosis is confirmed by 1 or more biopsies. Grocott-Gomori methenamine–silver nitrate stain shows septate branching hyphae of uniform width (see the discussion of aspergillosis in BCSC Section 5, *Neuro-Ophthalmology*). Therapy consists of aggressive surgical excision of all infected tissues and administration of antifungal agents, including polyenes (amphotericin B, liposomal amphotericin B), azoles (eg, itraconazole, voriconazole), echinocandins (caspofungin), and pyrimidine analogues (flucytosine), or a combination thereof.

Chronic necrotizing aspergillosis is an indolent infection resulting in slow destruction of the sinuses and adjacent structures. Although the prognosis is much better than that for acute fulminant disease, intraorbital and intracranial extension can still occur and result in significant morbidity.

Chronic, localized noninvasive aspergillosis also involves the sinuses and occurs in immunocompetent patients who may not have a history of atopic disease. Often, there is a history of chronic sinusitis, and the proliferation of fungal organisms results in a tightly packed fungus ball. This type of aspergillosis is characterized by a lack of either inflammation or bone erosion.

Allergic aspergillosis sinusitis occurs in immunocompetent patients with nasal polyposis and chronic sinusitis. Patients may have peripheral eosinophilia; elevated total immunoglobulin E (IgE), fungus-specific IgE, and immunoglobulin G (IgG) levels; or positive skin test results for fungal antigens. CT imaging reveals mottled areas of increased attenuation on nonenhanced images, corresponding to thick allergic mucin within the sinus. Bone erosion and remodeling, while often present, do not signify tissue invasion. MRI may be more specific, showing signal void areas on T2-weighted scans. Sinus biopsy reveals thick, peanut butter–like or green mucus, with histologic examination showing numerous eosinophils, eosinophil degradation products, and extramucosal fungal hyphae. Treatment consists of endoscopic sinus debridement as well as systemic and topical corticosteroids. Up to 17% of patients with allergic fungal sinusitis initially present with orbital signs.

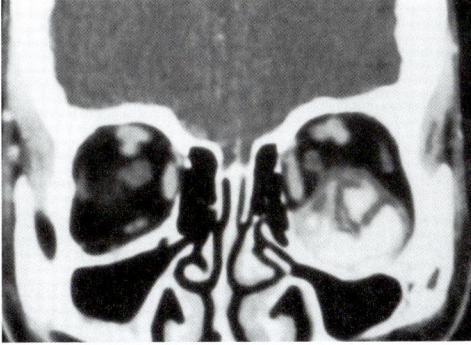

Figure 4-6 Coronal CT scan demonstrates a hydatid cyst of the left inferior rectus muscle. *(Courtesy of Don O. Kikkawa, MD.)*

Carter KD, Graham SM, Carpenter KM. Ophthalmic manifestations of allergic fungal sinusitis. *Am J Ophthalmol.* 1999;127(2):189–195.

Klapper SR, Lee AG, Patrinely JR, Stewart M, Alford EL. Orbital involvement in allergic fungal sinusitis. *Ophthalmology.* 1997;104(12):2094–2100.

Pushker N, Meel R, Kashyap S, Bajaj MS, Sen S. Invasive aspergillosis of orbit in immunocompetent patients: treatment and outcome. *Ophthalmology.* 2011;118(9):1886–1891.

Parasitic Diseases

Parasitic diseases of the orbit generally occur in developing countries. *Trichinosis*, caused by ingestion of the nematode *Trichinella spiralis*, may produce inflammation of the eyelids and extraocular muscles, resulting from larval migration. *Echinococcosis*, caused by the dog tapeworm *Echinococcus granulosus*, may manifest as a hydatid cyst within the orbit (Fig 4-6). Rupture of the cyst, which contains tapeworm larvae, may cause progressive inflammation and a severe immune response. *Taenia solium,* the pork tapeworm, may also encyst within the orbit and progressively enlarge to cause a condition known as *cysticercosis.*

Noninfectious Inflammation

Thyroid Eye Disease

Thyroid eye disease (TED; also known as *Graves ophthalmopathy, thyroid-associated orbitopathy,* and other terms) represents an autoimmune inflammatory disorder with characteristic clinical signs (Figs 4-7, 4-8, 4-9, 4-10). Originally described as part of the triad of

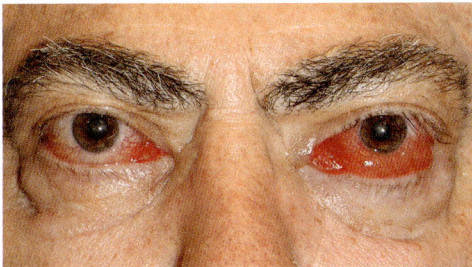

Figure 4-7 Active thyroid eye disease (TED) in a patient demonstrating bilateral chemosis, conjunctival injection, and caruncular edema. *(Courtesy of Bobby S. Korn, MD, PhD.)*

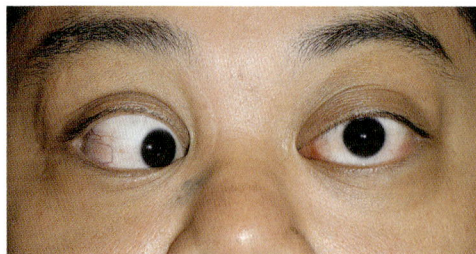

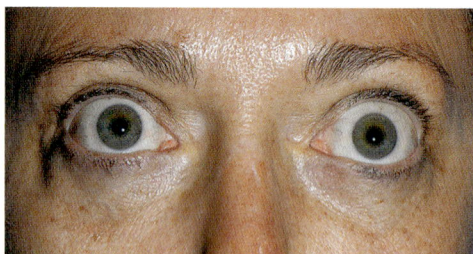

Figure 4-8 Restrictive strabismus causing marked esotropia in a patient with relative enlargement of the right medial rectus muscle. *(Courtesy of Bobby S. Korn, MD, PhD.)*

Figure 4-9 A patient with TED demonstrates bilateral upper and lower eyelid retraction, proptosis, and lateral flare. *(Courtesy of Bobby S. Korn, MD, PhD.)*

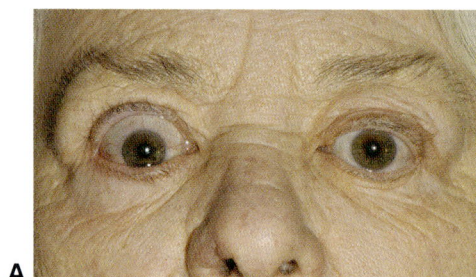

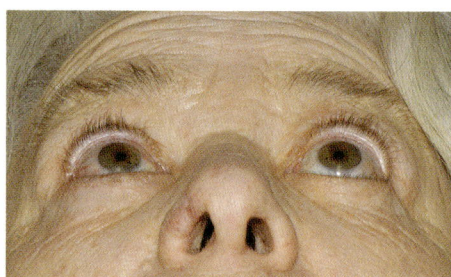

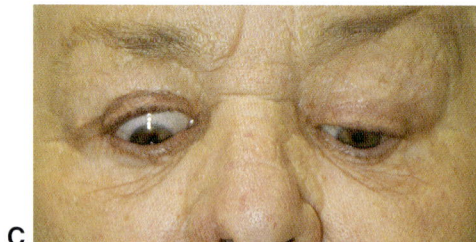

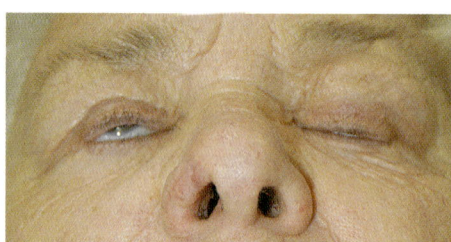

Figure 4-10 A patient with asymmetric TED. **A,** Right upper eyelid retraction. **B,** Left relative exophthalmos. **C,** Right upper lid lag with downgaze. **D,** Bilateral lagophthalmos with inferior corneal exposure on the right. *(Courtesy of Bobby S. Korn, MD, PhD.)*

Graves disease (orbital signs, hyperthyroidism, and pretibial myxedema), TED most often occurs in individuals with Graves hyperthyroidism. However, TED may also occur with Hashimoto thyroiditis (immune-induced hypothyroidism) or in the absence of thyroid dysfunction. The course of the eye disease does not necessarily parallel the activity of the thyroid gland or the treatment of thyroid abnormalities.

See Key Points 4-1.

> **KEY POINTS 4-1**
>
> **Thyroid eye disease (TED)** The following list highlights the essential points for the ophthalmologist to remember about TED.
>
> - Eyelid retraction is the most common clinical feature of TED (and TED is the most common cause of eyelid retraction).
> - TED is the most common cause of unilateral or bilateral proptosis.
> - TED may be markedly asymmetric.
> - TED is associated with hyperthyroidism in 90% of patients, but 6% of patients may be euthyroid.
> - Severity of TED usually does not parallel serum levels of triiodo-thyronine (T_3) or free thyroxine (T_4).
> - TED is up to 6 times as common in women as in men.
> - Smoking is associated with increased risk and severity of TED.
> - Urgent care may be required for optic neuropathy or severe prop-tosis with corneal decompensation.
> - If surgery is needed, the usual order is orbital decompression, fol-lowed by strabismus surgery, followed by eyelid retraction repair (see Chapter 7 in this volume).
> - Radiotherapy may prevent optic neuropathy and may improve some aspects of TED, but its role remains controversial.

Diagnosis

The diagnosis of TED is made when 2 of the following 3 signs are present:

1. Concurrent or recently treated immune-related thyroid dysfunction:

   a. Graves hyperthyroidism
   b. Hashimoto thyroiditis
   c. Presence of circulating thyroid antibodies without a coexisting dysthyroid state (partial consideration given): thyroid-stimulating hormone–receptor (TSH-R) antibodies, thyroid-binding inhibitory immunoglobulins, thyroid-stimulating immunoglobulins, antimicrosomal antibodies

2. Typical ocular signs:

   a. Chemosis and/or caruncular edema (see Fig 4-7)
   b. Restrictive strabismus in a typical pattern (see Fig 4-8)
   c. Unilateral or bilateral eyelid retraction with typical lateral flare (see Fig 4-9)
   d. Unilateral or bilateral proptosis (in comparison with old photos of the patient)
   e. Compressive optic neuropathy
   f. Fluctuating eyelid edema and/or erythema

3. Radiographic evidence of TED: unilateral or bilateral fusiform enlargement any of the rectus muscles and/or the levator muscle complex (Figs 4-11, 4-12).

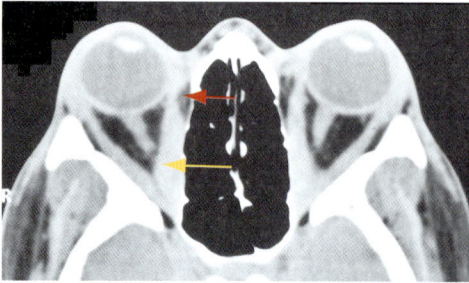

Figure 4-11 TED. Axial orbital CT scan shows characteristic fusiform extraocular muscle enlargement *(yellow arrow)* that spares the tendons *(red arrow)*. *(Courtesy of Julian D. Perry, MD.)*

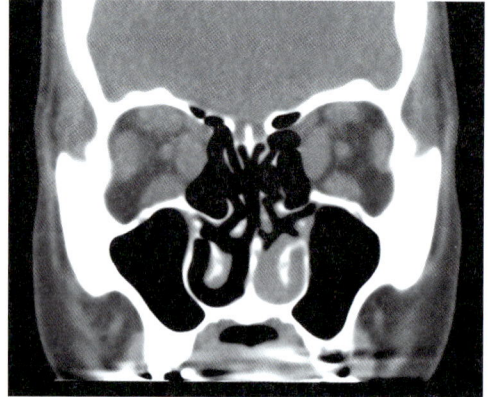

Figure 4-12 Coronal orbital CT scan shows bilateral enlargement of extraocular muscles in TED. *(Courtesy of Keith D. Carter, MD.)*

Serologic testing, using serum thyroid-stimulating hormone (TSH), triiodothyronine (T_3), and free thyroxine (T_4) levels, is well established in the diagnosis of thyroid disease. However, the usefulness of these tests in monitoring TED treatment and progression is unclear, because the systemic disease and the eye disease are discordant.

Tests of autoimmune function may be helpful in evaluating disease activity and severity. TSH-R antibody testing can be performed by measuring all immunoglobulins targeting the TSH-R (eg, the thyrotropin-binding inhibitory immunoglobulin [TBII] test) or by measuring only the stimulating antibodies (eg, the thyroid-stimulating immunoglobulin [TSI] assay).

These tests may help identify the cause of the thyroid disease and may help identify patients at high risk for TED; however, results should be interpreted with caution because the diagnosis of TED is based mainly on clinical findings. Thyroid peroxidase antibody testing has replaced antimicrosomal antibody testing; however, the presence of this antibody does not correlate with TED activity or severity or TSI levels. Similarly, thyroglobulin antibody levels do not correlate with TED. Insulin-like growth factor I (IGF-I) antibody levels may represent a future area of serologic testing for TED; however, no current recommendations exist.

Patients presenting with only orbital signs require observation for other orbital diseases or the development of a dysthyroid state.

Mourits MP, Prummel MF, Wiersinga WM, Koornneef L. Clinical activity score as a guide in the management of patients with Graves' ophthalmopathy. *Clin Endocrinol (Oxf)*. 1997;47(1):9–14.

Srinivasan A, Kleinberg TT, Murchison AP, Bilyk JR. Laboratory investigations for diagnosis of autoimmune and inflammatory periocular disease: Part II. *Ophthalmic Plast Reconstr Surg*. 2017;33(1):1–8.

Pathogenesis

Orbital fibroblasts, through the expression of characteristic surface receptors, gangliosides, and proinflammatory genes, play an active role in modulating the inflammatory process. Unlike fibroblasts from other body sites, orbital fibroblasts express CD40 receptors, which are generally found on B cells. When engaged by T-cell–bound CD154, several fibroblast pro-inflammatory cytokines are upregulated, including interleukin-6 (IL-6) and interleukin-8 (IL-8), as well as prostaglandin E2, increasing synthesis of hyaluronan and glycosaminoglycan (GAG). This upregulation of orbital fibroblast GAG synthesis represents an essential aspect of the pathology of TED, and it occurs at a rate 100 times that of abdominal fibroblasts from the same patient. Therapeutic levels of corticosteroids dampen the upregulation cascade.

Orbital fibroblasts, which are embryologically derived from the neural crest lineage, possess developmental plasticity. A subpopulation of orbital fibroblasts appears capable of undergoing adipocyte differentiation, contributing to the expansion of orbital fat that predominates in some patients.

A circulating immunoglobulin that recognizes and activates the insulin-like growth factor I receptor (IGF-IR) expressed on the surface of orbital fibroblasts of individuals with Graves disease may stimulate orbital fibroblasts to secrete GAGs, cytokines, and chemoattractants. These latter signaling families may contribute to orbital inflammation and congestion.

Kazim M, Goldberg RA, Smith TJ. Insights into the pathogenesis of thyroid-associated orbitopathy: evolving rationale for therapy. *Arch Ophthalmol.* 2002;120(3):380–386.

Naik V, Khadavi N, Naik MN, et al. Biologic therapeutics in thyroid-associated ophthalmopathy: translating disease mechanism into therapy. *Thyroid.* 2008;18(9):967–971.

Tsui S, Naik V, Hoa N, et al. Evidence for an association between thyroid-stimulating hormone and insulin-like growth factor 1 receptors: a tale of two antigens implicated in Graves' disease. *J Immunol.* 2008;181(6):4397–4405.

Epidemiology

A 1996 epidemiologic study of white patients with TED in the United States determined that the overall age-adjusted incidence per 100,000 population per year was 16 cases for women compared with 3 cases for men. The peak incidences occurred in the age groups 40–44 years and 60–64 years in women and 45–49 years and 65–69 years in men. Development of TED is up to 7 times as likely for smokers when compared to nonsmokers.

Clinical features

Among patients with TED, about 90% have Graves hyperthyroidism, 6% are euthyroid, 3% have Hashimoto thyroiditis, and 1% have primary hypothyroidism. A close temporal relationship exists between the development of hyperthyroidism and the development of TED: in about 20% of patients, the diagnoses are made at the same time, and in about 60% of patients, the eye disease occurs within 1 year of onset of the thyroid disease. For patients who have no history of abnormal thyroid function or regulation at the time TED is diagnosed, the risk for development of thyroid disease is about 25% within 1 year and 50% within 5 years. Although hyperthyroidism is present or will develop in most patients with TED, only about 30% of patients with autoimmune hyperthyroidism will develop TED.

Pretibial myxedema accompanies TED in about 4% of patients. Acropachy (soft-tissue swelling and periosteal changes affecting the distal extremities, principally fingers and toes) accompanies TED in about 1% of patients. Both are associated with a poor prognosis for the orbitopathy. Myasthenia gravis occurs in fewer than 1% of patients and should be considered when ptosis accompanies TED.

The most frequent presenting ocular symptoms and signs of TED are a dull, deep orbital pain or discomfort (30% of patients), lid lag with downgaze (unilateral or bilateral, 50%; see Fig 4-10), and upper eyelid retraction (unilateral or bilateral, 75%). Symptomatic dysthyroid optic neuropathy is present in less than 2% of eyes at the time of diagnosis of TED.

Upper eyelid retraction occurs in more than 90% of patients during their clinical course (see Fig 4-9); exophthalmos (unilateral or bilateral) in 60%; restrictive extraocular myopathy in 40%; and optic neuropathy (unilateral or bilateral) in 5%. Only 5% of patients develop the complete constellation of these 4 classic findings and hyperthyroidism. Some degree of diplopia is reported by about 17% of patients, lacrimation or photophobia by 15%–20% of patients, and blurred vision by 7% of patients.

Bartley GB, Fatourechi V, Kadrmas EF, et al. Clinical features of Graves' ophthalmopathy in an incidence cohort. *Am J Ophthalmol.* 1996;121(3):284–290.

Treatment and prognosis

TED is a self-limiting disease that on average lasts 1 year in nonsmokers and between 2 and 3 years in smokers. After the active disease plateaus, a quiescent "burnt-out" phase that follows Rundle's curve ensues (Fig 4-13). Reactivation of inflammation occurs in 5%–10% of patients over their lifetime.

Although several clinical scoring systems to guide TED evaluation and treatment exist, including NO SPECS, Clinical Activity Score (CAS), and VISA, no system prevails. The CAS and VISA systems each assign points for various findings; the CAS adds extra parameters for follow-up visits and the VISA uses the same scale for both initial and follow-up visits. Treatment of patients with TED follows a stepwise and graded approach based on symptoms, clinical examination, and ancillary testing (Tables 4-3, 4-4).

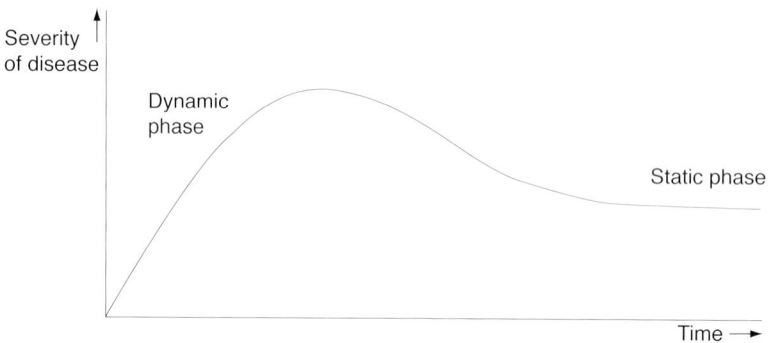

Figure 4-13 Rundle's curve as applied to the typical course of TED.

Table 4-3 VISA and CAS Inflammatory Scoring Systems

VISA: Presence of each sign/symptom receives 1–2 points as noted (maximum score of 10). Patients with sum scores <4/10 are managed conservatively, while patients with scores >5/10 or with evidence of inflammatory progression are managed more aggressively.

Swelling of caruncle (1 point)

Conjunctival chemosis behind the gray line (1 point); extends anterior to gray line (2 points)

Conjunctival erythema (1 point)

Eyelid erythema (1 point)

Eyelid swelling without redundant tissues (1 point); causing palpebral skin bulging or festoon (2 points)

Retrobulbar pain at rest (1 point)

Retrobulbar pain with movement (1 point)

CAS: Presence of each sign/symptom receives 1 point. A sum score of >3/7 at first examination or >4/10 at subsequent exams defines active ophthalmopathy.

Initial examination (maximum score of 7 points)
Ocular or retrobulbar pain

Pain with eye movement

Eyelid erythema

Eyelid swelling

Conjunctival chemosis

Conjunctival erythema

Swelling/erythema of caruncle

Subsequent examination (maximum score of 10 points, combining initial findings with parameters below)
>2-mm increase in proptosis

Impaired ductions in any 1 direction >8 degrees

>1-line decrease in Snellen visual acuity chart

Data from Mourits MP, Prummel MF, Wiersinga WM, Koornneef L. Clinical activity score as a guide in the management of patients with Graves' ophthalmopathy. *Clin Endocrinol (Oxf).* 1997;47(1):9–14.

Most patients with TED in the active phase require only smoking cessation and supportive care, including use of topical ocular lubricants. The following may also be helpful:

- topical cyclosporine, which may reduce ocular surface irritation
- a reduced-salt diet and sleeping with the head of the bed elevated, which may limit orbital edema
- wearing wraparound sunglasses, which may relieve exposure and dry eye symptoms
- temporary prism glasses, which may help maintain binocular fusion

In addition, selenium supplementation may improve the course of disease, especially in patients heralding from selenium-deficient regions. Neurotoxins can temporarily improve upper eyelid retraction by weakening the eyelid elevators. Neurotoxins can also be used to treat restrictive strabismus by weakening affected extraocular muscle(s).

Severe orbital inflammation may mandate early intervention to improve corneal exposure, globe subluxation, or optic neuropathy. Therapies generally attempt to decrease orbital

---

Table 4-4 Management of Thyroid Eye Disease

Mild disease
  Observation
  Patient education and lifestyle changes
    Smoking cessation
    Salt restriction
    Elevation of head of bed
    Use of sunglasses
  Ocular surface lubrication
  Establishment of a euthyroid state
  Oral selenium

Moderate disease
  Topical cyclosporine
  Eyelid taping at night
  Moisture goggles or chambers
  Prism glasses or selective ocular patching
  Moderate-dose oral corticosteroid therapy

Severe disease
  High-dose intravenous corticosteroid therapy
  Surgical orbital decompression (followed by strabismus surgery and/or eyelid surgery)
  Periocular radiotherapy

Refractory disease
  Steroid-sparing immunomodulators

---

congestion and inflammation (eg, glucocorticoids, biologics, radiotherapy), mechanically protect the cornea (eg, tarsorrhaphy), expand the orbital bony volume (eg, bony orbital decompression), or reduce orbital soft tissue volume (eg, fatty orbital decompression).

Establishing the euthyroid state represents a mainstay of therapy. Hyperthyroidism is most commonly treated with antithyroid drugs and sometimes with radioactive iodine (RAI). In some patients, RAI treatment may worsen TED, presumably because the TSH-R antigen release incites an enhanced immune response. In addition, hypothyroidism occurring after RAI treatment may exacerbate TED via stimulation of TSH-R. Exacerbation of TED after RAI treatment may occur more commonly in hyperthyroid patients with severe, active TED, those with elevated T_3 levels, and smokers. Oral glucocorticoid treatment tapered over 3 months may limit TED progression in patients with risk factors such as these, but it is not indicated for patients without preexisting TED and without risk factors. Another strategy, termed *block-and-replace therapy* (eg, with iodine 131, methimazole, and thyroxine) reduces exacerbation of eye findings by limiting posttreatment TSH spikes. A third strategy, usually reserved for patients whose disease is refractory to RAI or those with severe TED, involves thyroidectomy, which creates hypothyroidism without extended antigen release.

Patients with active TED featuring compressive optic neuropathy or other significant activity based on scoring systems (eg, VISA, CAS) may benefit from IV glucocorticoid treatment. Typical regimens vary from 500 mg to 1 g methylprednisolone weekly for 6–12 weeks, with a maximum dose of approximately 6 g in most cases and up to 8 g in severe cases. Hepatic function should be checked before administration and monitored throughout treatment due to potentially fatal hepatotoxicity. For oral glucocorticoids, which are now less commonly used than they were in the past, the usual starting dose is 1 mg/kg prednisone for 2–4 weeks until a clinical response is apparent. The dose is then reduced as rapidly as possible, based on the clinical response of optic nerve function. Although effective, high-dose glucocorticoids are associated with an extensive list of potential systemic adverse effects, limiting their long-term use. Refractory cases of optic neuropathy and vision-threatening exposure keratopathy may require additional treatments, such as orbital radiotherapy or decompressive surgery.

Some reports suggest that treatment with fractionated orbital radiotherapy improves compressive optic neuropathy and other signs of TED in some patients, possibly by inducing terminal differentiation of fibroblasts and killing tissue-bound monocytes, which play an important role in antigen presentation. Recent evidence has suggested it may provide a protective effect against the development of optic neuropathy. Given the biologic effects of radiation, it is likely more useful in the active phase of the disease. Although radiation has been used for decades, a wealth of data exists to both support and refute its use, with and without the use of glucocorticoids, for many signs and symptoms of TED. Radiation therapy carries a rare risk of exacerbating diabetic retinopathy or other ischemic retinopathies.

Treatment with rituximab may affect the clinical course of TED by blocking the CD20 receptor on B lymphocytes; however, it does not appear to target the central mechanisms of the disease, and most clinicians currently use this only as a second-line therapy in select cases. Tocilizumab, a monoclonal IL-6 antibody, may reduce inflammatory signs and even TSI via an upstream effect on the inflammatory cycle. A variety of other anti-inflammatory, antimetabolite, and biologic agents have been employed with limited success.

In a recent clinical trial, teprotumumab, a human monoclonal antibody inhibitor of IGF-IR, reduced exophthalmos and the CAS in patients with active ophthalmopathy. Teprotumumab may specifically target the autoimmune process underlying TED. This new therapeutic agent appears well tolerated; hyperglycemia in patients with diabetes mellitus represents the main adverse effect.

In patients with active TED, orbital decompression treats optic neuropathy and severe exposure keratopathy that is refractory to medical therapy. In the postinflammatory phase of the condition, the first stage of surgical rehabilitation is decompression to address disfiguring or symptomatic proptosis. Preoperative CT imaging details the relative contributions of extraocular muscle enlargement and fat expansion to the proptosis (see Figs 4-11, 4-12). Patients with more enlargement of the orbital fat compartment (type I orbitopathy) may benefit from more fatty decompression, whereas patients with more extraocular muscle enlargement (type II orbitopathy) may benefit from more bony decompression. Fat and bone removal can be combined, graded, and tailored to achieve different amounts of proptosis reduction while minimizing adverse effects, such as diplopia, hypoglobus, and sinusitis. See Chapter 7 for further discussion of orbital decompression.

Because decompression may produce or worsen diplopia, it should precede strabismus surgery, which may help restore single vision in patients with intractable diplopia in primary gaze or in the reading position. Prisms represent another option for patients with relatively comitant strabismus or for patients with a small deviation after strabismus surgery.

Surgery to recess the rectus muscles can change eyelid position, so strabismus surgery typically precedes eyelid repositioning surgery. Levator and/or Müller muscle recession improves upper eyelid retraction to decrease corneal exposure and help improve appearance. The lower eyelids can be repositioned as well, typically by recessing the eyelid retractors, with or without a spacer graft or during a midface-lift. Finally, the last stage of surgery includes redraping of the eyelid skin and subcutaneous tissues. These techniques often address redundant skin and fatty tissues in addition to concomitant and independent periocular aging changes.

Elective orbital decompression, strabismus surgery, and eyelid retraction repair are usually not considered until achieving a euthyroid state with stable ophthalmic signs for at least 6 to 9 months.

Fortunately, treatment usually mitigates vision loss from optic neuropathy and prism glasses typically treat persistent diplopia. Subjectively, however, more than 50% of patients believe that their eyes look abnormal, and 38% of patients are dissatisfied with the appearance of their eyes. Thus, although significant long-term functional impairment from TED remains uncommon, the disease leaves lasting psychological and aesthetic sequelae.

Bartalena L, Marcocci C, Bogazzi F, et al. Relation between therapy for hyperthyroidism and the course of Graves' ophthalmopathy. *N Engl J Med.* 1998;338(2):73–78.

Chundury RV, Weber AC, Perry JD. Orbital radiation therapy in thyroid eye disease. *Ophthalmic Plast Reconstr Surg.* 2016;32(2):83–89.

Dolman PJ, Rootman J. VISA classification for Graves orbitopathy. *Ophthalmic Plast Reconstr Surg.* 2006;22(5):319–324.

Smith TJ, Kahaly GJ, Ezra DG, et al. Teprotumumab for thyroid-associated ophthalmopathy. *N Engl J Med.* 2017;376(18):1748–1761.

Vasculitis

The vasculitides represent type III hypersensitivity reactions to circulating immune complexes leading to infiltration of vessel walls by inflammatory cells. Orbital involvement usually leads to significant morbidity and is typically associated with systemic vasculitis. The following discussion focuses mainly on the orbital manifestations of the vasculitides. See also BCSC Section 1, *Update on General Medicine*; Section 5, *Neuro-Ophthalmology*; and Section 9, *Uveitis and Ocular Inflammation*.

Giant cell arteritis

Although it is not typically thought of as an orbital disorder, giant cell arteritis (GCA; also called *temporal arteritis*) involves inflammation of the orbital vessels. The vasculitis affects the aorta, vertebral arteries, and branches of the external and internal carotid arteries; however, it typically spares the intracranial carotid artery branches, which lack an elastic lamina. Vision loss may occur from central retinal artery occlusion or ischemic optic neuropathy, and diplopia may result from ischemic dysfunction of associated cranial nerves. Systemic manifestations include headache, scalp tenderness, jaw claudication, and constitutional symptoms.

The combined sensitivity of erythrocyte sedimentation rate (ESR) and C-reactive protein testing may be as high as 99%, and thrombocytosis (platelet count) greater than 400×10^3 μL supports the diagnosis. However, temporal artery biopsy represents the gold standard for diagnosis (Video 4-1). Biopsies may contain intervals of normal tissue between affected segments, and discordant biopsy may occur after bilateral biopsy. For these reasons, bilateral biopsy and longer specimens have been advocated by some; however, no consensus exists.

VIDEO 4-1 Temporal artery biopsy.
Courtesy of Julian D. Perry, MD, and Alexander D. Blandford, MD.
Access all Section 7 videos at www.aao.org/bcscvideo_section07.

Because serologic testing may be negative in some cases, and because devastating progression may occur without treatment, administration of high-dose corticosteroids should begin as soon as possible when GCA is suspected. Tocilizumab, a monoclonal interleukin-6 receptor antibody, can induce and maintain remission with a shorter corticosteroid taper. Risks associated with biopsy include scarring, hemorrhage, and cranial nerve VII frontal branch injury that produces paralytic lagophthalmos or brow ptosis, especially if nerve injury occurs proximal to its course over the zygoma.

Stone JH, Tuckwell K, Dimonaco S, et al. Trial of tocilizumab in giant-cell arteritis. *N Engl J Med*. 2017;377(4):317–328.

Granulomatosis with polyangiitis

Granulomatosis with polyangiitis (GPA, formerly known as Wegener granulomatosis), is a multisystem disease characterized by necrotizing granulomatous inflammation and vasculitis of small- to medium-sized vessels. Although the disease often affects the respiratory and renal systems, it can affect any body site. Orbital involvement occurs in 45%–60% of patients with GPA and represents the most common ophthalmologic manifestation of the disease.

GPA typically presents clinically as either a systemic and generalized disease or in a more limited form. The generalized form may produce sinusitis with or without bone erosion, tracheobronchial necrotic and stenotic lesions, cavitary lung lesions, and glomerulonephritis (Fig 4-14). It is unclear whether the limited form of the disease represents a distinct clinical entity or is just a subtype of the general form. Either form can extend from the surrounding sinuses to involve the orbit and nasolacrimal drainage system, but the limited form causes approximately two-thirds of orbital GPA cases.

Histologic examination, especially in cases of isolated orbital involvement, may not always show the classic triad of vasculitis, granulomatous inflammation (with or without giant cells), and tissue necrosis. Often, only 1 or 2 of these findings are present on extrapulmonary biopsies.

Although their exact pathogenic role remains unclear, antineutrophil cytoplasmic autoantibodies (ANCAs) are strongly associated with certain vasculitides, including GPA. Testing for ANCAs distinguishes 2 types of immunofluorescence patterns.

Diffuse granular fluorescence within the cytoplasm (c-ANCA) is highly specific for GPA. This pattern is caused by autoantibodies directed against proteinase-3, which can then be measured by enzyme-linked immunosorbent assay (ELISA).

Fluorescence surrounding the nucleus (p-ANCA) is an artifact of ethanol fixation and can be caused by autoantibodies against many different target antigens. This finding

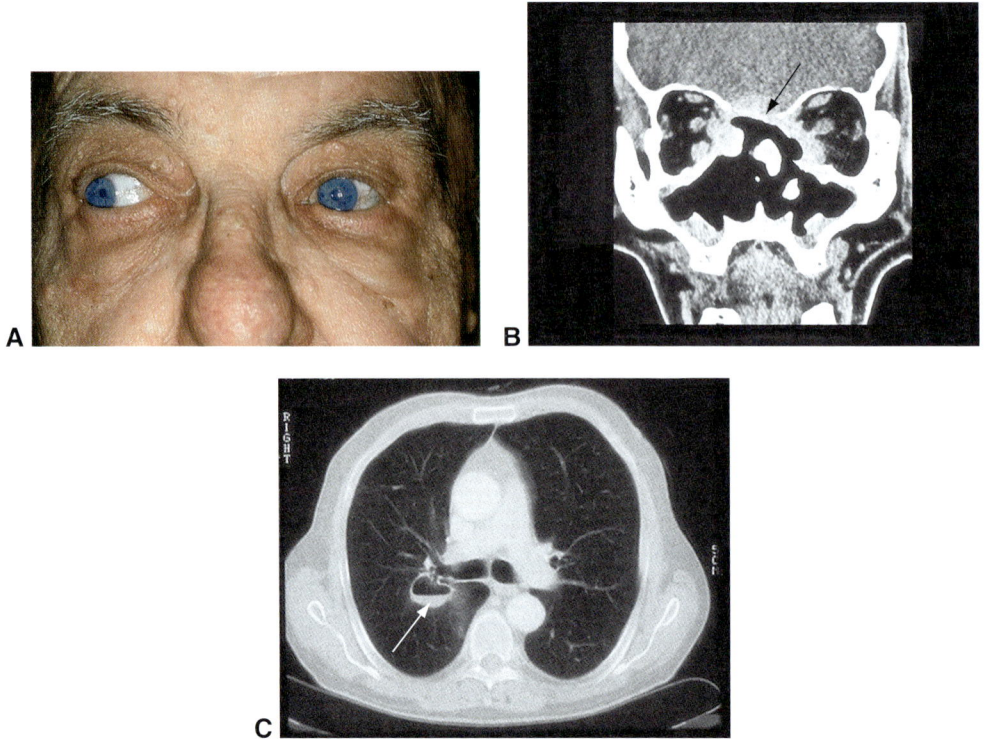

Figure 4-14 Granulomatosis with polyangiitis (GPA). **A,** Photograph of a patient with restrictive strabismus of the left eye due to inflammatory tissue extending into the medial aspects of the orbit. **B,** Coronal CT scan shows extensive destruction of the nasal and sinus cavities with inflammatory tissue extending into orbits and brain *(arrow)*. **C,** CT of chest shows cavitary lung lesions *(arrow)*. *(Courtesy of Jeffrey A. Nerad, MD.)*

is therefore nonspecific and needs to be confirmed by ELISA for ANCA reacting with myeloperoxidase (MPO-ANCA). MPO-ANCA testing has moderate specificity for small-vessel vasculitis but may return a positive result in patients with nonvasculitic diseases such as rheumatoid arthritis, sarcoidosis, or systemic lupus erythematosus.

Although highly specific for GPA, c-ANCA tests possess less sensitivity, especially in cases of isolated sino-orbital GPA and in inactive disease. Unlike c-ANCA–positive disease, p-ANCA–positive disease rarely affects the eye and orbit. Absolute levels of ANCA do not define disease severity or activity, and the use of titers to monitor for response to therapy, remission, and relapse remains controversial.

Treatment of GPA relies on remission-induction therapy, often using cytotoxic agents (eg, cyclophosphamide) and corticosteroids, followed by remission-maintenance therapy, often using methotrexate, azathioprine, and corticosteroids. Long-term treatment with TMP-SMX appears to suppress disease activity in some patients, and rituximab may help induce remission, although relapses are common regardless of treatment. Patients require care coordination from a rheumatologist, because both GPA and its treatment can produce life-threatening effects.

Polyarteritis nodosa

Polyarteritis nodosa (PAN) is a multisystem disease in which small- and medium-sized arteries are affected by inflammation characterized by the presence of neutrophils and eosinophils, with necrosis of the muscularis layer. Although PAN may affect multiple organ systems, the disease rarely produces orbital inflammation. Ophthalmic manifestations more commonly result from retinal and choroidal infarction.

Sarcoidosis

Sarcoidosis, which is characterized by collections of noncaseating granuloma, can affect any organ, most commonly the lungs. It may also affect the orbit. In America, the disease occurs 3 to 4 times as frequently in individuals of African descent as in those of European or Asian descent.

Within the orbit, the disease most frequently affects lacrimal gland, typically bilaterally. Gallium scanning, although nonspecific, shows lacrimal gland involvement in 80% of patients with systemic sarcoidosis, although only 7% of patients demonstrate clinically detectable lacrimal gland enlargement. Subconjunctival nodules (Fig 4-15A, B) and other orbital soft tissues, including the extraocular muscles and optic nerve, are involved only in rare cases. Infrequently, there is sinus involvement, with associated lytic bone lesions invading into the adjacent orbit. The disease may also affect the nasolacrimal drainage system, producing nasolacrimal duct obstruction.

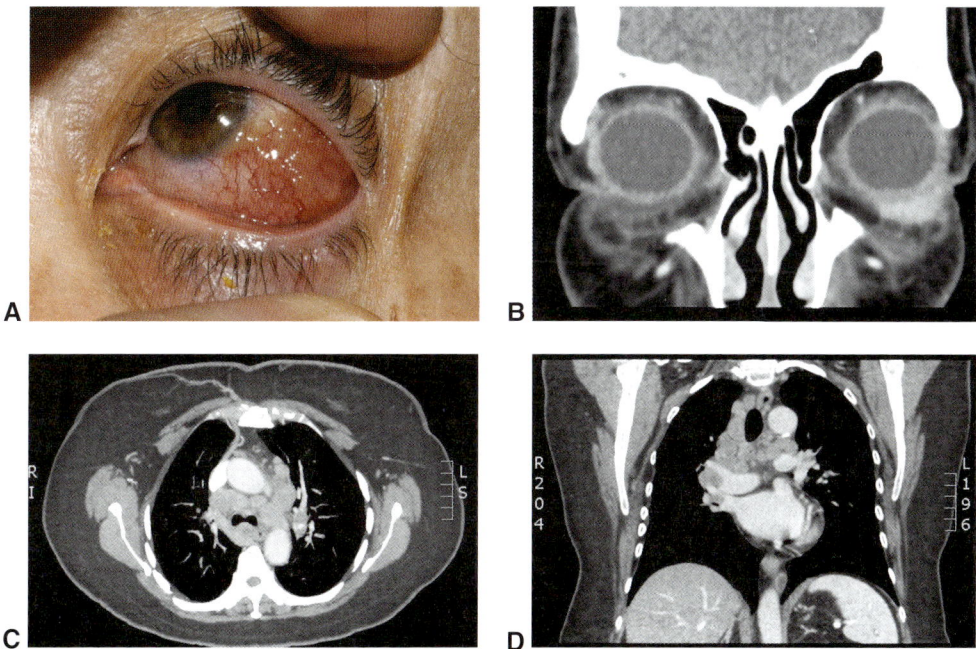

Figure 4-15 Sarcoidosis. **A,** Sarcoidosis presenting in a patient as left subconjunctival nodules. **B,** Orbital coronal CT scan shows the lesion in the anterior orbit. **C** and **D,** CT scans of the chest show bilateral hilar adenopathy. *(Courtesy of Bobby S. Korn, MD, PhD.)*

Chest radiography, CT, or gallium scans may detect hilar adenopathy or pulmonary infiltrates (Fig 4-15C, D). Serologic testing may show elevated levels of angiotensin-converting enzyme (ACE), lysozyme, and calcium. ACE is produced by the epithelioid cells and macrophages found in sarcoid granulomas, so the ACE level reflects the mass of granulomas in the body and the severity of sarcoidosis.

Regardless of serologic and imaging findings, when possible, it may be best to confirm the diagnosis with tissue biopsy. Biopsy of an affected lacrimal gland or of a suspicious conjunctival lesion may establish the diagnosis; however, random conjunctival biopsies have a low yield. Bronchoscopy with bronchial washing and biopsy may confirm pulmonary involvement. Histologic examination reveals noncaseating collections of epithelioid histiocytes in a granulomatous pattern, with mononuclear cells often appearing at the periphery of the granuloma.

Isolated orbital lesions can occur without associated systemic disease; this condition is called orbital sarcoidosis. Interestingly, patients with either isolated or systemic sarcoidosis involving the orbit rarely develop intraocular involvement and vice versa.

See BCSC Section 5, *Neuro-Ophthalmology,* and Section 9, *Uveitis and Ocular Inflammation,* for more extensive discussion and clinical photographs of sarcoidosis.

Immunoglobulin G4–Related Disease

Immunoglobulin G4–related disease (IgG4-RD) is a fibroinflammatory disorder that may affect 1 or more organs (Fig 4-16). Orbital disease may occur alone or with systemic disease, either synchronously or metachronously. Within the orbit, the disease most commonly

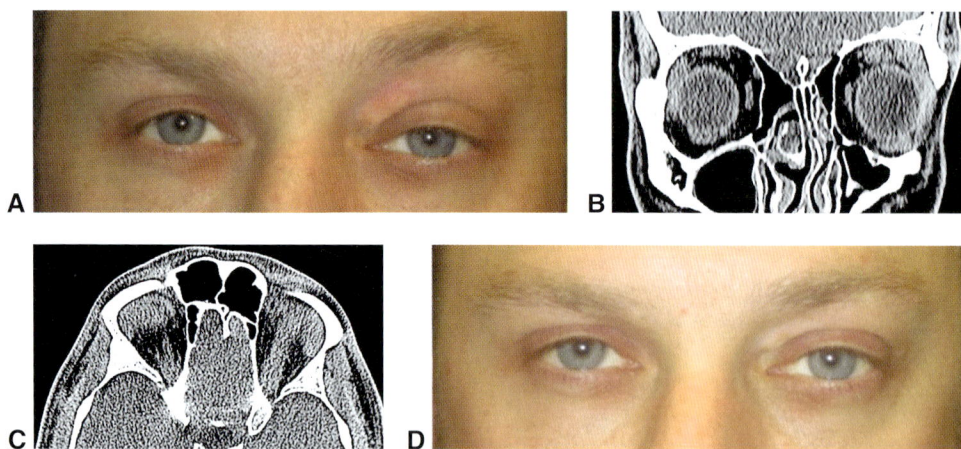

Figure 4-16 Immunoglobulin G4–related disease (IgG4-RD) of the lacrimal gland. **A,** Photograph of a patient with left-sided proptosis. **B** and **C,** Axial and coronal CT imaging studies, respectively, show enlargement of the left lacrimal gland region. **D,** Photograph shows patient improvement after immunosuppressive treatment. *(Courtesy of Julian D. Perry, MD, and Alexander D. Blandford, MD.)*

affects the lacrimal gland, and orbital involvement occurs in common patterns, including the following:

- enlargement of the orbital nerves (typically the infraorbital), extraocular muscles, and lacrimal gland, often with sinusitis, peripheral eosinophilia, and systemic involvement
- sclerosing dacryoadenitis (unilateral or bilateral)
- sclerosing orbital inflammation without dacryoadenitis

Histologic examination shows lymphoplasmacytic infiltrates with large numbers of immunoglobulin G4 (IgG4)-positive plasma cells, storiform fibrosis, obliterative phlebitis, and eosinophil infiltration. A consensus statement set the minimum number of IgG4-positive plasma cells for the lacrimal gland at greater than 100 per high-power field; however, many published series report smaller numbers of cells. In most cases, the ratio of IgG4-to-IgG plasma cells is greater than 40%. Given the spectrum of histologic findings, the diagnosis requires integrating clinical, imaging, and histopathologic criteria.

About half of patients with the orbital disease will also have disease in other organs. Rheumatological evaluation often includes examination for salivary gland, lymph node, lung, liver, and retroperitoneal involvement using various imaging studies, including CT, MRI, and CT-PET (positron emission tomography) scanning. Serologic testing may show peripheral eosinophilia and elevated IgG4 levels.

Treatment includes the use of corticosteroids and other immunosuppressants and biologic agents, including rituximab. Another monoclonal antibody that targets CD19 shows promise to treat this condition as well.

Immunoglobulin G4–related disease comprises a significant proportion of what was previously labeled nonspecific orbital inflammation; thus, biopsy of orbital inflammatory lesions should routinely include an examination for features of IgG4-RD. With greater understanding of inflammatory disease, other conditions previously labeled nonspecific orbital inflammation may be elucidated.

McNab AA, McKelvie P. IgG4-related ophthalmic disease. Part I: background and pathology. *Ophthalmic Plast Reconstr Surg.* 2015;31(2):83–88.

McNab AA, McKelvie P. IgG4-related ophthalmic disease. Part II: clinical aspects. *Ophthalmic Plast Reconstr Surg.* 2015;31(3):167–178.

Nonspecific Orbital Inflammation

Diagnosis of nonspecific orbital inflammation (NSOI, also known as idiopathic orbital inflammation) remains a diagnosis of exclusion, made only after all specific causes of inflammation have been eliminated. The condition is characterized by a polymorphous lymphoid infiltrate with varying degrees of fibrosis, without a known local or systemic cause.

Although controversial, the pathogenesis of NSOI appears to be immune-mediated due to its association with systemic immunologic disorders, including Crohn disease, systemic lupus erythematosus, rheumatoid arthritis, diabetes mellitus, myasthenia gravis, and ankylosing spondylitis. In addition, NSOI typically responds rapidly to treatment with corticosteroids and other immunosuppressive agents, indicating a cell-mediated component.

The symptoms and clinical findings in NSOI vary, depending on the degree and anatomical location of the inflammation. In order of frequency, NSOI tends to occur in the 5 following orbital locations or patterns:

- extraocular muscles *(myositis)*
- lacrimal gland *(dacryoadenitis)*
- anterior orbit (eg, *scleritis*)
- orbital apex
- throughout the orbit (as diffuse inflammation)

Although it is usually limited to the orbit, NSOI may also extend into the adjacent sinuses or intracranial space. Deep, boring pain occurs in many cases; pain associated with ocular movement suggests myositis. Symptoms of vision impairment may occur with involvement of the optic nerve or posterior sclera. Signs include extraocular muscle restriction, proptosis, conjunctival inflammation, chemosis, and erythema and edema of the eyelid (Fig 4-17).

Diagnosis

Imaging studies such as CT, MRI, and ultrasonography reveal enlargement of affected tissues and may show other characteristic findings. Up to 50% of cases show thickening of

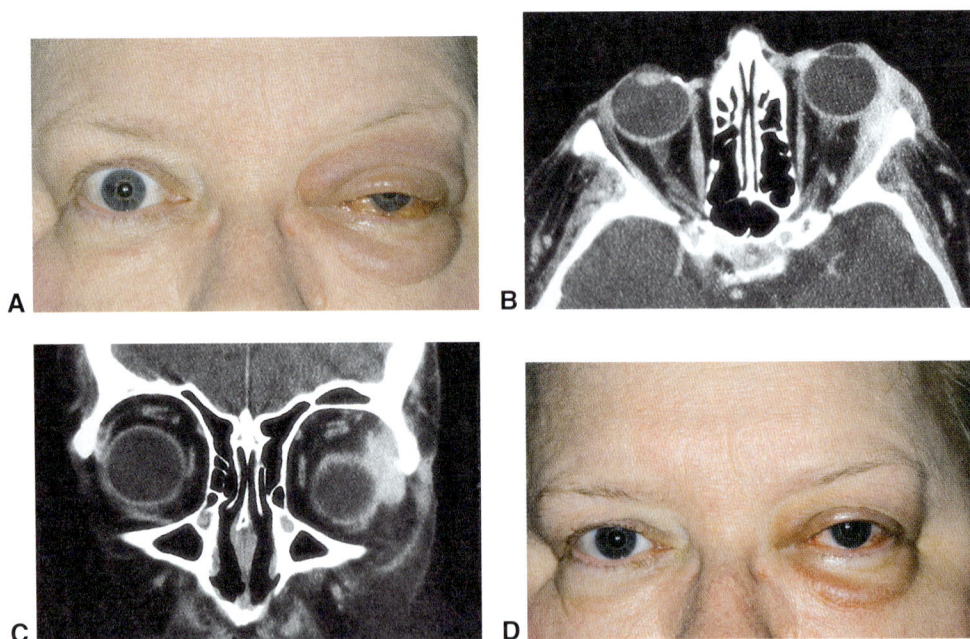

Figure 4-17 Nonspecific orbital inflammation (NSOI). **A,** Photograph of a patient presenting with acute onset of inflammation of the left eyelid, proptosis, pain, and left lateral rectus paresis. **B,** Axial CT scan shows left-eye proptosis and hazy inflammatory swelling of lateral rectus and lacrimal gland, suggestive of a diagnosis of NSOI. **C,** Coronal CT scan shows inflammatory process adjacent to the lateral rectus. **D,** Photograph shows marked improvement of inflammatory changes in the patient after a 48-hour course of oral prednisone. *(Parts A and D courtesy of Keith D. Carter, MD; parts B and C courtesy of Robert C. Kersten, MD.)*

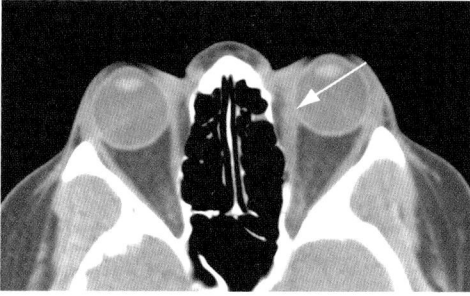

Figure 4-18 Axial CT scan shows myositis of the left medial rectus muscle with involvement of the tendon *(arrow)*. *(Courtesy of Bobby S. Korn, MD, PhD.)*

the extraocular muscle tendon insertions (Fig 4-18), in contrast with TED, which typically spares the muscle insertions. Involvement of the retrobulbar fat pad may produce fat stranding, and tendonitis may produce contrast enhancement of the sclera. B-scan ultrasonography often shows an acoustically hollow area that corresponds to an edematous Tenon capsule (T-sign).

A prompt initial response to high-dose (1 mg/kg oral prednisone or equivalent) systemic corticosteroids supports the diagnosis; this response is observed in most myositic cases and in about 80% of nonmyositic cases. However, inflammation associated with other orbital processes (eg, metastases, lymphoma, ruptured dermoid cysts, infections) may also improve with systemic corticosteroid administration. In 1 study, 50% of biopsied inflammatory lacrimal gland lesions were associated with systemic disease, including GPA, sclerosing inflammation, Sjögren syndrome, sarcoidal reactions, and autoimmune disease.

Given the low morbidity associated with biopsy, the possibility of other orbital processes responding to treatment with corticosteroids, and the high incidence of systemic disease involving the lacrimal gland, many experts recommend diagnostic biopsy of all nonmyositic lesions not attached to the optic nerve. Surgical debulking of idiopathic dacryoadenitis during the biopsy procedure may carry a therapeutic as well as a diagnostic benefit.

In cases of myositis, lesions attached to the optic nerve and lesions involving the orbital apex may produce characteristic clinical and radiographic findings to strongly support the presumed diagnosis, and the risk associated with biopsy may outweigh the risk of a missed diagnosis.

Not all patients with NSOI present with the classic signs and symptoms; some patients present with atypical pain, limited inflammatory signs, or a fibrotic variant called *sclerosing NSOI*. Simultaneous bilateral orbital inflammation in adults suggests the possibility of systemic vasculitis. Any diagnostic uncertainty mandates a thorough systemic evaluation.

In children with NSOI, approximately one-third of cases present bilaterally and approximately one-half present with systemic signs, such as headache, fever, vomiting, abdominal pain, and lethargy. Uveitis, elevated ESR levels, and eosinophilia are also more common in children with NSOI. Pediatric NSOI is not generally associated with systemic disorders.

On histologic examination, NSOI is characterized by a pleomorphic cellular infiltrate consisting of lymphocytes, plasma cells, and eosinophils with variable degrees of reactive fibrosis. The sclerosing subtype of NSOI demonstrates a predominance of fibrosis with sparse cellular inflammation. Hypercellular lymphoid proliferations represent clinical and histologic entities that are different from NSOI.

Mombaerts I, Bilyk JR, Rose GE, et al; Expert Panel of the Orbital Society. Consensus on diagnostic criteria of idiopathic orbital inflammation using a modified Delphi approach. *JAMA Ophthalmol.* 2017;135(7):769–776.

Treatment

As previously mentioned, initial therapy for NSOI consists of systemic corticosteroids, with a typical initial daily adult dosage of 1 mg/kg prednisone. Acute cases generally respond rapidly, with abrupt resolution of pain. Steroid taper begins after maximal clinical response; it should proceed more slowly below about 40 mg/day and even slower below 20 mg/day, based on the clinical response. Rapid reduction of systemic steroids may allow for recurrence. Some investigators believe that pulse-dosed IV dexamethasone followed by oral prednisone may produce clinical improvement when oral prednisone alone fails to control the inflammation. Sclerosing NSOI responds poorly to steroids and to low-dose fractionated radiotherapy; it typically requires more aggressive immunosuppression with agents such as cyclosporine, methotrexate, or cyclophosphamide.

Mombaerts I, Rose GE, Garrity JA. Orbital inflammation: biopsy first. *Surv Ophthalmol.* 2016;61(5):664–669.

Rootman J. *Orbital Disease: Present Status and Future Challenges.* Boca Raton, FL: CRC Press; 2005:1–13.

CHAPTER **5**

Orbital Neoplasms
and Malformations

▶ *This chapter includes a related video, which can be accessed by scanning the QR code provided in the text or going to www.aao.org/bcscvideo_section07.*

Highlights

- The orbit is a rigid, confined space, and lesions that originate in or infiltrate the orbit often present with ophthalmic manifestations.
- Pathology can occur in any orbital tissue, including bone, vasculature, nerve, muscle, and gland.
- Careful history provides diagnostic clues, as certain lesions present more commonly in different age groups.
- Imaging of the orbit and surrounding sinuses and intracranial cavity helps guide diagnosis and management.
- Understanding the hemodynamics of vascular lesions is critical for safe and effective treatment.

Vascular Tumors, Malformations, and Fistulas

Infantile (Capillary) Hemangioma

Infantile (capillary) hemangiomas are common primary benign tumors of the orbit in children (Fig 5-1). These lesions present at birth or within the first few weeks of life.

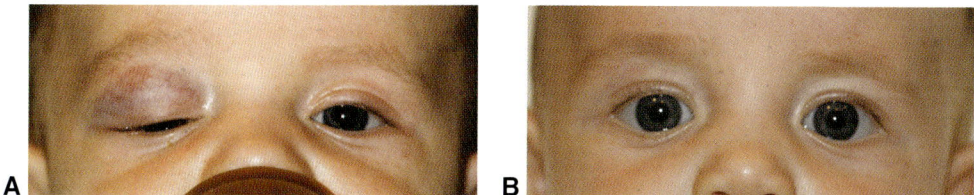

Figure 5-1 Infantile (capillary) hemangioma. **A,** Infantile hemangioma involving the right upper eyelid. **B,** Marked regression of lesion 6 weeks after initiation of propranolol therapy. *(Courtesy of William R. Katowitz, MD.)*

71

They enlarge dramatically over the first 6–12 months and begin to involute after the first year of life; 75% of lesions resolve by the age of 3–7 years. Female sex, low birth weight, prematurity, and maternal chorionic villus sampling are associated with infantile hemangiomas.

Congenital infantile hemangiomas may be superficial—in which case they involve the skin and appear as a bright red, soft mass with a dimpled texture—or they may be subcutaneous and bluish. Hemangiomas located deeper within the orbit may present as a progressively enlarging mass without any overlying skin change. Magnetic resonance imaging (MRI) may help to distinguish infantile hemangiomas from other vascular malformations by demonstrating characteristic fine intralesional vascular channels and high blood flow. Color Doppler ultrasound imaging is a reliable and inexpensive imaging tool for diagnosing these lesions, often showing numerous blood vessels within the mass and abundant blood flow.

In the periocular area, infantile hemangiomas occur most commonly in the superonasal quadrant of the orbit and the medial upper eyelid (see also the section Congenital Eyelid Lesions in Chapter 10). They may be associated with hemangiomas on other parts of the body; lesions that involve the neck can compromise the airway and lead to respiratory obstruction, and multiple large visceral lesions can produce thrombocytopenia *(Kasabach-Merritt syndrome)*.

Management

Most lesions regress spontaneously, requiring only observation with refractive correction and amblyopia therapy. The main ocular complications of infantile hemangiomas are amblyopia, strabismus, and anisometropia. Although disruption of vision or severe disfigurement may require therapy, treatment can be deferred until it is clear that such complications may develop.

For infantile hemangiomas that require therapy, β-blockers are the first-line treatment. Topical timolol gel treats superficial tumors and has limited systemic adverse effects. Oral propranolol treats deeper lesions and offers fewer adverse effects than systemic steroids, although life-threatening hypotension, bradycardia, and hypoglycemia can occur in rare instances. Oral β-blocker treatment should be initiated under the guidance of a pediatrician, so the patient can be monitored for systemic adverse effects. Lesions that do not respond adequately to β-blockers may require treatment with steroids, administered topically, by local injection, or orally (see the section Congenital Eyelid Lesions in Chapter 10). Adverse effects of steroid injection include skin necrosis, subcutaneous fat atrophy, and retinal embolic vision loss. Steroid treatment by any route in infants may produce hypothalamic-pituitary-adrenal axis suppression, systemic growth retardation, and a variety of other metabolic adverse effects.

Surgical excision with meticulous hemostasis may be considered for active-phase lesions refractory to steroids or for some smaller or subcutaneous nodular lesions. Pulsed-dye laser therapy can improve superficial components of the hemangioma. Radiation therapy has also been used, but it can lead to cataract formation, bony hypoplasia, and future malignancy. Sclerosing solutions are not recommended, as they can cause severe scarring. Residual lesions that remain after involution or treatment can be removed surgically.

Chambers CB, Katowitz WR, Katowitz JA, Binenbaum G. A controlled study of topical 0.25% timolol maleate gel for the treatment of cutaneous infantile capillary hemangiomas. *Ophthalmic Plast Reconstr Surg.* 2012;28(2):103–106.

Fridman G, Grieser E, Hill R, Khuddus N, Bersani T, Slonim C. Propranolol for the treatment of orbital infantile hemangiomas. *Ophthalmic Plast Reconstr Surg.* 2011;27(3):190–194.

Lymphatic Malformation

Pure lymphatic malformations (LMs; previously called *lymphangiomas*) are low-flow orbital lesions resulting from disruption of the initially pluripotent vascular anlage, which leads to aberrant development and congenital malformation. LMs can also occur in the conjunctiva (Fig 5-2A), eyelids, oropharynx (Fig 5-2B), or sinuses. In the orbit, LMs usually become apparent in the first or second decade of life. They can be described as *macrocystic* (cysts ≥2 cm), *microcystic* (cysts ≤2 cm), or *mixed macrocystic/microcystic*. LMs cannot be decompressed and do not distend with a Valsalva maneuver. However, they may enlarge

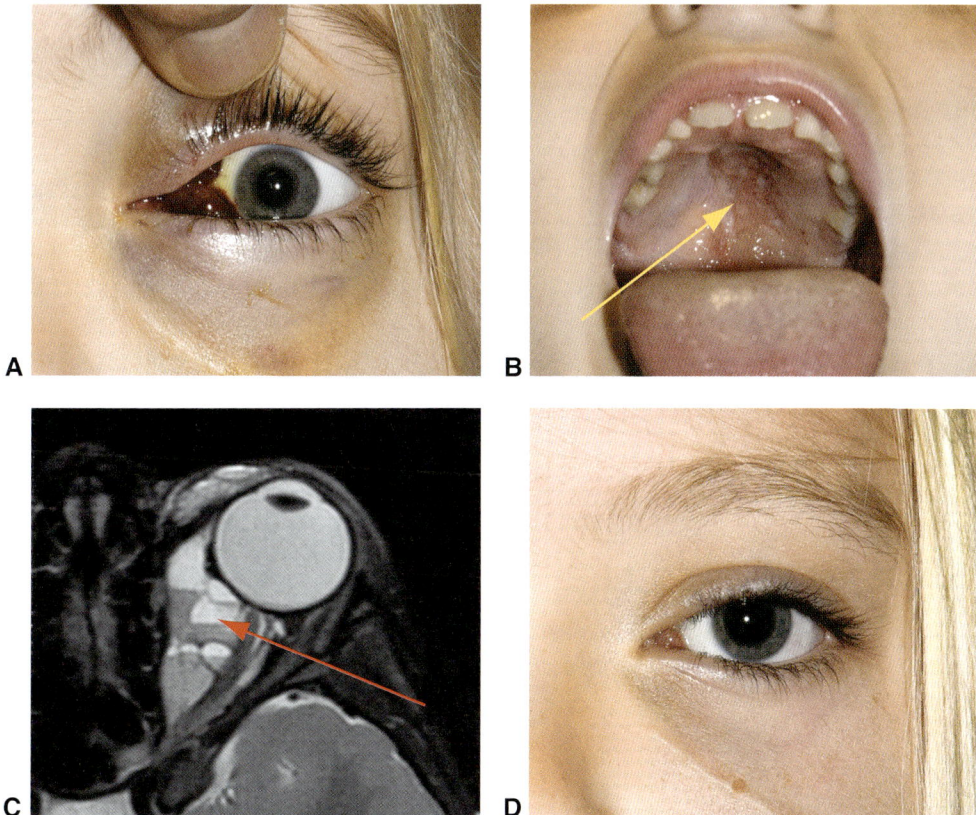

Figure 5-2 Lymphatic malformation. **A,** External photograph shows lymphatic malformation presenting as a hemorrhagic subconjunctival mass. **B,** Involvement of the hard palate *(arrow).* **C,** T2-weighted axial MRI shows multiple saccular lesions with serum and blood fluid levels *(arrow)* medial to the optic nerve. **D,** External photograph after injection with bleomycin. *(Courtesy of Bobby S. Korn, MD, PhD.)*

during upper respiratory tract infections, and they may present with sudden proptosis caused by spontaneous intralesional hemorrhage *(chocolate cysts).*

The natural history of LMs is variable; some are localized and progress slowly, whereas others may diffusely infiltrate orbital structures and enlarge inexorably. MRI may show pathognomonic features (multiple grapelike cystic lesions with fluid–fluid layering of serum and red blood cells), confirming the diagnosis (Fig 5-2C).

LMs are characterized by their hemodynamic properties, and classification schemes continue to evolve. Some LMs possess a significant venous flow component and have clinical characteristics that overlap with venous malformations (VMs, discussed later in this chapter); these lesions are termed *combined lymphatic venous malformations.* Treatment depends on the hemodynamic flow characteristics of the lesion.

Histologically, pure LMs are characterized by serum-filled channels lined by flat endothelial cells that have immunostaining patterns consistent with lymphatic capillaries. Scattered follicles of lymphoid tissues are found in the interstitium. These lesions have an infiltrative pattern and are not encapsulated.

Management

Treatment of LM is challenging for several reasons: the vascular channels are typically not amenable to endovascular approaches, the infiltrative nature of the lesion often involves vital orbital structures, significant hemorrhage may occur during surgery, and recurrence is common. Observation is a reasonable approach for lesions that are asymptomatic and not amblyogenic. If treatment is warranted, debulking of the lesion combined with use of intralesional sclerosing agents, either percutaneous or intraoperatively, may be successful. Sclerosants include morrhuate sodium, bleomycin (Fig 5-2D), polidocanol, OK-432, thrombosing agents such as fibrin glue, and embolizing agents such as cyanoacrylate glues and ethylene vinyl alcohol copolymer.

Acute hemorrhage complicated by optic neuropathy or corneal ulceration may respond to ultrasound-guided aspiration of blood through a hollow-bore needle or by open surgical exploration. While mild hematomas may resolve spontaneously, the mass effect of such hemorrhages can persist due to bleeding within dead-end lymphatic channels.

Noncontiguous intracranial vascular malformations have been reported to occur in up to 25% of patients with orbital LMs. These lesions have a low rate of spontaneous hemorrhage and are not treated prophylactically.

Distensible Venous Malformation

Distensible venous malformations of the orbit, previously known as *orbital varices*, are low-flow lesions that enlarge with a Valsalva maneuver. Patients may exhibit enophthalmos at rest, when the lesion is not engorged. Proptosis that increases when the patient's head is dependent or after a Valsalva maneuver suggests the presence of a venous malformation (Fig 5-3A, C). Apart from the inducible proptosis, the ophthalmic examination is often unremarkable, with symmetric intraocular pressures (IOPs), lack of conjunctival vessel engorgement, and no reflux of blood in the Schlemm canal. The diagnosis can be confirmed with imaging such as MRI (Fig 5-3D) or contrast-enhanced rapid spiral computed tomography (CT) during a Valsalva maneuver or other means of decreasing venous

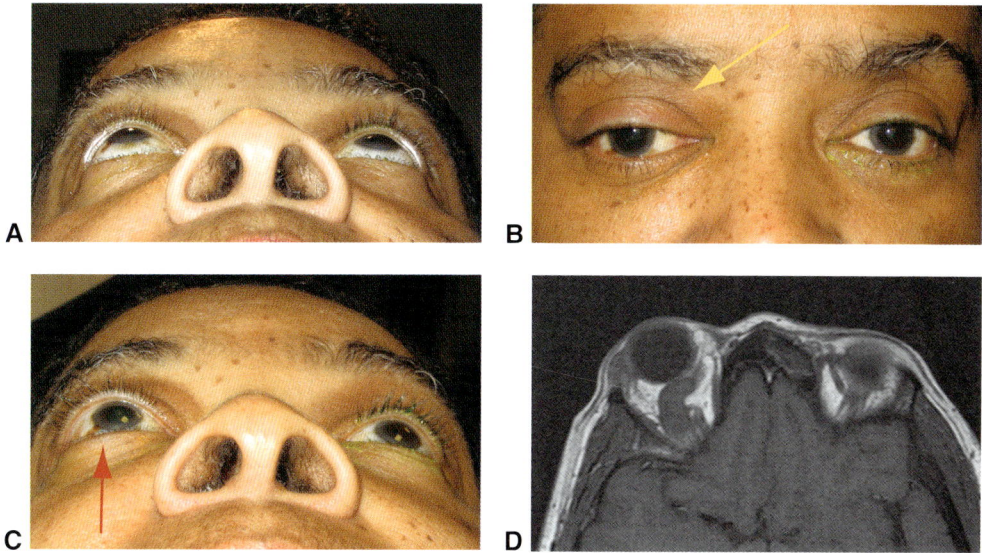

Figure 5-3 Distensible venous malformation. **A,** Mild proptosis resulting from venous malformation of the right orbit. **B,** Fullness of the right superior orbit *(arrow)*. Note the absence of dilated corkscrew conjunctival vessels. **C,** After Valsalva maneuver, proptosis of the right globe increases *(arrow)*. **D,** T1-weighted axial MRI shows a venous malformation of the superior ophthalmic vein. *(Courtesy of Bobby S. Korn, MD, PhD.)*

return; cases show characteristic enlargement of the engorged veins. Phleboliths may be present on imaging.

Management

Management is usually conservative, with observation of relatively asymptomatic lesions. Biopsy should be avoided because of the risk of hemorrhage. Surgery is reserved for patients who have significant pain or in whom the malformation causes vision-threatening compressive optic neuropathy. Complete surgical excision is difficult, as these lesions often intertwine with normal orbital structures and directly communicate with the abundant venous reservoir in the cavernous sinus. Treatment of highly symptomatic lesions typically consists of combined embolization and excision. Sclerosants, injected either percutaneously or directly through an open approach, are an additional treatment option. However, orbital compartment syndrome may occur, requiring urgent decompression.

Cavernous Venous Malformation

Cavernous venous malformations (CVMs) are nondistensible, low-flow vascular lesions previously known as *cavernous hemangiomas*. They are the most common type of primary orbital lesion in adults, typically presenting in the fourth and fifth decades of life. Women represent 60% of cases, and circulating estrogen and progesterone levels may play a role in clinical progression, with growth sometimes accelerating during pregnancy.

CVMs typically produce slowly progressive, painless proptosis (Fig 5-4A). Other findings may include retinal striae, hyperopia, optic nerve compression, increased IOP, and

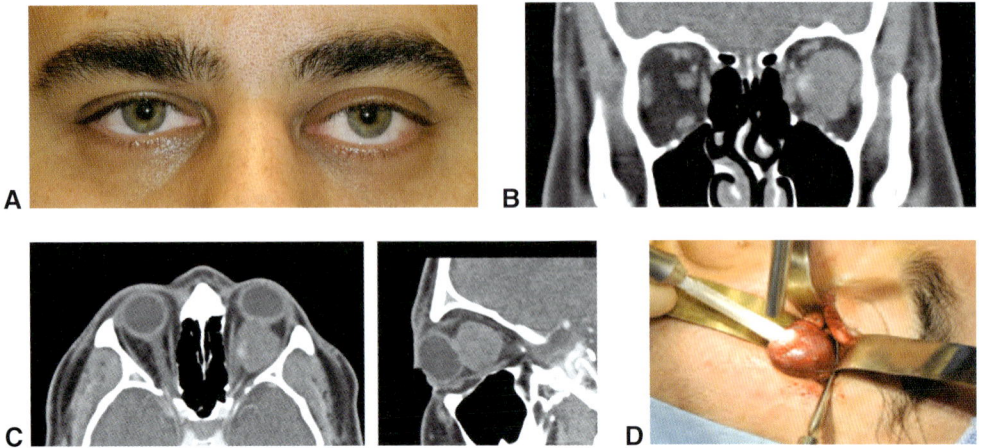

Figure 5-4 Cavernous venous malformation (CVM). **A,** Proptosis of the left eye as a result of CVM. **B,** Coronal computed tomography (CT) scans show a well-circumscribed lesion the muscle cone. **C,** Axial *(left)* and sagittal *(right)* CT scans show the mass. **D,** Intra-operative traction with a cryoprobe facilitates complete removal of the mass. *(Courtesy of Bobby S. Korn, MD, PhD.)*

strabismus. Contrast-enhanced orbital imaging shows a stippled pattern in the early phase of contrast that develops into homogeneous staining in the late phase. The lesion appears as a well-circumscribed mass that can have an intraconal and/or extraconal component (Fig 5-4B, C). Chronic lesions may contain radiodense phleboliths. Arteriography and venography typically do not aid in the diagnosis as these lesions have very limited communication with the systemic circulation.

On histologic examination, CVMs are encapsulated and composed of large cavernous spaces with walls of smooth muscle containing red blood cells.

Management

Treatment consists of complete surgical excision if the lesion compromises visual function, causes significant proptosis, or demonstrates substantial growth. The growth potential of a CVM is not predictable at the time of diagnosis or following incomplete resection; in rare cases, these lesions may involute spontaneously.

Because they are encapsulated and relatively isolated from the surrounding tissue, CVMs are often easier to remove than many other orbital tumors. Coronal imaging helps determine the position of the CVM relative to the optic nerve, and the surgical approach is dictated by the location of the lesion. Deeper lesions may be attached to vital (and sometimes vascular) structures within the orbital apex, so their complete excision may not always warrant the risks. Radiotherapy can be considered for lesions located deep within the orbital apex.

Calandriello L, Grimaldi G, Petrone G, et al. Cavernous venous malformation (cavernous hemangioma) of the orbit: current concepts and a review of the literature. *Surv Ophthalmol.* 2017;62(4):393–403.

Hill RH 3rd, Shiels WE 2nd, Foster JA, et al. Percutaneous drainage and ablation as first line therapy for macrocystic and microcystic orbital lymphatic malformations. *Ophthalmic Plast Reconstr Surg.* 2012;28(2):119–125.

Rootman J, Heran MK, Graeb DA. Vascular malformations of the orbit: classification and the role of imaging in diagnosis and treatment strategies. *Ophthalmic Plast Reconst Surg.* 2014;30(2):91–104.

Arteriovenous Malformation

Arteriovenous malformations (AVMs) are high-flow developmental anomalies that, like venous malformations, result from vascular dysgenesis. They are characterized by rapid arterial flow through the nidus into the draining venous circulation and often occur at choke anastomotic zones. Dilated corkscrew episcleral vessels and pulsatile proptosis may be present, and vascular steal or shunting from the orbit may produce ischemic changes. Noninvasive imaging supports the diagnosis, with CT revealing diffuse enhancement and MRI showing flow voids (Fig 5-5).

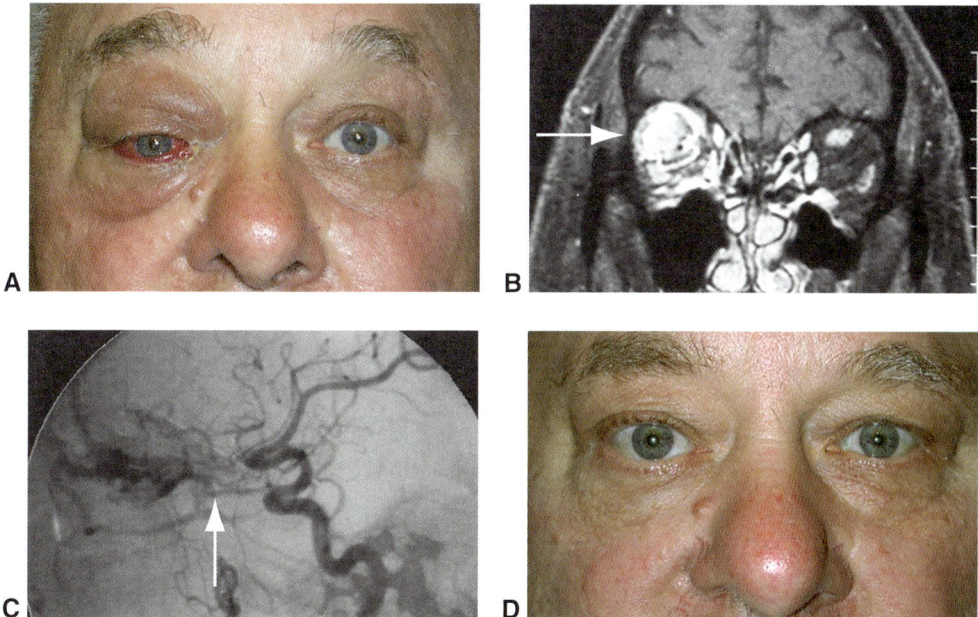

Figure 5-5 Arteriovenous malformation. **A,** Arteriovenous malformation in the right eye causing proptosis and arterialization of conjunctival vessels. **B,** T1-weighted, gadolinium-enhanced MRI shows enhancing superolateral nidus of lesion *(arrow)*. **C,** Angiogram shows enlarged ophthalmic artery *(arrow)*. **D,** Proptosis and arterialized vessels resolved after embolization and excision of nidus. *(Courtesy of Julian D. Perry, MD, and Alexander D. Blandford, MD.)*

Management

AVMs gradually enlarge as they recruit more arterial feeders. They often require treatment, which involves preoperative selective angiography with embolization followed by resection of the nidus. Failure to completely resect the nidus may allow recurrence; however, complete resection of the nidus may not be possible without significant morbidity. Exsanguinating arterial hemorrhage can occur with surgical intervention, especially in unsuspected lesions without preoperative embolization.

Arteriovenous Fistula

Arteriovenous fistulas are acquired lesions characterized by abnormal direct communication between an artery and a vein without flow through an intervening capillary bed. An arteriovenous fistula may be caused by trauma or degeneration. There are 2 forms, direct and indirect (dural). *Direct carotid-cavernous fistulas* are characterized by a connection between the internal carotid artery and the cavernous sinus; they typically occur after trauma that creates a tear or hole in a branch artery of the internal carotid within the cavernous sinus. They may also be caused iatrogenically, for example, during neurosurgical or neuroradiologic procedures.

Direct carotid-cavernous fistulas possess high blood flow and may produce characteristic tortuous epibulbar vessels, as well as pulsatile proptosis and an audible bruit. Ischemic ocular damage results from diversion of arterialized blood into the venous system, which causes venous outflow obstruction (Fig 5-6A). This in turn leads to elevated IOP, choroidal effusions, blood in the Schlemm canal, and nongranulomatous anterior uveitis. Ocular motility abnormalities can result from either congestion within the orbit or increased pressure in the cavernous sinus. The latter can cause compression of cranial nerves III, IV, or,

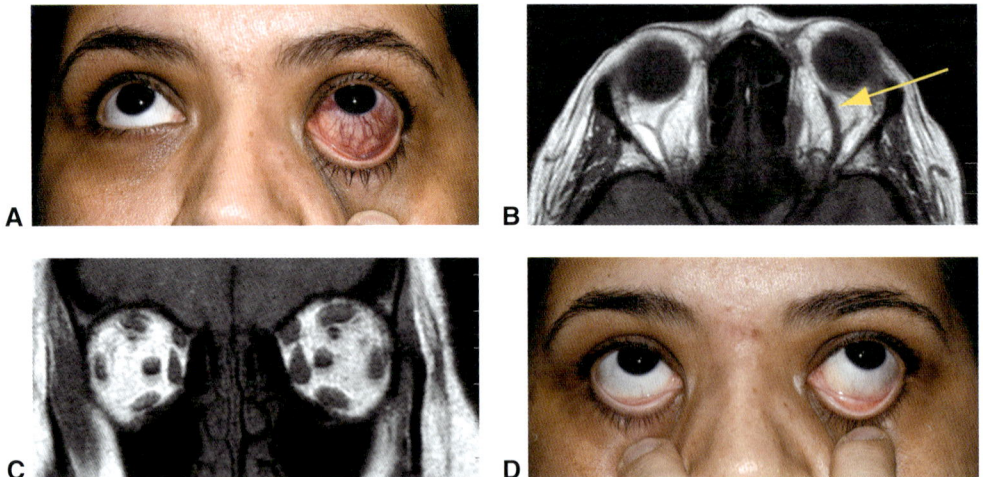

Figure 5-6 Carotid-cavernous fistula. **A,** Carotid-cavernous fistula presenting with left proptosis and arterialization of the conjunctival and episcleral vessels. **B,** T1-weighted axial MRI shows an enlarged left superior ophthalmic vein *(arrow).* **C,** T1-weighted coronal MRI shows diffuse enlargement of the superior oblique and all 4 rectus muscles in the left orbit. **D,** External photograph after endovascular closure of the carotid-cavernous fistula. *(Courtesy of Bobby S. Korn, MD, PhD.)*

most commonly, VI, with associated extraocular muscle palsies. CT scans may show diffuse enlargement of some or all of the extraocular muscles resulting from venous engorgement and a characteristically enlarged superior ophthalmic vein (Fig 5-6B, C).

Indirect (dural) carotid-cavernous fistulas are characterized by a connection between meningeal branches of the internal and/or external carotid artery and the cavernous sinus. These fistulas most commonly develop as a degenerative process in older patients with systemic hypertension, vascular disease, and/or atherosclerosis. Because dural fistulas generally have lower rates of blood flow than direct carotid-cavernous fistulas, their onset can be insidious, with only mild orbital congestion, proptosis, and pain. Arterialization of the conjunctival veins causes chronic red eye. Increased episcleral venous pressure results in asymmetric elevation of IOP on the affected side, and patients with chronic fistulas are at risk for glaucomatous damage to the optic nerve head.

Magnetic resonance angiography (MRA) may be helpful in diagnosing arteriovenous fistulas, with fewer associated adverse effects than conventional angiography (eg, stroke). However, conventional angiography possesses more sensitivity than MRA and remains the gold standard for diagnosis.

Management

The decision to treat an arteriovenous fistula is based on weighing the severity of symptoms against the risks associated with intervention. Because they are high-flow lesions, direct carotid-cavernous fistulas usually require intervention. Small indirect carotid-cavernous fistulas often close spontaneously and may initially be observed. However, because even these lesions may result in intracranial hemorrhage, some investigators have recommended more aggressive management of indirect fistulas.

Intervention typically involves an endovascular treatment (coils or glue) to block the fistula (Fig 5-7). Transvenous access is used to reach dural fistulas, while direct carotid-cavernous fistulas are generally treated via a transarterial approach. Occasionally, a transvenous approach by transcutaneous canalization of the superior ophthalmic vein is employed for embolization, which may require an orbitotomy to directly access the vein.

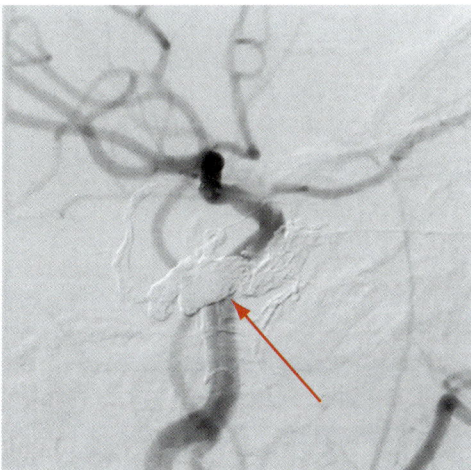

Figure 5-7 Closure of carotid-cavernous fistula by endovascular coiling *(arrow). (Courtesy of Bobby S. Korn, MD, PhD.)*

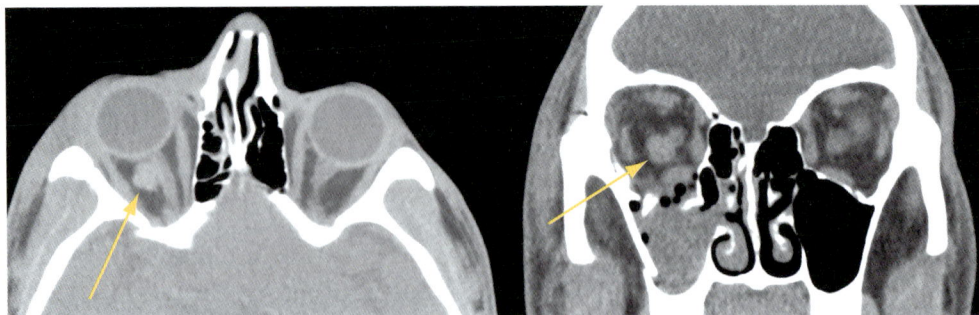

Figure 5-8 CT scan shows an intraconal orbital hemorrhage *(arrows)* associated with a zygo-maticomaxillary complex fracture. *(Courtesy of Bobby S. Korn, MD, PhD.)*

See BCSC Section 5, *Neuro-Ophthalmology,* for additional discussion of carotid-cavernous fistulas.

Stacey AW, Gemmete JJ, Kahana A. Management of orbital and periocular vascular anomalies. *Opthalmic Plast Reconstr Surg.* 2015;31(6):427–436.

Orbital Hemorrhage

An orbital hemorrhage may result from trauma, surgery, or spontaneous bleeding from vascular malformations (Fig 5-8). In rare instances, a spontaneous hemorrhage may be caused by a sudden increase in venous pressure (eg, due to a Valsalva maneuver). A spontaneous orbital hemorrhage almost always occurs in the superior subperiosteal space. It should be allowed to resorb unless there is associated visual compromise, in which case urgent drainage is indicated. Also see the section Orbital Compartment Syndrome in Chapter 6.

Neural Tumors

The neural tumors that may involve the orbit include optic nerve gliomas, neurofibromas, meningiomas, and schwannomas.

Optic Nerve Glioma

Optic nerve gliomas are uncommon, usually benign tumors that occur predominantly in children in the first decade of life (Fig 5-9). The chief clinical feature is gradual, painless, unilateral axial proptosis associated with vision loss and an afferent pupillary defect. Other ocular findings may include optic atrophy, optic nerve head swelling, nystagmus, and strabismus. The chiasm is involved in roughly half of cases of optic nerve glioma. Intracranial involvement may be associated with intracranial hypertension as well as decreased function of the hypothalamus and pituitary gland. Up to half of optic nerve gliomas are associated with neurofibromatosis (NF). In patients with NF, the gliomas often proliferate in the subarachnoid space, while those occurring in patients without NF usually expand within the optic nerve substance without invading the dura mater.

Optic nerve gliomas can usually be diagnosed by means of orbital imaging. CT and MRI typically show fusiform enlargement of the optic nerve, often with stereotypical kinking of

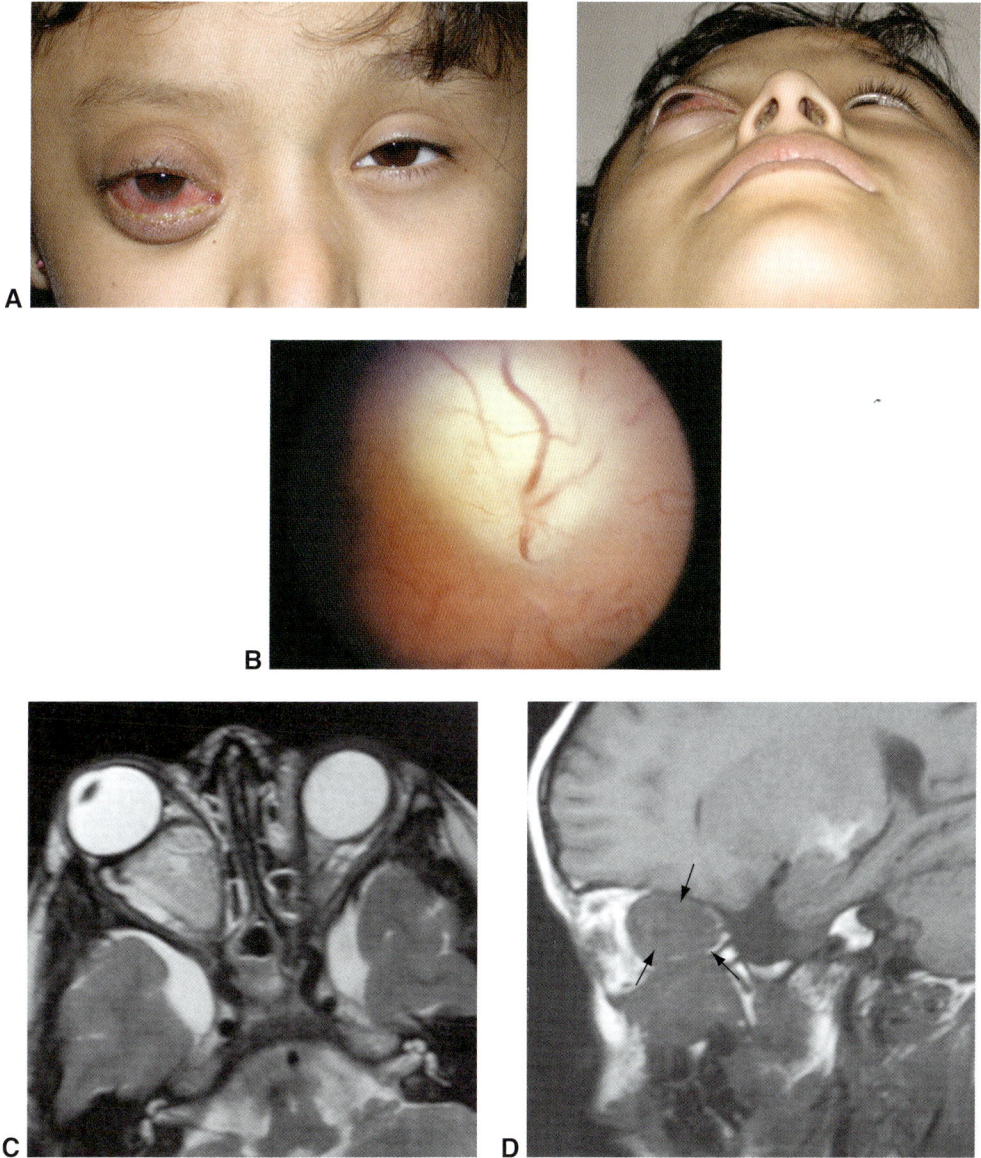

Figure 5-9 Optic nerve glioma. **A,** Right optic nerve glioma. The patient has severe proptosis with exposure and light perception vision. **B,** Funduscopic view. Note swollen optic nerve head with obscured margins. **C,** T2-weighted axial MRI shows glioma extending into the optic canal. **D,** Sagittal MRI shows a heterogeneous mass *(arrows)* in the apex of the orbit. *(Parts A, C, and D courtesy of Raymond Douglas, MD; part B courtesy of Roger A. Dailey, MD.)*

the nerve. MRI may also show cystic degeneration, if present, and may be more accurate than CT in defining the extent of an optic canal lesion and intracranial disease.

Because neuroimaging is frequently diagnostic, it is usually unnecessary to perform a biopsy of a suspected lesion. Moreover, obtaining tissue from an appropriate site may be challenging: biopsy of the optic nerve itself may produce additional loss of visual field or vision, while a specimen from a too-peripheral portion of the nerve may inadvertently capture reactive meningeal hyperplasia adjacent to the glioma and lead to a misdiagnosis of fibrous meningioma. Gross pathology of resected tumors reveals a smooth, fusiform intradural lesion. On microscopic examination, benign tumors in children are considered to be juvenile pilocytic (hairlike) astrocytomas. Other histologic findings include arachnoid hyperplasia, mucosubstance, and Rosenthal fibers (see the discussion of the pathologic features of glioma in BCSC Section 4, *Ophthalmic Pathology and Intraocular Tumors*).

Malignant optic nerve gliomas (glioblastomas) are very rare and tend to affect adult males. Initial signs and symptoms of malignant gliomas include severe retro-orbital pain, unilateral or bilateral vision loss, and, typically, massive swelling and hemorrhage of the optic nerve head (pallor may also be observed with posterior lesions). Despite treatment, including high-dose radiotherapy and chemotherapy, these tumors usually result in death within 6–12 months.

Management

The treatment of nonmalignant optic nerve gliomas is controversial. Although most cases remain stable or progress very slowly, leading some authors to consider them benign hamartomas, the occasional case behaves aggressively. There are rare reports of spontaneous regression of optic nerve and visual pathway gliomas. Cystic enlargement of the lesions leading to sudden vision loss can occur even without true cellular growth. A treatment plan must be carefully individualized for each patient. Factors affecting therapeutic decisions include the tumor's growth characteristics, extent of optic nerve and chiasmal involvement as determined by clinical and radiographic evaluation, vision in the involved and uninvolved eyes, presence or absence of concomitant neurologic or systemic disease, and history of previous treatment. The following options may be considered.

Observation only Presumed optic nerve glioma, particularly with good vision on the involved side, may be carefully followed if the radiographic evidence is characteristic of this type of tumor and the glioma is confined to the orbit. Because visual function does not directly correlate with glioma size or growth, follow-up should include precise measurements of optic nerve function in addition to serial imaging studies. Many patients maintain good vision and never require surgery.

Surgical excision Rapid intraorbital tumor growth may prompt surgical resection in an effort to isolate the tumor from the optic chiasm and thus prevent chiasmal invasion. To obtain tumor-free surgical margins, the surgeon uses a transcranial approach. Surgical excision of a tumor confined to the orbit may also be considered if it causes severe proptosis with corneal exposure or unacceptable cosmesis. Removal through an intracranial approach may also be indicated at the time of initial diagnosis or after a short period of observation if the tumor involves the prechiasmal intracranial portion of the optic nerve. Complete excision is possible if the tumor ends 2–3 mm anterior to the chiasm.

Chemotherapy Combination chemotherapy using dactinomycin, vincristine, etoposide, and other agents has been reported to be effective in patients with progressive chiasmal-hypothalamic gliomas. Chemotherapy may delay the need for radiation therapy and thus reduce deleterious effects on long-term intellectual development and endocrine function in children. However, chemotherapy may carry long-term risks of blood-borne cancers.

Radiation therapy Radiation therapy is typically considered if the tumor cannot be resected (usually lesions of the chiasm or optic tract) and if symptoms, particularly neurologic, progress after chemotherapy. It may also be considered after surgical excision if reliable radiographic studies document subsequent growth of the tumor in the chiasm or if chiasmal and optic tract involvement is extensive. Because of potentially debilitating adverse effects (including intellectual disability, growth retardation, secondary tumors, and malignant transformation within the radiation field), radiation is generally reserved as a last resort for children who have not completed growth and development.

See additional discussion of optic nerve glioma in BCSC Section 5, *Neuro-Ophthalmology.*

Glass LR, Canoll P, Lignelli A, Ligon AH, Kazim M. Optic nerve glioma: case series with review of clinical, radiologic, molecular, and histopathologic characteristics. *Ophthalmic Plast Reconstr Surg.* 2014;30(5):372–376.

Neurofibroma

Neurofibromas are tumors composed chiefly of proliferating Schwann cells within the nerve sheaths. Axons, endoneural fibroblasts, and mucin are also noted on histologic examination. *Plexiform neurofibromas* consist of diffuse proliferations of Schwann cells within nerve sheaths, and they usually occur in cases of neurofibromatosis 1 (NF1). They are well-vascularized infiltrative lesions, making complete surgical excision difficult. *Discrete neurofibromas* are less common than the plexiform type and can usually be excised without recurrence. In either instance, surgery is limited to tumors that compromise vision or produce disfigurement.

Neurofibromatosis 1

Patients with neurofibromas are evaluated for neurofibromatosis. Also known as *von Recklinghausen disease,* NF1 is inherited through an autosomal dominant gene with incomplete penetrance. Because NF1 is characterized by the presence of hamartomas involving the skin, eye, central nervous system, and viscera, it is classified as a phakomatosis. NF1 is the most common phakomatous disorder; its significant orbital features include plexiform neurofibromas of the lateral aspect of the upper eyelid resulting in an S-shaped contour of the eyelid margin (Fig 5-10), pulsatile proptosis (Video 5-1) secondary to sphenoid bone

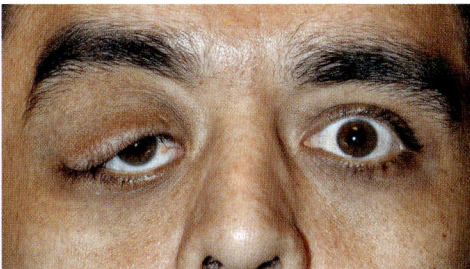

Figure 5-10 Neurofibromatosis 1 presenting with a plexiform neurofibroma of the right upper eyelid in S-shaped configuration. *(Courtesy of Bobby S. Korn, MD, PhD.)*

aplasia, and optic nerve glioma. See BCSC Section 6, *Pediatric Ophthalmology and Strabismus,* for further discussion of neurofibromatosis and other phakomatoses.

VIDEO 5-1 Patient with NF1 presenting with pulsatile proptosis from sphenoid wing aplasia.
Courtesy of Bobby S. Korn, MD, PhD.
Access all Section 7 videos at www.aao.org/bcscvideo_section07.

Rasool N, Odel JG, Kazim M. Optic pathway glioma of childhood. *Curr Opin Ophthalmol.* 2017;28(3):289–295.

Meningioma

Meningiomas are invasive tumors that arise from the arachnoid villi. Orbital meningiomas usually originate intracranially along the sphenoid wing, with secondary extension through the bone into the orbit (Fig 5-11), the superior orbital fissure, or the optic canal; or they may arise primarily in the orbital portion of the optic nerve sheath. Ophthalmic manifestations are related to the location of the primary tumor. Meningiomas arising near the sella and optic nerve cause early visual field defects and optic nerve edema or optic atrophy. Tumors arising near the pterion (the posterior end of the parietosphenoid fissure, at the lateral portion of the sphenoid bone) often produce a mass in the temporal fossa and may be associated with proptosis or nonaxial displacement of the globe (see Fig 5-11A, B). Eyelid edema (especially of the lower eyelid) and chemosis are common. Interestingly, although primary optic nerve sheath meningiomas can, in rare cases, produce axial proptosis with preserved vision, depending on their anatomic location, some meningiomas can cause early profound vision loss without any proptosis.

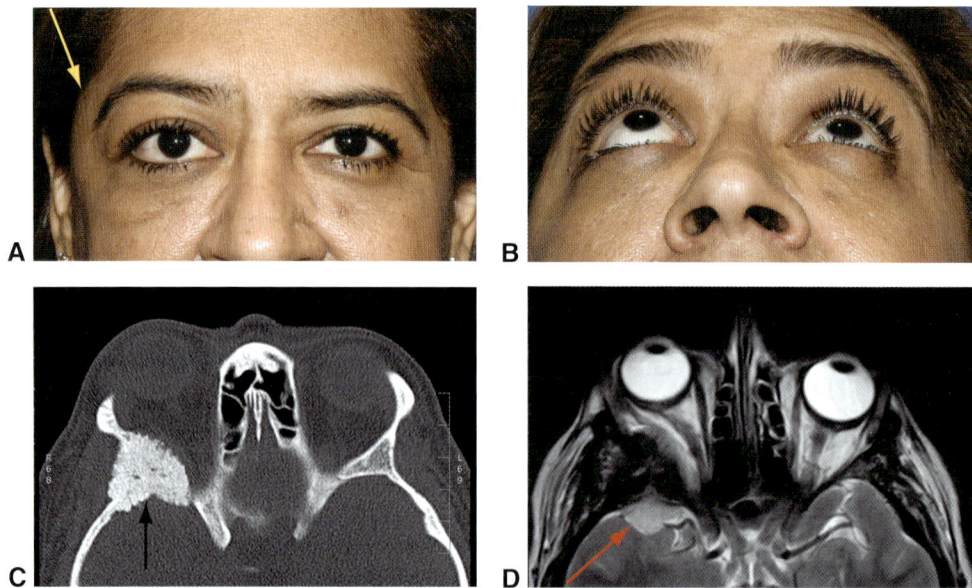

Figure 5-11 Sphenoid wing meningioma. **A,** External photograph shows right temporal fullness *(arrow).* **B,** Worm's eye view shows right proptosis. CT **(C)** and MRI **(D)** show hyperostosis of the sphenoid bone *(arrow)* from the associated meningioma *(arrow). (Courtesy of Bobby S. Korn, MD, PhD.)*

Sphenoid wing meningiomas produce hyperostosis of the involved bone (see Fig 5-11C) and hyperplasia of associated soft tissues. Contrast-enhanced MRI helps define the extent of meningiomas along the dura (see Fig 5-11D). The presence of a *dural tail* (reactive thickening of the dura adjacent to the meningioma) helps distinguish a meningioma from fibrous dysplasia.

Primary orbital meningiomas usually originate in the arachnoid of the optic nerve sheath. They occur most commonly in women in their third or fourth decade of life. Symptoms usually include a gradual, painless, unilateral loss of vision. Examination typically shows decreased vision and a relative afferent pupillary defect. Proptosis and ophthalmoplegia may also be present. The optic nerve head may appear normal, atrophic, or swollen; and tortuous vessels may be visible (Fig 5-12A, B). Occasionally, optic nerve sheath meningiomas are present bilaterally, or meningiomas occur ectopically in the orbit; these are associated with neurofibromatosis.

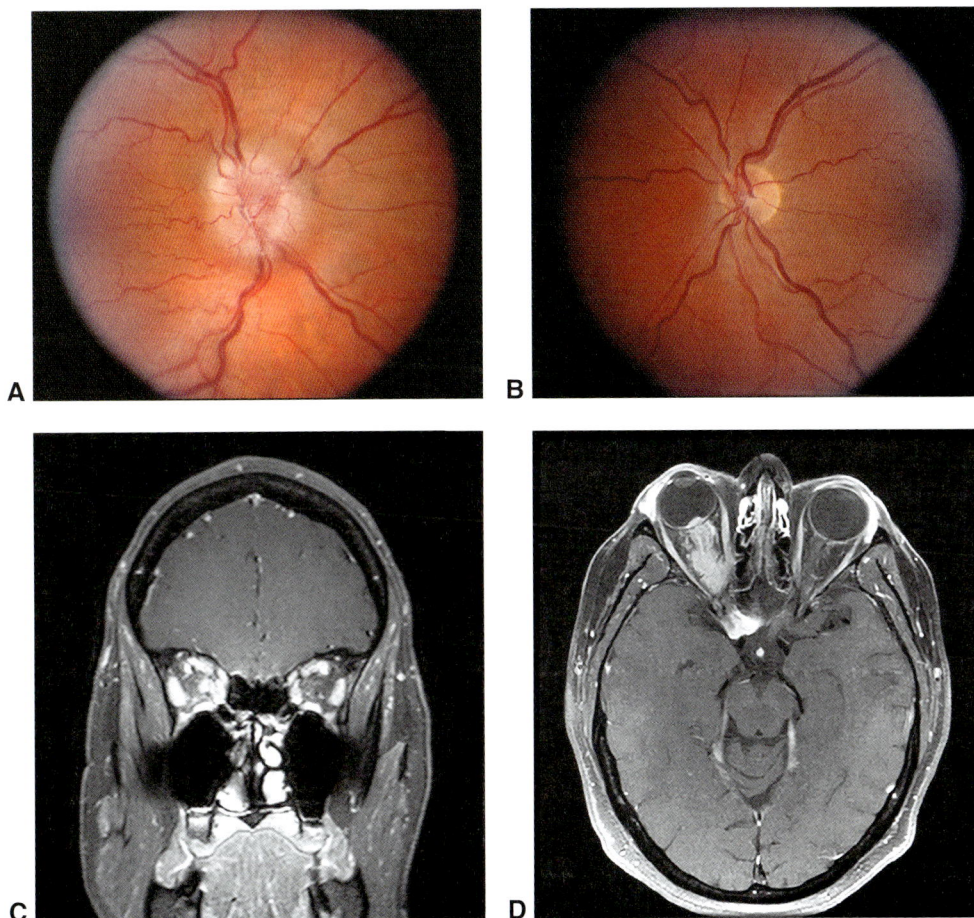

Figure 5-12 Optic nerve sheath meningioma. **A,** Swollen right optic nerve with tortuous arteries and dilated veins. **B,** Normal left optic nerve. Coronal **(C)** and axial **(D)** T1-weighted, gadolinium-enhanced MRI scans show optic nerve sheath meningioma. Note enlargement of the optic nerve sheath. *(Courtesy of Wayne Cornblath, MD.)*

Optic nerve sheath meningiomas can usually be diagnosed by means of imaging characteristics. Both CT and MRI show diffuse tubular enlargement of the optic nerve with contrast enhancement (Fig 5-12C, D). In some cases, CT can show calcification within the meningioma, referred to as *tram-tracking*. MRI reveals a fine pattern of enhancing striations emanating from the lesion in a longitudinal fashion. These striations represent the infiltrative nature of what otherwise appears to be an encapsulated lesion. As with sphenoid wing meningiomas, dural extension through the optic canal into the intracranial space can be seen on MRI.

Malignant meningioma is rare and results in rapid tumor growth that is not responsive to surgical resection, radiotherapy, or chemotherapy. On histologic examination, malignant meningiomas are indistinguishable from the more common benign group.

Management

Sphenoid wing meningioma Sphenoid wing meningiomas are typically observed until they cause functional deficits, such as profound proptosis, compressive optic neuropathy, motility impairment, or cerebral edema. Treatment includes resection of the tumor through a combined approach to the intracranial and orbital component. Complete surgical resection is not always practical because of tumor extension beyond the surgical field. Rather, the goal of surgery is to reverse the volume-induced compressive effects of the lesion. Postoperative radiotherapy may be used to reduce the risk of further growth and spread of the residual tumor, or patients can be followed clinically and with serial MRI scans.

Optic nerve sheath meningioma Treatment of optic nerve sheath meningiomas in the orbit also must be individualized. Both the amount of vision loss and the presence of intracranial extension are important factors in treatment planning. Observation is indicated if vision is minimally affected and no intracranial extension is present. If the tumor is confined to the orbit and vision loss is significant or progressive, radiation therapy should be considered. Fractionated stereotactic radiotherapy often results in stabilization or improvement of visual function. If the patient is observed or treated with radiation, periodic MRI examination is used to carefully monitor for possible posterior or intracranial extension. With rare exceptions, attempts to surgically excise optic nerve sheath meningiomas result in irreversible vision loss due to compromise of the optic nerve blood supply. Thus, surgery is reserved for patients with severe vision loss and profound proptosis. In such cases, the optic nerve is excised with the tumor, from the back of the globe to the chiasm, if preoperative MRI suggests that complete resection is possible.

Shapey J, Sabin HI, Danesh-Meyer HV, Kaye AH. Diagnosis and management of optic nerve sheath meningiomas. *J Clin Neurosci.* 2013;20(8):1045–1056.

Schwannoma

Schwannomas, sometimes known as *neurilemomas,* are proliferations of Schwann cells that are encapsulated by perineurium. These tumors have a characteristic biphasic pattern of solid areas with nuclear palisading *(Antoni A pattern)* and myxoid areas *(Antoni B pattern).* These tumors are usually well encapsulated and can be excised with relative ease.

Hypercellular schwannomas sometimes recur even after what was thought to be complete removal, but they seldom undergo malignant transformation.

Mesenchymal Tumors

Rhabdomyosarcoma

Rhabdomyosarcoma is the most common primary orbital malignancy of childhood. The average age of onset is 5–7 years. The classic clinical picture is that of a child with sudden onset and rapid progression of unilateral proptosis. However, patients in their early teens may experience a less dramatic course, with gradually progressive proptosis developing over weeks to more than a month. There is often a marked adnexal response with edema and discoloration of the eyelids. Ptosis and strabismus may also be present. A mass may be palpable, particularly in the superonasal quadrant of the eyelid, and it may cause proptosis if sufficiently large (Fig 5-13A, B). However, the tumor may be retrobulbar, may involve any quadrant of the orbit, and may in rare cases arise from the conjunctiva. If the patient has an unrelated history of trauma to the orbital area, this can lead to a delay in diagnosis and treatment.

If a rhabdomyosarcoma is suspected, the workup should proceed urgently. CT and MRI can be used to define the location and extent of the tumor (Fig 5-13C). A biopsy should be performed, usually through an anterior orbitotomy approach (Fig 5-13D). If the lesion is focal and has a pseudocapsule, it may be possible to completely remove the tumor. If this

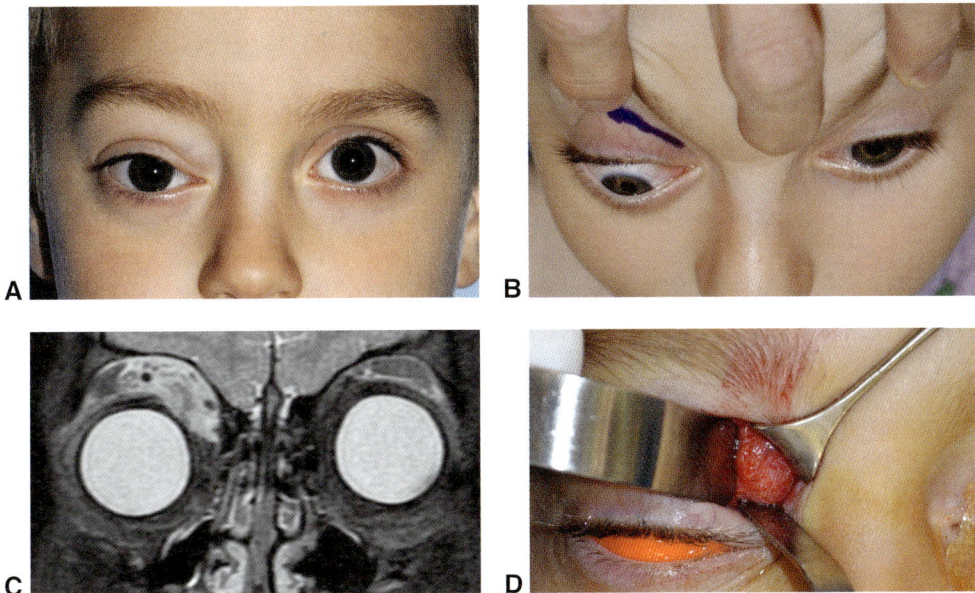

Figure 5-13 Orbital rhabdomyosarcoma. Lesion presenting as a right upper eyelid mass causing **(A)** inferolateral globe displacement and **(B)** proptosis. **C,** T2-weighted MRI shows a mass in the right superonasal quadrant. **D,** Anterior orbitotomy through the upper eyelid provided tissue for pathologic analysis. *(Courtesy of Bobby S. Korn, MD, PhD.)*

is not practical, there is some indication that the smaller the volume of residual tumor, the more effective is the combination of adjuvant radiation and chemotherapy in achieving a cure. In diffusely infiltrating rhabdomyosarcoma, a large biopsy specimen should be obtained to provide adequate tissue for frozen sections, permanent light-microscopy sections, electron microscopy, and immunohistochemistry. Cross-striations are often not visible on light microscopy and may be more readily apparent on electron microscopy.

The physician should palpate the cervical and preauricular lymph nodes of a patient with orbital rhabdomyosarcoma to evaluate for regional metastases. Chest radiography, bone marrow aspiration and biopsy, and lumbar puncture should be performed to search for more distant metastases. Sampling of the bone marrow and cerebrospinal fluid is best performed, if possible, with the patient under anesthesia at the time of the initial orbital biopsy.

Rhabdomyosarcomas arise from undifferentiated pluripotent mesenchymal elements in the orbital soft tissues, not from the extraocular muscles. They may be grouped into the following 4 categories:

- *Embryonal.* This is by far the most common type, accounting for more than 80% of cases. The embryonal form is typically found in the superonasal quadrant of the orbit. The tumor is composed of loose fascicles of undifferentiated spindle cells, only a minority of which show cross-striations in immature rhabdomyosarcomas on trichrome staining. Embryonal rhabdomyosarcomas are associated with a good 5-year survival rate (94%).
- *Alveolar.* This form typically occurs in the inferior orbit and accounts for 9% of orbital rhabdomyosarcomas. The tumor displays regular compartments composed of fibrovascular strands in which rounded rhabdomyoblasts either line up along the connective tissue strands or float freely in the alveolar spaces. This is the most malignant form of rhabdomyosarcoma; the 5-year survival rate for the alveolar subtype is 65%.
- *Pleomorphic.* Pleomorphic rhabdomyosarcoma is the least common and best-differentiated form overall, most frequently affecting young adults. In this type, many of the cells are straplike or rounded, and cross-striations are easily visualized with trichrome stain. The pleomorphic variety has the best prognosis (5-year survival rate of 97%).
- *Botryoid.* This rare variant of embryonal rhabdomyosarcoma appears grapelike. It is not found in the orbit as a primary tumor; rather, the botryoid variant occurs only through secondary extension from the paranasal sinuses or the conjunctiva. Rhabdomyosarcoma that occurs in the head and neck region outside the orbit, including the sinus cavities, has a lower 5-year survival rate (50%–71%) than rhabdomyosarcoma in the orbit, likely because tumors in the head and neck region produce fewer signs and symptoms.

Crist W, Gehan EA, Ragab AH, et al. The Third Intergroup Rhabdomyosarcoma Study. *J Clin Oncol.* 1995;13(3):610–630.

Management

Before 1965, the standard treatment for orbital rhabdomyosarcoma was orbital exenteration, and the survival rate was poor. After 1965, radiation therapy and systemic chemotherapy became the mainstays of primary treatment, based on the guidelines set forth by the Intergroup Rhabdomyosarcoma Study Group. Exenteration is reserved for recurrent cases. The total dose of local radiation varies from 4500 to 6000 cGy, given over a period of 6 weeks. The goal of systemic chemotherapy is to eliminate microscopic cellular metastases. With radiation and chemotherapy, survival rates are better than 90% if the orbital tumor has not invaded or extended beyond the bony orbital walls. Adverse effects of radiation are common in children and include cataract, radiation dermatitis, and bony hypoplasia if orbital development has not been completed.

See also BCSC Section 6, *Pediatric Ophthalmology and Strabismus.*

Raney RB, Walterhouse DO, Meza JL, et al. Results of the Intergroup Rhabdomyosarcoma Study Group D9602 protocol, using vincristine and dactinomycin with or without cyclophosphamide and radiation therapy, for newly diagnosed patients with low-risk embryonal rhabdomyosarcoma: a report from the Soft Tissue Sarcoma Committee of the Children's Oncology Group. *J Clin Oncol.* 2011;29(10):1312–1318.

Miscellaneous Mesenchymal Tumors

Tumors of fibrous connective tissue, cartilage, and bone are uncommon lesions that may involve the orbit. It is likely that a number of these mesenchymal tumors were classified incorrectly before the availability of immunohistochemical staining, which has allowed them to be differentiated accurately.

Fibrous histiocytoma is the most common of these tumors. Characteristically, it is very firm and displaces normal structures. Both fibroblastic and histiocytic cells in a storiform (matlike) pattern are found in these locally aggressive tumors. Less than 10% have metastatic potential. This tumor is sometimes difficult to distinguish, clinically and histologically, from a solitary fibrous tumor.

A solitary fibrous tumor (Fig 5-14) is composed of spindle-shaped cells that are strongly positive for CD34 and STAT 6 on immunohistochemical studies. These lesions, some of which were previously termed *hemangiopericytomas*, are uncommon, encapsulated, hypervascular, and hypercellular; they often appear in midlife. They can occur anywhere in the orbit; and they may recur, undergo malignant degeneration, or metastasize if incompletely excised. They may resemble cavernous hemangiomas on both CT and MRI, but they appear bluish intraoperatively. On histologic examination, these tumors are unique in that microscopically "benign" lesions may recur and metastasize, whereas microscopically "malignant" lesions may remain localized. Treatment consists of complete excision.

Fibrous dysplasia (Fig 5-15) is a benign developmental disorder of bone that may involve a single region or be polyostotic. CT shows hyperostotic bone, and MRI shows the lack of dural enhancement that distinguishes this condition from meningioma. When associated with cutaneous pigmentation and endocrine disorders, the condition is known as *Albright syndrome.* Resection or debulking is performed when the lesion causes disfigurement or vision loss due to stricture of the optic canal.

Osteomas (Fig 5-16) are benign tumors that can involve any of the periorbital sinuses. CT scans show dense hyperostosis with well-defined margins. The lesions can produce proptosis, compressive optic neuropathy, and orbital cellulitis secondary to obstructive sinusitis.

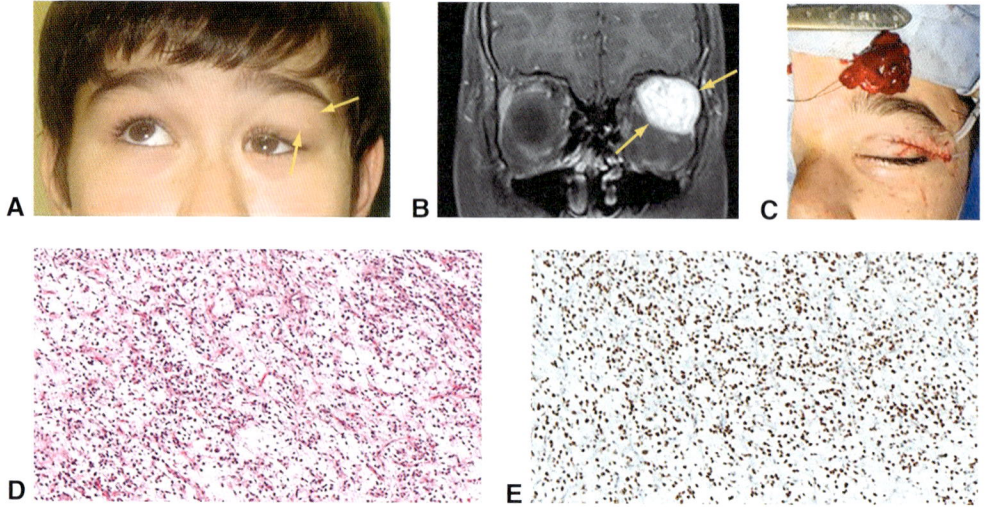

Figure 5-14 Solitary fibrous tumor. **A,** Solitary fibrous tumor *(arrows)* producing hypoglobus. **B,** T1-weighted, gadolinium-enhanced MRI shows superolateral enhancing lesion *(arrows).* **C,** Intraoperative appearance demonstrates high vascularity of the tumor. **D,** Spindle cell neoplasm with myxoid background in a "patternless pattern" with extensive vasculature (original magnification ×200, hematoxylin-eosin [H&E] stain). **E,** Predominant STAT-6 immunostaining positivity (original magnification ×200). Brown areas represent STAT-6 immunohistochemical positivity. *(Courtesy of Julian D. Perry, MD, and Alexander D. Blandford, MD.)*

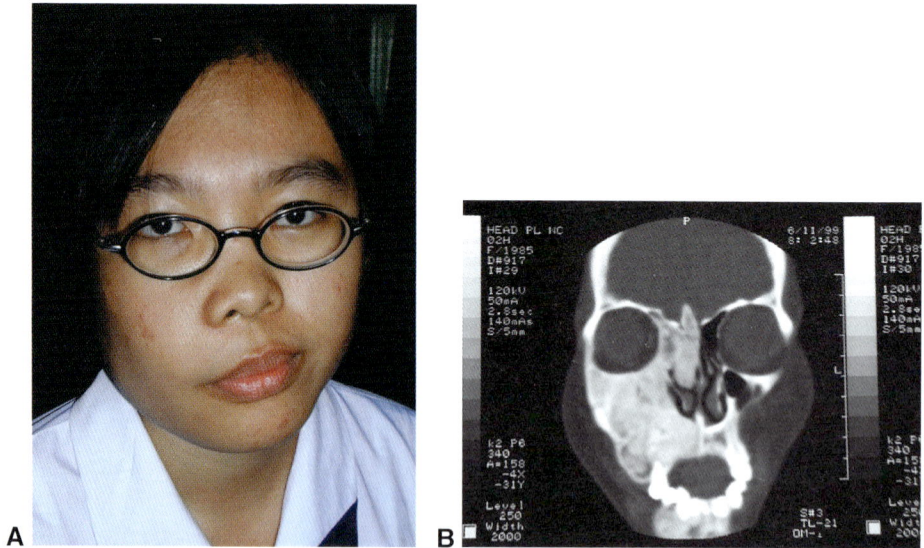

Figure 5-15 Fibrous dysplasia. **A,** Facial asymmetry. **B,** CT scan shows characteristic hyperostosis of involved facial bones. *(Courtesy of Jerry Popham, MD.)*

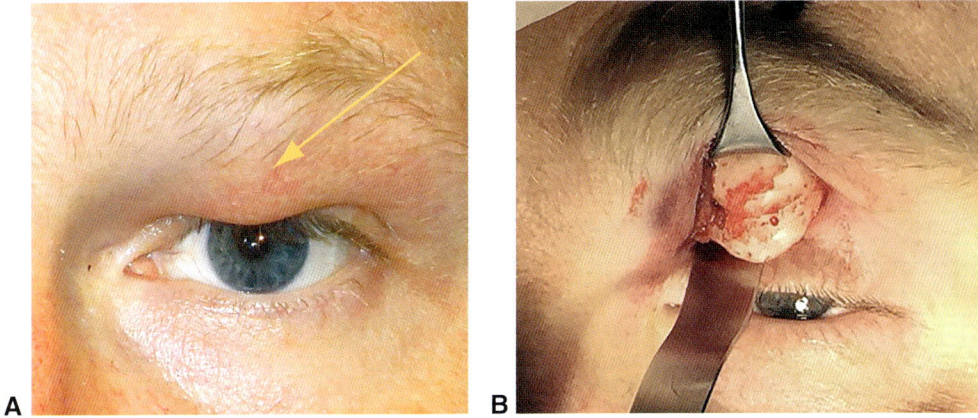

Figure 5-16 Osteoma. **A,** External photograph shows a firm, immobile lesion along the superior orbit *(arrow)*. **B,** Intraoperative view shows osteoma arising from the frontal bone. *(Courtesy of Julian D. Perry, MD, and Alexander D. Blandford, MD.)*

Most are incidental, slow-growing lesions that require no treatment. Complete excision is advised when the tumor is symptomatic.

Malignant mesenchymal tumors such as *liposarcoma, fibrosarcoma, chondrosarcoma,* and *osteosarcoma* rarely appear in the orbit. When chondrosarcomas and osteosarcomas are present, they usually destroy normal bone and demonstrate characteristic calcifications in radiographs and CT scans. Children with a history of bilateral retinoblastoma are at higher risk for osteosarcoma, chondrosarcoma, or fibrosarcoma, even if they have not been treated with therapeutic radiation.

> Katz BJ, Nerad JA. Ophthalmic manifestations of fibrous dysplasia: a disease of children and adults. *Ophthalmology.* 1998;105(12):2207–2215.

Lymphoproliferative Disorders

Lymphoid Hyperplasia and Lymphoma

Lymphoproliferative lesions of the ocular adnexa constitute a heterogeneous group of neoplasms that are defined by clinical, histologic, immunologic, molecular, and genetic characteristics. Lymphoproliferative neoplasms account for more than 20% of all orbital tumors.

The vast majority of orbital lymphoproliferative lesions are non-Hodgkin lymphoma (NHL). In the United States, the incidence of NHL in all anatomic sites has been increasing, and it is one of the most common malignancies affecting the orbit. Workers with long-term exposure to bioactive solvents and reagents are at increased risk for NHL, as are older adults and individuals with chronic autoimmune diseases.

Identification and classification of lymphoproliferative disorders

Non-Hodgkin lymphoma encompasses a heterogeneous group of malignancies and includes many subtypes. The Revised European-American Lymphoma Classification applies immunophenotypic and genetic features to identify distinct clinicopathologic NHL entities, including extranodal sites such as the orbit. The World Health Organization's classification elaborates on this approach. Orbital extranodal disease appears to represent a biological continuum and behaves unpredictably. By molecular genetic studies, approximately 90% of orbital lymphoproliferative disease is monoclonal, and 10% is polyclonal; however, both types of lesions may involve prior, concurrent, or future systemic spread. Approximately 20%–30% of periocular lymphoproliferative lesions have a history of previous or concomitant systemic disease, and an additional 30% develop it over 5 years. The risk of systemic disease remains elevated for decades after the original lesion is diagnosed, regardless of the initial lesion's location in the orbit or its clonality.

The risk of having or developing systemic NHL is lowest for conjunctival lesions, greater for orbital lesions, and highest for lesions arising in the eyelid. Lymphoid lesions developing in the fossa of the lacrimal gland may carry a greater risk of systemic disease than those occurring elsewhere in the orbit. Bilateral periocular involvement markedly increases the risk of systemic disease, but such involvement is not definitive evidence of systemic disease.

Most orbital lymphomas are derived from B cells (98%). T-cell lymphoma is rare and more lethal. B-cell lymphoma is divided into Hodgkin and non-Hodgkin tumors, with the former rarely metastasizing to the orbit. The 4 most common types of orbital lymphomas are presented in order below:

- *Extranodal marginal zone B-cell lymphoma, EMZL* (also known as *mucosa-associated lymphoid tissue,* or *MALT*). EMZL accounts for approximately 57% of orbital lymphomas and is associated with upregulation of nuclear factor κB (NF-κB). NF-κB is a major transcription factor that is involved in the innate and adaptive immunologic system. Inactivating mutations in the *A20* gene, an inhibitor of NF-κB, have also been noted in cases of EMZL. In the gastrointestinal tract, EMZL has been associated with *Helicobacter pylori* in gastric lymphomas where antimicrobial therapy has been shown to be effective. EMZL has been weakly associated with chlamydial infection, and antibiotic therapy is generally not recommended.

  EMZLs are low-grade malignancies, and 5%–15% of cases undergo spontaneous remission. However, systemic disease develops in at least 50% of patients at 10 years, and 15%–20% of cases undergo histologic transformation to a higher-grade lesion, usually of a large cell type. Such transformation usually occurs after several years and is not related to therapy.
- *Diffuse large B-cell lymphoma (DLBCL)* comprises 15% of orbital lymphomas. DLBCL also occurs in various intraocular compartments. It has been associated with multiple chromosomal translocations and alterations in the *BCL2, BCL6, MYC, EZH2,* and *MEF2B* genes.
- *Follicular lymphoma (FL).* This type of lymphoma represents a low-grade lesion with follicular centers and is the third-most-common orbital lymphoma (11%). The most common translocation associated with FL is t(14;18)(q32;q21), which results in high levels of the antiapoptotic protein BCL2.
- *Mantle cell lymphoma (MCL)* accounts for 8% of orbital lymphomas. Translocation t(11;14)(q13;q32) that is associated with overexpression of CCND1 (Cyclin D-1) is classically seen with MCL.

See also BCSC Section 4, *Ophthalmic Pathology and Intraocular Tumors.*

Swerdlow SH, Campo E, Pileri SA, et al. The 2016 revision of the World Health Organization classification of lymphoid neoplasms. *Blood.* 2016;127(20):2375–2390.

Clinical presentation

The typical lymphoproliferative lesion presents as a gradually progressive, painless mass, resulting in proptosis, a visible periocular mass, or ptosis (Fig 5-17). These tumors are often located anteriorly in the orbit or beneath the conjunctiva, where they may show the typical salmon-patch appearance (Fig 5-18). Lymphoproliferative lesions, whether benign or malignant, usually mold to surrounding orbital structures rather than invading them; consequently, disturbances of extraocular motility or visual function are unusual. Reactive lymphoid hyperplasia and low-grade lymphomas often have a history of slow expansion over a period of months to years. Regional lymph nodes should be palpated during the clinical examination.

Diagnosis

Orbital imaging reveals a characteristic puttylike molding of the tumor to normal structures (see Fig 5-17B). Bone erosion or infiltration is usually not seen except with high-grade malignant lymphomas. Up to 50% of orbital lymphoproliferative lesions arise in the fossa

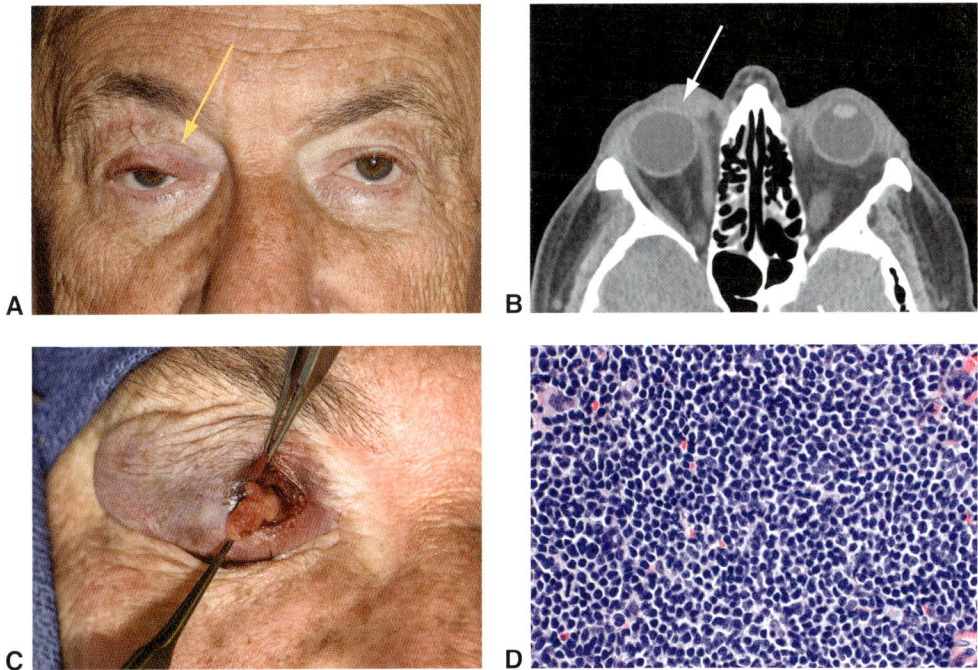

Figure 5-17 Lymphoproliferative lesion. **A,** Ptosis of the right upper eyelid and fullness *(arrow)* in the superior orbit. **B,** Axial CT scan shows a homogeneous mass *(arrow)* with characteristic molding along the globe. **C,** Incisional biopsy through an anterior orbitotomy approach via the upper eyelid crease. **D,** H&E stain of this hypercellular lesion is consistent with B-cell lymphoma. *(Courtesy of Bobby S. Korn, MD, PhD.)*

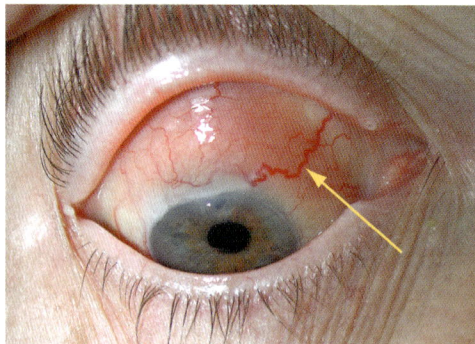

Figure 5-18 Lymphoproliferative lesion presenting as a salmon-patch subconjunctival lesion. Note the prominent feeder vessel *(arrow)* overlying the lesion. *(Courtesy of Bobby S. Korn, MD, PhD.)*

of the lacrimal gland. Lymphomas in the retrobulbar fat may appear more infiltrative. Approximately 17% of orbital lymphoid lesions occur bilaterally, but this does not necessarily indicate the presence of extraorbital disease.

For all lymphoproliferative lesions, an open biopsy is preferred to obtain an adequate tissue specimen. A portion of the tissue should be placed in a suitable fixative for light microscopy, and the majority should be sent fresh to a molecular diagnostics laboratory for possible flow cytometry, immunohistochemistry, and genomic analysis. Fine-needle aspiration biopsy may establish all but the morphologic characteristics of the lesion. Conjunctival biopsy for follicular conjunctivitis can sometimes reveal a lymphoproliferative lesion.

Both reactive lymphoid hyperplasia and malignant lymphoma are hypercellular proliferations with sparse or absent stromal components. Light microscopy may reveal a histologic continuum from reactive lymphoid hyperplasia to low-grade lymphoma to higher-grade malignancy; it may not by itself adequately characterize a given lesion. In such cases, immunopathology and molecular diagnostic studies aid in further categorization.

Malignant lymphomas are thought to represent clonal expansions of abnormal precursor cells. Immunologic identification of lymphocyte cell-surface markers can classify tumors as containing B cells or T cells. Specific monoclonal antibodies directed against surface light-chain immunoglobulins are used to determine whether the cells represent monoclonal (ie, malignant) proliferations.

Genetic analysis has shown that most lymphoproliferative lesions that appear to be immunologically polyclonal actually harbor small monoclonal proliferations of B lymphocytes. However, the finding of monoclonality, by either immunophenotype or molecular genetics, does not predict which tumors will ultimately result in systemic disease.

Management

Because there is considerable overlap among the various lymphoproliferative lesions in terms of clinical presentation and behavior, all patients with hypercellular lymphoid lesions (whether monoclonal or polyclonal) should be examined by an oncologist. Depending on the histologic type of the lesion, the examination may include a general physical examination, a complete blood count, a bone marrow biopsy, CT and/or MRI imaging, a positron emission tomography scan, and serum immunoprotein electrophoresis. The patient should be reexamined periodically because systemic lymphoma may develop many years after the occurrence of an isolated orbital lymphoid neoplasm.

For EMZL and FL, radiotherapy usually results in good outcomes, with 10-year survival rates of 92% and 71%, respectively. DLBCL and MCL have a poorer prognosis, with 10-year survival rates of 41% and 32%, respectively. Treatment of non-EMZL more often involves chemotherapy and immunomodulation in addition to radiotherapy. The optimal dose of radiation has not been established, with published amounts ranging from 20–40 Gy in fractionated doses. A surgical cure is usually not possible because of the infiltrative nature of lymphoid tumors. Alternative treatments include targeted therapies such as rituximab for CD20-positive lymphomas.

The management of low-grade lymphoid lesions that have already undergone systemic dissemination is somewhat controversial, because indolent lymphomas are generally refractory to chemotherapy and are associated with long-term survival, even if untreated. Many oncologists take a watchful waiting approach and treat only symptomatic disease.

Andrew NH, Coupland SE, Pirbhai A, Selva D. Lymphoid hyperplasia of the orbit and ocular adnexa: A clinical pathologic review. *Surv Ophthalmol.* 2016;61(6):778–790.

Olsen TG, Holm, F, Mikkelsen LH, et al. Orbital lymphoma—an international multicenter retrospective study. *Am J Ophthalmol.* 2019;199:44–57.

Yen MT, Bilyk JR, Wladis EJ, Bradley EB, Mawn LA. Treatments for ocular adnexal lymphoma. A report by the American Academy of Ophthalmology. *Ophthalmology.* 2018;125(1):127–136.

Plasma Cell Tumors

Lesions composed predominantly of mature plasma cells may be plasmacytomas or localized plasma cell–rich masses. Multiple myeloma should be ruled out, particularly if there is bone destruction or any immaturity or mitotic activity of the plasmacytic elements. Some lesions are composed of lymphocytes and lymphoplasmacytoid cells, with the combined properties of both lymphocytes and plasma cells. Plasma cell tumors display the same spectrum of clinical involvement as do lymphoproliferative lesions but are much less common.

Histiocytic Disorders

Langerhans cell histiocytosis (formerly called *histiocytosis X*) is a collection of rare disorders of the mononuclear phagocytic system (Fig 5-19). These disorders are thought to result from abnormal immune regulation. All subtypes are characterized by an accumulation of proliferating dendritic histiocytes. The disease occurs most commonly in children, with a peak incidence between 5 and 10 years of age, and it varies in severity, from benign lesions with spontaneous resolution to chronic dissemination that results in death. Older names representing the various manifestations of histiocytic disorders *(eosinophilic granuloma of bone, Hand-Schüller-Christian disease,* and *Letterer-Siwe disease)* are being replaced by the terms *unifocal* and *multifocal eosinophilic granuloma of bone* and *diffuse soft tissue histiocytosis.*

If sufficiently large, the mass may cause proptosis (see Fig 5-19A, B). Younger children more often present with significant overlying soft-tissue inflammation; they are also more

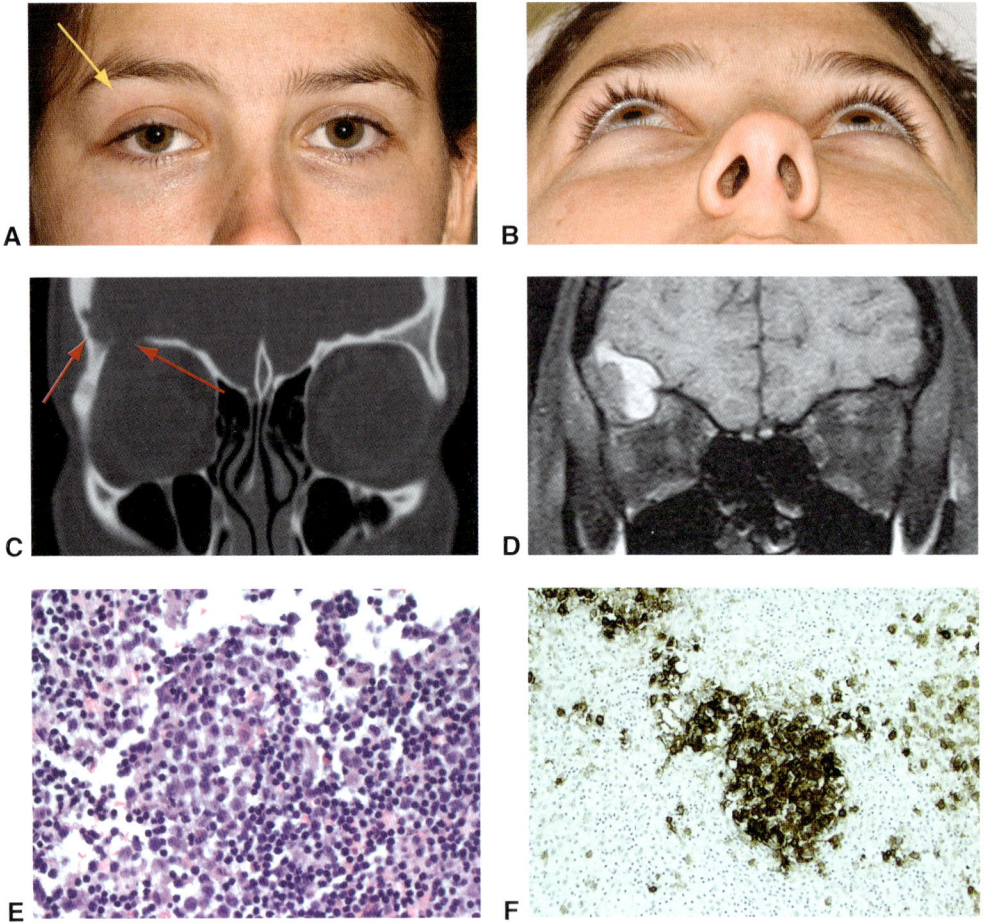

Figure 5-19 Langerhans cell histiocytosis. **A,** 18-year-old woman with ptosis of the right upper eyelid, fullness *(arrow),* and inferior globe displacement. **B,** Worm's-eye view demonstrates 2 mm of proptosis of the right eye. **C,** Coronal CT scan shows lytic erosion of the superotemporal orbital bone *(arrows).* **D,** Coronal MRI scan shows the soft tissue with an intracranial and intraorbital component. **E,** H&E stain of the lesion demonstrates numerous foamy histiocytes. **F,** Immunohistochemistry with CD1a antibody confirms the diagnosis of Langerhans cell histiocytosis. *(Courtesy of Bobby S. Korn, MD, PhD.)*

likely to have multifocal or systemic involvement. Even if the initial workup shows no evidence of systemic dissemination, younger patients require regular observation for possible development of multiorgan disease. The most frequent presentation in the orbit is a lytic defect best noted on CT imaging (see Fig 5-19C), usually affecting the superotemporal orbit or sphenoid wing and causing relapsing episodes of orbital inflammation, often initially misdiagnosed as infectious orbital cellulitis. MRI imaging aids in visualization of the soft-tissue component (see Fig 5-19D). Histopathology shows foamy histiocytes with abundant eosinophilic cytoplasm and irregular nuclei that are immunoreactive for antibodies against CD1a (see Fig 5-19E, F).

Management

Histiocytic disorders have a reported survival rate of only 50% in patients who are younger than 2 years at presentation; if the disease develops after age 2, the survival rate rises to 87%. Treatment of localized orbital disease consists of confirmatory biopsy with debulking, which may be followed by intralesional steroid injection or low-dose radiation therapy. Spontaneous remission has also been reported. Although destruction of the orbital bone may be extensive at the time of presentation, the bone usually reossifies completely. Children with systemic disease are treated aggressively with chemotherapy.

Esmaili N, Harris GJ. Langerhans cell histiocytosis of the orbit: spectrum of disease and risk of central nervous system sequelae in unifocal cases. *Ophthalmic Plast Reconstr Surg.* 2016;32(1):28–34.

Xanthogranuloma

Adult xanthogranuloma of the adnexa and orbit is often associated with systemic manifestations. These manifestations are the basis for classification into the following 4 syndromes, presented in their order of frequency.

- *Necrobiotic xanthogranuloma (NBX).* This disorder is characterized by the presence of subcutaneous lesions in the eyelids and anterior orbit; lesions may also occur throughout the body. Although skin lesions are seen in all 4 syndromes, those occurring in NBX have a propensity for ulceration and fibrosis. Systemic findings frequently include paraproteinemia and multiple myeloma.
- *Adult-onset asthma with periocular xanthogranuloma (AAPOX).* This syndrome includes periocular xanthogranuloma, asthma, lymphadenopathy, and, often, increased levels of immunoglobulin G.
- *Erdheim-Chester disease (ECD).* The most devastating of the adult xanthogranulomas, ECD (Fig 5-20) is characterized by dense, progressive, recalcitrant fibrosclerosis of the orbit and internal organs, including the mediastinum; the pericardium; and the pleural, perinephric, and retroperitoneal spaces. Whereas xanthogranuloma of the orbit and adnexa tends to be anterior in NBX, AAPOX, and AOX, it is often diffuse in ECD and leads to vision loss. Bone involvement is common, and the syndrome often is fatal, despite aggressive therapies.
- *Adult-onset xanthogranuloma (AOX).* AOX is an isolated xanthogranulomatous lesion without systemic involvement. *Juvenile xanthogranuloma* is a separate non-Langerhans histiocytic disorder that occurs as a self-limited, corticosteroid-sensitive, and usually focal subcutaneous disease of childhood. See BCSC Section 6, *Pediatric Ophthalmology and Strabismus,* for additional discussion of juvenile xanthogranuloma.

Satchi K, McNab AA, Godfrey T, Prince HM. Adult orbital xanthogranuloma successfully treated with rituximab. *Ophthalmology.* 2014;121(8):1664–1665.

Sivak-Callcott JA, Rootman J, Rasmussen SL, et al. Adult xanthogranulomatous disease of the orbit and ocular adnexa: new immunohistochemical findings and clinical review. *Br J Ophthalmol.* 2006;90(5):602–608.

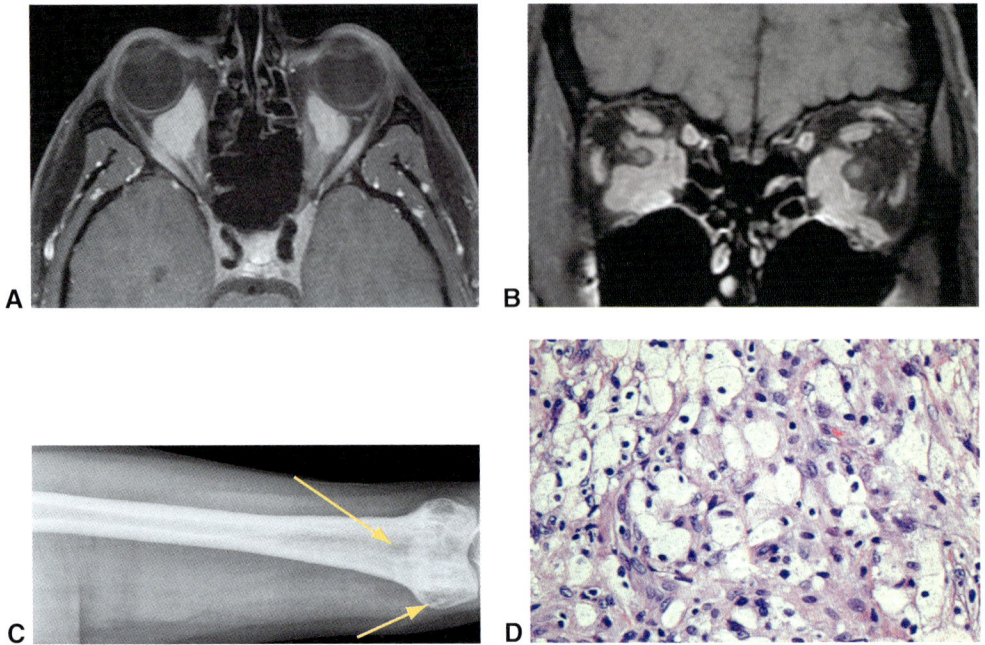

Figure 5-20   Erdheim-Chester disease. T1-weighted MRI axial **(A)** and coronal **(B)** views show diffuse infiltration of a mass in the intraconal space bilaterally. **C,** X-ray of the femur shows lytic bone lesions *(arrows)*. **D,** H&E stain of the lesion demonstrates numerous foamy histiocytes. *(Courtesy of Don O. Kikkawa, MD.)*

Lacrimal Gland Tumors

Most lacrimal gland masses represent nonspecific inflammation *(dacryoadenitis)*. They present with acute inflammatory signs and usually respond to anti-inflammatory medication (see the section Nonspecific Orbital Inflammation in Chapter 4). Of those lacrimal gland tumefactions not presenting with inflammatory signs and symptoms, the majority are lymphoproliferative disorders (discussed previously). Up to 50% of orbital lymphomas develop in the fossa of the lacrimal gland. Only a minority of lacrimal fossa lesions are epithelial neoplasms of the lacrimal gland.

Imaging is helpful in evaluating lesions in the lacrimal gland region. Inflammatory and lymphoid proliferations in the lacrimal gland tend to cause it to expand diffusely and appear elongated, whereas epithelial neoplasms tend to appear as isolated globular masses. Inflammatory and lymphoproliferative lesions usually mold around the globe, but epithelial neoplasms tend to displace and indent it. The bone of the lacrimal fossa is remodeled in response to a slowly growing benign epithelial lesion of the lacrimal gland; however, lymphoproliferative lesions typically do not cause bony changes.

Epithelial Tumors of the Lacrimal Gland

Approximately 50% of epithelial tumors are benign mixed tumors *(pleomorphic adenomas)*, and about 50% are carcinomas. Approximately half of the carcinomas are adenoid cystic carcinomas, and the remainder are malignant mixed tumors, primary adenocarcinomas, mucoepidermoid carcinomas, or squamous carcinomas.

Pleomorphic adenoma

Pleomorphic adenoma is the most common epithelial tumor of the lacrimal gland. This tumor usually occurs in adults during the fourth or fifth decade of life and affects slightly more men than women. Patients present with a progressive, painless inferior and medial displacement of the globe with axial proptosis (Fig 5-21A). Symptoms usually persist for more than 12 months.

A firm, lobular mass may be palpated near the superolateral orbital rim, and orbital imaging often reveals enlargement or expansion of the fossa of the lacrimal gland. On imaging, the lesion appears well circumscribed but may have a slightly nodular configuration (Fig 5-21B, C).

Microscopically, pleomorphic adenomas have a varied cellular structure consisting primarily of a proliferation of benign epithelial cells and a stroma composed of spindle-shaped cells with occasional cartilaginous, mucinous, or even osteoid degeneration or metaplasia. Because of this variability, the term *benign mixed tumor* is sometimes used. The lesion is circumscribed by a pseudocapsule.

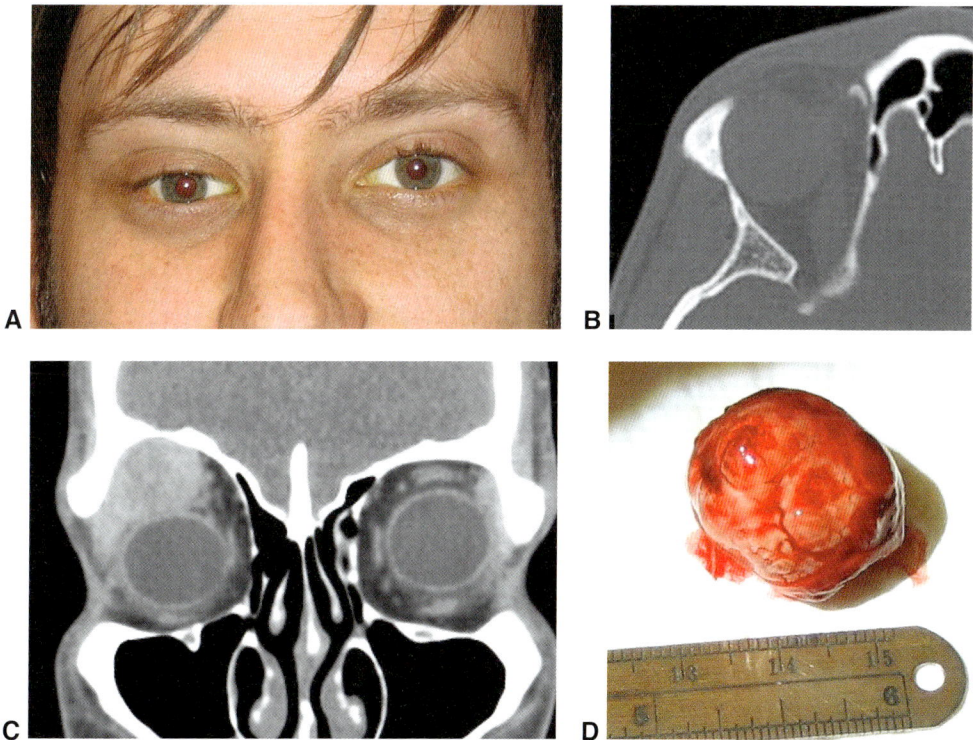

Figure 5-21 Pleomorphic adenoma. **A,** Adult male with inferomedial displacement of the right globe. **B,** Axial CT scan shows a well-circumscribed mass in the superotemporal orbit with no lytic erosion of the bone. **C,** Coronal CT shows the mass displacing the right globe inferiorly and medially. **D,** The mass was completely removed with the pseudocapsule intact through a lateral orbitotomy approach. *(Courtesy of Eric A. Steele, MD.)*

Management Treatment is complete removal of the pleomorphic adenoma with its pseudocapsule and a surrounding margin of orbital tissue (Fig 5-21D). Surgery should be performed without a preliminary biopsy: in an early study, the recurrence rate was 32% when the capsule was incised for direct biopsy. In recurrences, the risk of malignant degeneration into carcinoma ex pleomorphic adenoma is 10% per decade.

Chawla B, Kashyap S, Sen S, et al. Clinicopathologic review of epithelial tumors of the lacrimal gland. *Ophthalmic Plast Reconstr Surg.* 2013;29(6):440–445.

Adenoid cystic carcinoma

Adenoid cystic carcinoma (ACC) is the most common malignant epithelial tumor of the lacrimal gland. This highly malignant carcinoma may cause pain because of perineural invasion and bone destruction. The relatively rapid course, with a history of generally less than 1 year, and early onset of pain help differentiate ACC from pleomorphic adenoma, which is painless and characteristically exhibits progressive proptosis for more than a year. The tumor usually extends into the posterior orbit because of its capacity to infiltrate and its lack of true encapsulation.

Microscopically, this tumor is composed of deceptively benign-appearing cells that grow in tubules, solid nests, or a Swiss-cheese pattern. The basaloid morphology is associated with worse survival than the cribriform variant. Infiltration of the orbital tissues, including perineural invasion, is often seen in microscopic sections.

Malignant mixed tumor

These lesions are histologically similar to pleomorphic adenomas (benign mixed tumors), but they have areas of malignant change, usually poorly differentiated adenocarcinomas. They typically arise from a long-standing primary pleomorphic adenoma or from a pleomorphic adenoma that has recurred after initial incomplete excision or violation of the pseudocapsule (see the section "Pleomorphic adenoma"). An increase in growth rate is a hallmark of malignant degeneration.

Management of malignant lacrimal gland tumors

Suspicion of a malignant lacrimal gland tumor warrants biopsy with permanent histologic confirmation. Traditional treatment is centered around orbital exenteration or radical orbitectomy followed by radiotherapy; however, the survival benefit of exenteration remains unproven. Other treatment strategies include neoadjuvant intra-arterial chemotherapy followed by exenteration or eye-sparing surgery followed by radiation (typically proton) therapy. Despite these measures, ascending perineural extension often develops, usually leading to death from intracranial extension or, less commonly, from systemic metastases (managed by local resection) a decade or more after the initial presentation.

Tse DT, Kossler AL, Feuer WJ, Benedetto PW. Long-term outcomes of neoadjuvant intra-arterial cytoreductive chemotherapy for lacrimal gland adenoid cystic carcinoma. *Ophthalmology.* 2013;120(7):1313–1323.

Woo KI, Kim YD, Sa HS, Esmaeli B. Current treatment of lacrimal gland carcinoma. *Curr Opin Ophthalmol.* 2016;26(5):449–456.

Nonepithelial Tumors of the Lacrimal Gland

The vast majority of nonepithelial lesions of the lacrimal gland represent lymphoid prolif-eration or inflammations, discussed earlier in this chapter and in Chapter 4 of this volume.

Benign lymphocytic infiltrates may be seen in patients, particularly women, who have bilateral swelling of the lacrimal gland, producing a dry eye syndrome. This condition can occur insidiously or following a symptomatic episode of lacrimal gland inflammation. The enlargement of the lacrimal glands may not be clinically apparent. Biopsy specimens of the affected glands show a spectrum of lymphocytic infiltration, from scattered patches of lymphocytes to lymphocytic replacement of the lacrimal gland parenchyma with preserva-tion of the inner duct cells, which are surrounded by proliferating myoepithelial cells *(epi-myoepithelial islands)*. This combination of lymphocytes and epimyoepithelial islands has led some authors to designate this manifestation as a lymphoepithelial lesion. Some patients with lymphocytic infiltrates may also have systemic rheumatoid arthritis and, therefore, have classic Sjögren syndrome. These lesions may develop into low-grade B-cell lymphoma (see the section Lymphoproliferative Disorders). Associated dry eye symptoms may improve with the use of topical cyclosporine.

Shields JA, Shields CL, Epstein JA, Scartozzi R, Eagle RC Jr. Review: primary epithelial malignancies of the lacrimal gland: the 2003 Ramon L. Font lecture. *Ophthalmic Plast Reconstr Surg.* 2004;20(1):10–21.

Secondary Orbital Conditions

Secondary orbital tumors are those that extend into the orbit from contiguous structures, including the globe, the eyelids, the lacrimal drainage system, the sinuses, or the brain.

Globe and Eyelid Origin

Tumors and inflammations from within the eye (especially from choroidal melanomas and retinoblastomas) or from the eyelid (eg, sebaceous gland carcinoma, squamous cell carci-noma, and basal cell carcinoma) can invade the orbit. Primary eyelid tumors are discussed in Chapter 10. Retinoblastoma, choroidal melanoma, and other ocular neoplasms are cov-ered in BCSC Section 4, *Ophthalmic Pathology and Intraocular Tumors,* and Section 6, *Pedi-atric Ophthalmology and Strabismus.*

Yin VT, Pfeiffer ML, Esmaeli B. Targeted therapy for orbital and periocular basal cell carcinoma and squamous cell carcinoma. *Ophthalmic Plast Reconstr Surg.* 2013;29(2): 87–92.

Sinus Disease Affecting the Orbit

Tumors from the nose or the paranasal sinuses may secondarily invade the orbit. Proptosis and globe displacement are common. The diagnosis is made by imaging, which is ordered to include the base of the sinuses for proper evaluation.

Mucoceles and *mucopyoceles* of the sinuses (Fig 5-22) are cystic structures with pseu-dostratified ciliated columnar (respiratory) epithelium resulting from obstruction of the

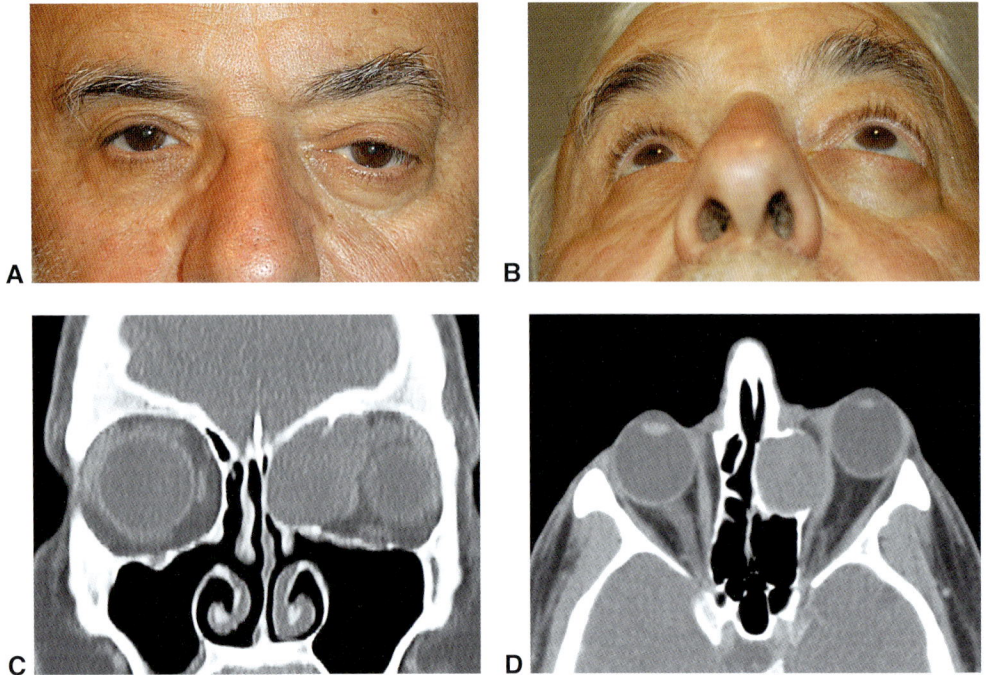

Figure 5-22 Mucocele. **A,** Photograph shows inferior and lateral displacement of the left globe. **B,** Worm's-eye view demonstrates left proptosis. Coronal **(C)** and axial **(D)** CT scans show a frontoethmoidal mucocele expanding laterally into the orbit. *(Courtesy of Bobby S. Korn, MD, PhD.)*

sinus excretory ducts. These lesions may invade the orbit by expansion and erosion of the bones of the orbital walls and cause globe displacement. In the case of mucoceles, the cysts are usually filled with thick mucoid secretions; in the case of mucopyoceles, they are filled with pus. Most mucoceles arise from the frontal and/or ethmoid sinuses. Surgical treatment includes evacuation of the mucocele and reestablishment of drainage of the affected sinus or obliteration of the sinus by mucosal stripping and packing with bone or fat.

Silent sinus syndrome is another orbital condition that results from sinus outflow pathology (Fig 5-23). Chronic subclinical sinusitis presumably causes thinning of the bones of the maxillary sinus, leading to collapse of the orbital floor and subsequent enophthalmos. This collapse may occur in association with a recent significant change in atmospheric pressure (eg, during airplane travel or scuba diving). Upper eyelid ptosis, deepening of the superior sulcus, and, occasionally, diplopia may occur. Treatment includes restoration of maxillary sinus aeration and reconstruction of the orbital floor. The entrapped maxillary sinus secretions are often sterile in nature.

Squamous cell carcinoma and *adenocarcinoma* of the sinuses may secondarily invade the orbit (Fig 5-24). These malignancies usually arise in the maxillary sinuses, followed by the nasopharynx or the oropharynx. Nasal obstruction, epistaxis, or epiphora may be associated with the growth of such tumors. Treatment is usually a combination of surgical excision and radiation therapy and often includes exenteration if the periorbita is traversed by tumor.

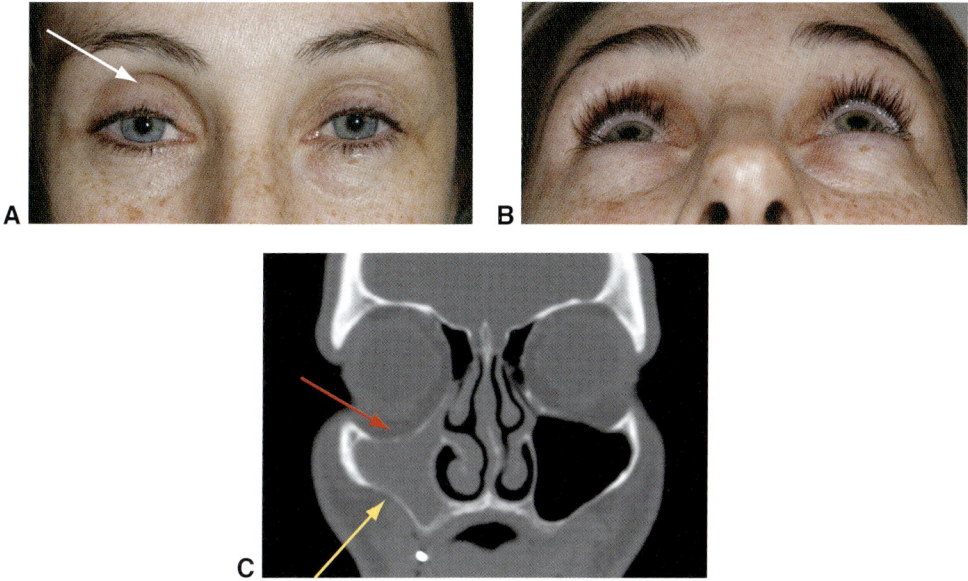

Figure 5-23 Silent sinus syndrome. **A,** External photograph shows ptosis of the right upper eyelid and deepening of the superior sulcus *(arrow).* **B,** Worm's-eye view shows enophthalmos of the right eye. **C,** Coronal CT scan shows inferior bowing of the orbital floor *(red arrow),* concave deformation the lateral wall of the maxillary sinus *(yellow arrow),* and opacification of the maxillary sinus consistent with silent sinus syndrome. *(Courtesy of Bobby S. Korn, MD, PhD.)*

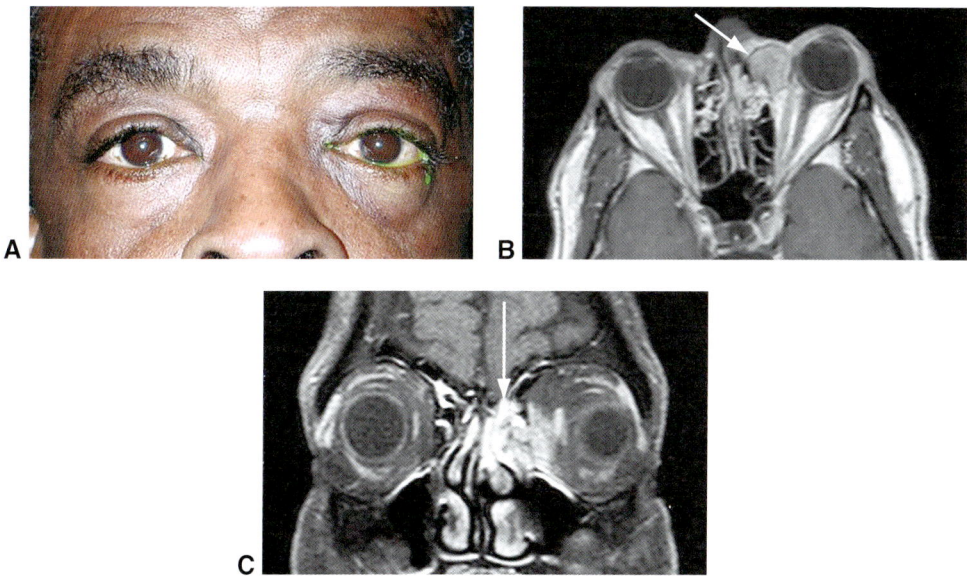

Figure 5-24 Ethmoid sinus squamous cell carcinoma. **A,** Photograph shows fullness of the medial canthal area overlying the mass. Axial **(B)** and coronal **(C)** T1-weighted MRI with gadolinium contrast reveals a mass in the ethmoid sinus eroding into the medial orbit. *(Courtesy of Julian D. Perry, MD, and Alexander D. Blandford, MD.)*

Nonepithelial tumors that can invade the orbit from the sinuses, nose, and facial bones include a wide variety of benign and malignant lesions. Among the most common are osteomas, fibrous dysplasia, and miscellaneous sarcomas.

Brown SJ, Hardy T, McNab AA. "Silent sinus syndrome" following orbital trauma: a case series and review of the literature. *Ophthalmic Plast Reconstr Surg.* 2017;33(3): 209–212.

Metastatic Tumors

Metastatic Tumors in Children

In children, distant tumors metastasize to the orbit more frequently than to the globe (in contrast to adults, who more frequently have metastases to the choroid). Tumors that can metastasize to the orbit in children include Burkitt lymphoma, leukemia, neuroblastoma, Ewing sarcoma, and Wilms tumor (nephroblastoma).

Leukemia

In advanced stages, leukemia may produce unilateral or bilateral proptosis. *Acute lymphoblastic leukemia* is the type of leukemia most likely to metastasize to the orbit. A primary leukemic orbital mass, called *granulocytic sarcoma* or *chloroma,* is a rare variant of myelogenous leukemia. Least common are metastases to the subarachnoid space of the optic nerve. These cases present with sudden vision loss and swelling of the optic nerve. They constitute an emergency and are treated with orbital radiotherapy.

Typically, orbital lesions present before blood or bone marrow signs of leukemia, which almost invariably follow within several months. Special stains for cytoplasmic esterase in the cells (Leder stain) indicate that they are granulocytic precursor cells. Chances for survival are improved if chemotherapy is instituted before the discovery of leukemic involvement in bone marrow or peripheral blood.

Neuroblastoma

Metastatic orbital neuroblastoma occurs in 10%–20% of cases and typically produces an abrupt ecchymotic proptosis that may be bilateral. A deposition of blood in the eyelids may lead to the mistaken impression of injury (Fig 5-25). Horner syndrome may also be evident in some cases. Commonly, bone destruction is apparent on CT, particularly in the lateral orbital wall or sphenoid marrow. Metastases typically occur late in the course of the disease, when the primary tumor can be detected readily in the abdomen, mediastinum, or neck. Treatment consists primarily of chemotherapy; radiotherapy is reserved for cases of impending vision loss due to compressive optic neuropathy. The survival rate of neuroblastoma is related to the patient's age at diagnosis. Patients diagnosed before 1 year of age have a significantly better prognosis (a 5-year survival of 85%) than children diagnosed after 1 year of age (5-year survival rate of 36%). Unfortunately, the average age of presentation of patients with orbital metastases is over 2 years of age. Congenital neuroblastoma of the cervical ganglia may produce an ipsilateral Horner syndrome with heterochromia.

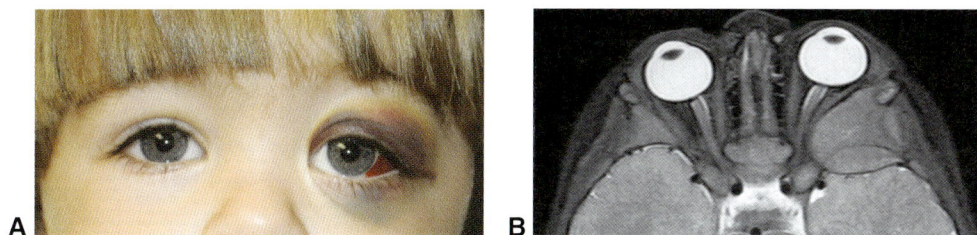

Figure 5-25 Metastatic neuroblastoma. **A,** Child with metastatic left orbital neuroblastoma. **B,** T2-weighted MRI shows a large infiltrating lesion of the left sphenoid wing extending into the orbital soft tissues and the temporal fossa. *(Courtesy of Bobby S. Korn, MD, PhD.)*

Aggarwal E, Mulay K, Honavar SG. Orbital extra-medullary granulocytic sarcoma: clinico-pathologic correlation with immunohistochemical features. *Surv Ophthalmol.* 2014;59(2):232–235.

Ahmed S, Goel S, Khandwala M, Agrawal A, Chang B, Simmons IG. Neuroblastoma with orbital metastasis: ophthalmic presentation and role of ophthalmologists. *Eye (Lond).* 2006;20(4):466–470.

Metastatic Tumors in Adults

Although virtually any cancer of the internal organs, hematopoietic system, or skin can metastasize to the orbit, most orbital metastases derive from lung, breast, and prostate tumors. The presence of pain, proptosis, inflammation, bone destruction, and early ophthalmoplegia suggests the possibility of metastatic carcinoma.

Some 75% of patients have a history of a known primary tumor, but orbital metastasis is the presenting sign of cancer in 25% of patients. The extraocular muscles are frequently involved because of their abundant blood supply. The second most common site is the bone marrow space of the sphenoid bone because of the relatively high volume of low-flow blood in this area (Fig 5-26). Lytic destruction of this part of the lateral orbital wall is highly suggestive of metastatic disease. Elevation of serum carcinoembryonic antigen levels also may

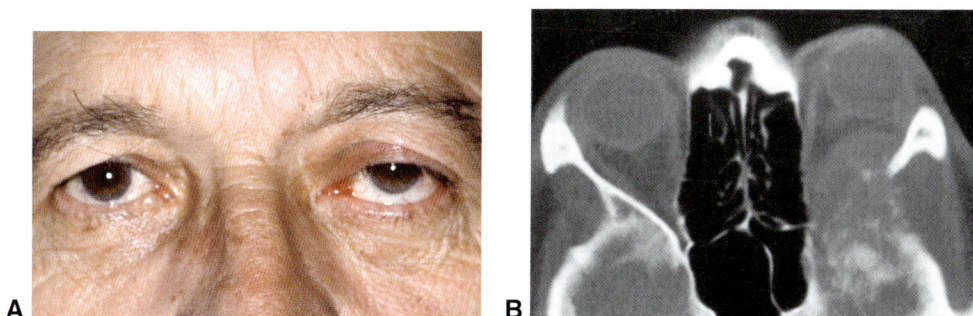

Figure 5-26 Metastatic prostate cancer. **A,** Left proptosis and orbital congestion in a patient with prostate carcinoma. **B,** CT scan shows a left posterior orbital mass with adjacent bony destruction, confirmed by biopsy to be metastatic prostate cancer. *(Courtesy of Roberta E. Gausas, MD.)*

suggest a metastatic process. Fine-needle aspiration biopsy can be performed in the office and may obviate the need for orbitotomy and open biopsy.

Breast carcinoma

The most common primary source of orbital metastases in women is breast cancer. Metastases may occur many years after the breast lesion has been removed; thus, the history should always include inquiries about previous cancer surgery. Breast metastasis to the orbit can elicit a fibrous response that causes enophthalmos and, possibly, restriction of ocular motility (Fig 5-27).

Some patients with breast cancer respond favorably to hormone therapy. This response usually correlates with the presence of estrogen and other hormone receptors in the tumor tissue. Estrogen receptor assay results from orbital metastases may differ from those of the primary lesion; thus, orbital tissue studies should include this assay. Hormone therapy is most likely to help patients whose tumors are receptor positive.

Bronchogenic carcinoma

The most frequent origin of orbital metastasis in men is bronchogenic carcinoma. The primary lesion may be quite small, and CT of suspicious lung lesions may be performed in patients suspected of having orbital metastases.

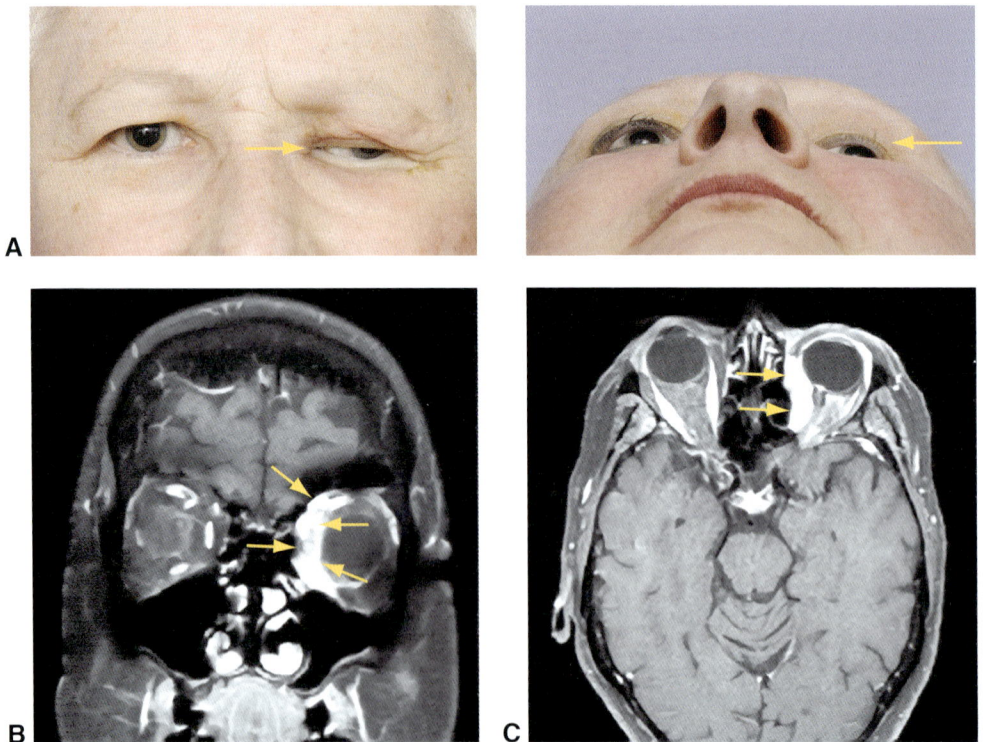

Figure 5-27 Metastatic breast carcinoma. **A,** Left enophthalmos *(arrows)* secondary to breast carcinoma metastasis to the orbit. Coronal **(B)** and axial **(C)** MRI images show medial infiltration of the orbit *(arrows)*. *(Courtesy of Hakan Demirci, MD.)*

Prostate carcinoma

Metastatic prostate carcinoma can produce a clinical picture resembling that of acute nonspecific orbital inflammation. Typically, an osteoblastic bone lesion is identified on imaging.

Management of Orbital Metastases

The treatment of metastatic tumors of the orbit is usually palliative, consisting of local radiation therapy. Some metastatic tumors, such as carcinoids and renal cell carcinomas, may be candidates for wide excision of the orbital lesion because patients may survive for many years following resection of isolated metastases. Consultation with the patient's oncologist is important for identifying candidates who might benefit from wide excision.

Bonavolontà G, Strianese D, Grassi P, et. al. An analysis of 2,480 space-occupying lesions of the orbit from 1976 to 2011. *Ophthalmic Plast Reconstr Surg.* 2013;29(2):79–86.

Garrity JA, Henderson JW, Cameron JD. *Henderson's Orbital Tumors.* 4th ed. Philadelphia: Lippincott Williams & Wilkins; 2007.

CHAPTER 6

Orbital Trauma

▶ *This chapter includes a related video, which can be accessed by scanning the QR code provided in the text or going to www.aao.org/bcscvideo_section07.*

Highlights

- Orbital trauma is amongst the most common emergency department consultations and is often accompanied by trauma of the facial bones and soft tissue.
- Additional injuries that may be observed in the setting of orbital trauma include orbital hemorrhage, retained foreign body, and optic neuropathy.
- Ophthalmic manifestations of orbital trauma may include decreased vision, intraocular injury, strabismus, and eyelid or globe malposition.
- An ophthalmic examination should be performed on all patients who have sustained orbital trauma as ocular injuries may also be present.

Midfacial (Le Fort) Fractures

Le Fort fractures involve the maxilla and are often complex and asymmetric (Figs 6-1, 6-2). By definition, Le Fort fractures extend posteriorly through the pterygoid plates. These fractures may be divided into 3 categories, although clinically they often do not conform precisely to these groupings:

- *Le Fort I* fractures are low transverse maxillary fractures above the teeth with no orbital involvement.
- *Le Fort II* fractures generally have a pyramidal configuration and involve the nasal, lacrimal, and maxillary bones as well as the medial orbital floor.
- *Le Fort III* fractures cause craniofacial disjunction, in which the entire facial skeleton is completely detached from the base of the skull and is suspended only by soft tissues. The orbital floor as well as the medial and lateral orbital walls are involved.

Treatment may include dental stabilization with arch bars and open reduction of the fracture with rigid fixation using titanium plating systems.

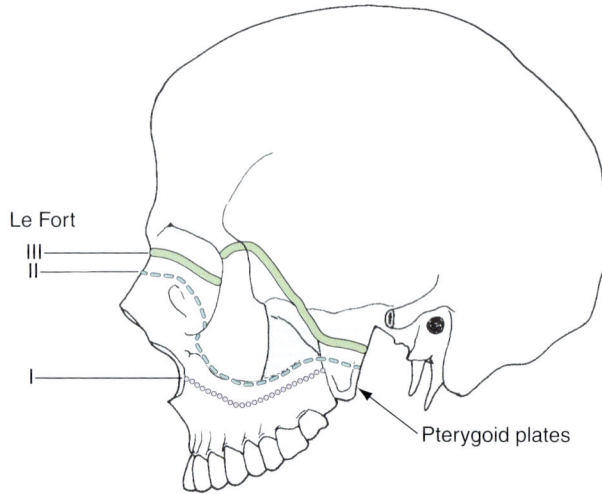

Figure 6-1 Le Fort fractures (lateral view). Note that all the fractures extend posteriorly through the pterygoid plates *(arrow)*. *(Modified with permission from Converse JM, ed.* Reconstructive Plastic Surgery: Principles and Procedures in Correction, Reconstruction, and Transplantation. *2nd ed. Philadelphia: Saunders; 1977:2.)*

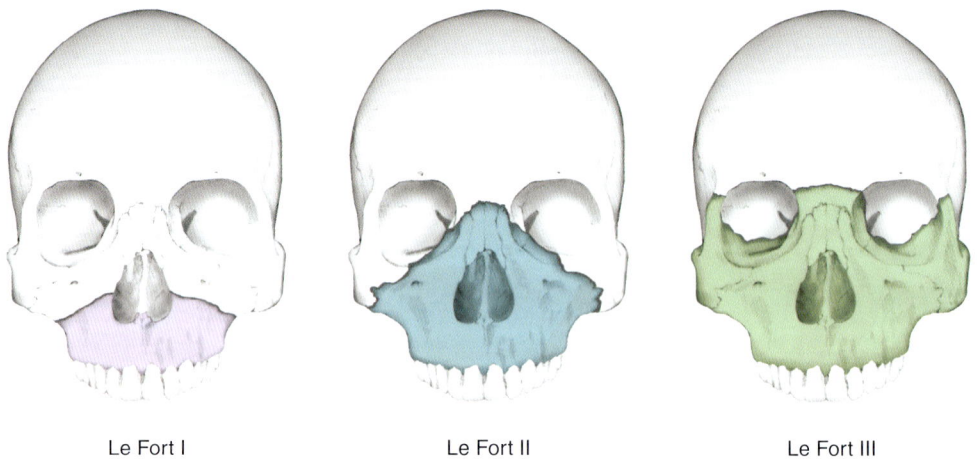

Le Fort I   Le Fort II   Le Fort III

Figure 6-2 Le Fort classification of midfacial fractures. Le Fort I, horizontal fracture of the maxilla, also known as Guérin fracture. Le Fort II, pyramidal fracture of the maxilla. Le Fort III, craniofacial disjunction. *(Modified with permission from Converse JM, ed.* Reconstructive Plastic Surgery: Principles and Procedures in Correction, Reconstruction, and Transplantation. *2nd ed. Philadelphia: Saunders; 1977:2. Illustration by Cyndie C. H. Wooley.)*

Orbital Fractures

Zygomatic Fractures

Zygomaticomaxillary complex (ZMC) fractures (Fig 6-3) are also referred to as *quadripod fractures* because the zygoma is usually fractured at 4 of its articulations with the adjacent bones: (1) frontozygomatic suture, (2) inferior orbital rim, (3) zygomatic arch, and (4) lateral wall

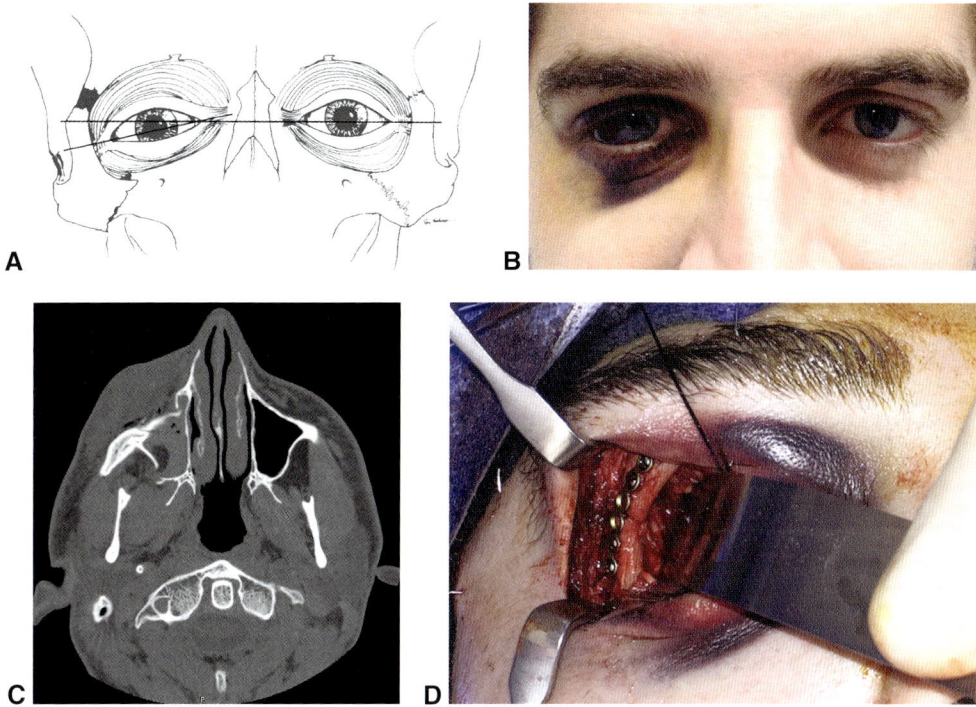

Figure 6-3 Zygomaticomaxillary complex (ZMC) fracture. **A,** ZMC, anterior view. Downward displacement of the globe and lateral canthus result from frontozygomatic separation and downward displacement of the zygoma and the floor of the orbit. **B,** Globe ptosis and lateral canthal dystopia result from depressed ZMC fracture. **C,** Axial computed tomography (CT) scan shows depression of malar prominence and telescoping of bone fragment into the maxillary sinus. **D,** Intraoperative view shows rigid plate fixation of supralateral orbital rim fracture that was performed in addition to fixation of the inferior rim and lateral maxillary buttress. *(Part A modified with permission from Converse JM, ed.* Reconstructive Plastic Surgery: Principles and Procedures in Correction, Reconstruction, and Transplantation. *2nd ed. Philadelphia: Saunders; 1977:2. Parts B–D courtesy of M. Reza Vagefi, MD.)*

of the maxillary sinus. ZMC fractures involve the orbital floor to varying degrees. If the zygoma is not significantly displaced, treatment may not be necessary. ZMC fractures can cause globe displacement, lateral canthal dystopia, cosmetic deformity, diplopia, and trismus (limitation of mandibular opening) due to fracture impingement on the coronoid process of the mandible.

When treatment is indicated, the best results are obtained with open reduction of the fracture and rigid plate fixation (see Fig 6-3D). Exact realignment and stabilization of the lateral maxillary buttress and the lateral orbital wall are essential for accurate fracture reduction and can be achieved through a combination of eyelid and buccal sulcus incisions. If the lateral maxillary buttress is only mildly displaced, complete reduction and fixation can be accomplished through an eyelid incision.

Orbital Apex Fractures

Orbital apex fractures usually occur in association with other fractures of the face, orbit, or skull and may involve the optic canal, superior orbital fissure, and structures that pass through them. Possible associated complications include traumatic optic neuropathy; cerebrospinal fluid leak; and carotid-cavernous fistula. Orbital computed tomography (CT) may demonstrate evidence of direct optic nerve injury with a fracture at or adjacent to the optic canal.

Orbital Roof Fractures

Orbital roof fractures are usually caused by blunt trauma or missile injuries. They are more common in young children, in whom the frontal sinus has yet to pneumatize. Because the ratio of the cranial vault to the midface is greater in children than in adults, frontal impact is more likely to occur with a fall. By contrast, frontal trauma in older individuals is partially absorbed by the frontal sinus, which diffuses the force and prevents extension of the fracture along the orbital roof. Complications of orbital roof fractures include intracranial injuries, cerebrospinal fluid rhinorrhea, pneumocephalus, pulsatile proptosis, subperiosteal hematoma, ptosis, and extraocular muscle imbalance. In roof fractures, the entrapment of extraocular muscles is rare, with most early diplopia resulting from hematoma, edema, or contusion of the orbital structures. In severely comminuted fractures, pulsating exophthalmos may occur as a delayed complication. Young children may develop nondisplaced linear roof fractures after fairly minor trauma, which may present with delayed ecchymosis of the upper eyelid. Most roof fractures do not require repair. Indications for surgery are generally neurosurgical, and treatment often involves a multidisciplinary team.

> Hink EM, Wei LA, Durairaj VD. Clinical features and treatment of pediatric orbit fractures. *Ophthalmic Plast Reconstr Surg.* 2014;30(2):124–131.

Medial Orbital Fractures

Naso-orbital-ethmoidal (NOE) fractures (Fig 6-4) usually result from the face striking a solid surface. These fractures commonly involve the frontal process of the maxilla, the lacrimal bone, and the ethmoid bones along the medial wall of the orbit. Patients characteristically have a depressed bridge of the nose and traumatic telecanthus. These fractures may be divided into 3 categories:

- Type I involve a central fragment of bone attached to canthal tendon.
- Type II are comminuted fractures of the central fragment.
- Type III involve a comminuted tendon attachment or an avulsed tendon.

Complications associated with NOE fractures include cerebral and ocular damage, severe epistaxis due to avulsion of the anterior ethmoidal artery, orbital hematoma, cerebrospinal fluid rhinorrhea, damage to the lacrimal drainage system, lateral displacement of the medial canthus, and associated fractures of the medial orbital wall and floor. Treatment is dependent on the type of fracture; it generally includes fracture reduction and microplate fixation. Transnasal wiring of the medial canthus is used less frequently, because microplates often allow precise bony reduction.

Indirect (blowout) fractures of the medial wall are frequently extensions of blowout fractures of the orbital floor. Isolated blowout fractures of the medial orbital wall may also occur. Surgical intervention is indicated in cases involving muscle and associated tissue

Type I

Type II

Type III

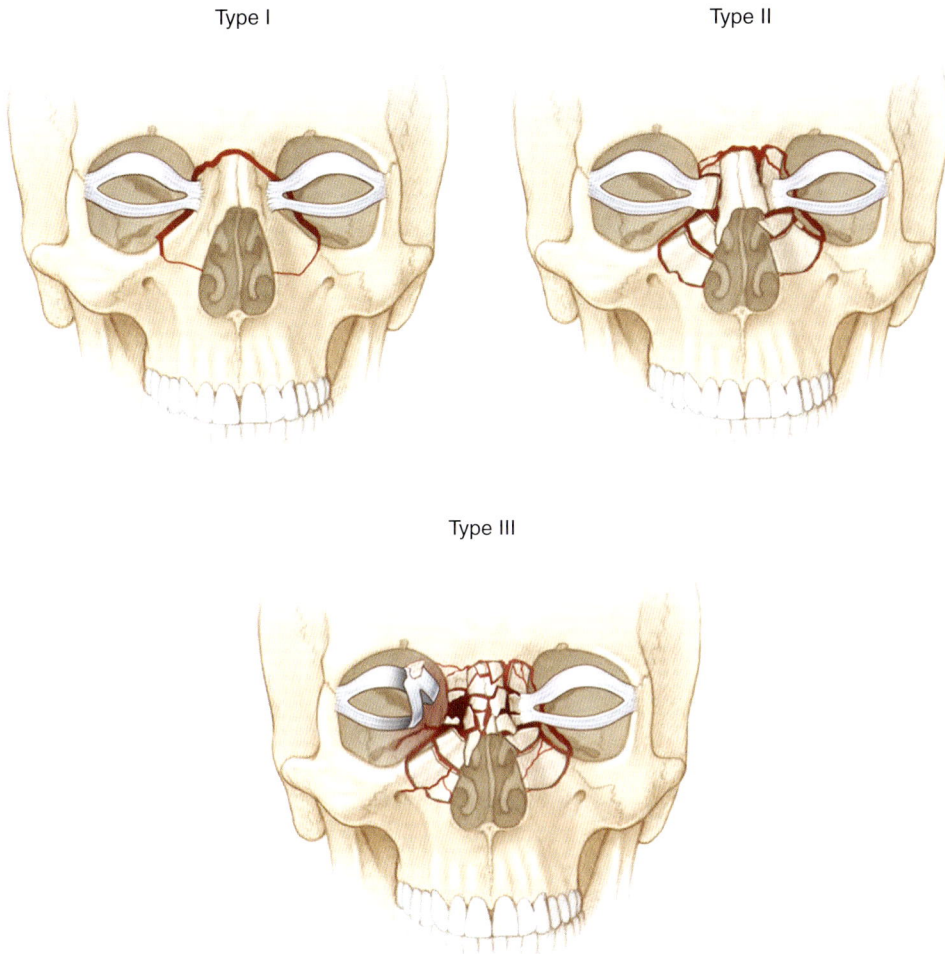

Figure 6-4 Naso-orbital-ethmoidal fractures result in traumatic telecanthus with rounding of the medial canthus. Types I–III are described according to the severity of the injury. *(Illustration by Christine Gralapp.)*

entrapment, persistent restrictive diplopia, and aesthetically unacceptable enophthalmos. Some surgeons choose to intervene on the basis of fracture size and believe the risk of enophthalmos is greatest when both the floor and the medial wall are fractured. However, determining the size of the fracture from imaging studies can be difficult. If surgery is required, the medial orbital wall can be approached by continuing the exploration of the floor superiorly along the medial wall via a lower eyelid or transconjunctival approach. An alternative approach is a medial orbitotomy through a retrocaruncular approach or, less commonly, a frontoethmoidal skin incision. See Chapter 7 in this volume for discussion of orbital surgery approaches.

Vicinanzo MG, McGwin G Jr, Allamneni C, Long JA. Interreader variability of computed tomography for orbital floor fracture. *JAMA Ophthalmol.* 2015;133(12):1393–1397.

Orbital Floor Fractures

Direct fractures of the orbital floor can extend from fractures of the inferior orbital rim, whereas indirect fractures of the orbital floor are not associated with fractures of the rim. Indications for repair of both fracture types are similar.

It is thought that orbital floor fractures are caused by 1 of 2 mechanisms or a combination of the 2. According to the hydraulic mechanism theory, blunt trauma rapidly occludes the orbital aperture, resulting in increased intraorbital pressure. This pressure causes the orbital bones to break or "blow out" at their weakest point along the posterior medial part of the floor, which comprises the maxillary bone. By contrast, according to the buckling mechanism theory, a striking object causes deformation of the inferior rim, resulting in forces that are transmitted and focused on the orbital floor, resulting in a blowout. Regardless of the mechanism, orbital contents may prolapse through the fracture into the maxillary sinus and sometimes become entrapped.

The diagnosis of a blowout fracture of the orbital floor is suggested by the patient's history, physical examination, and orbital imaging studies. There is often a history of the orbital aperture being struck by an object that is larger than its diameter (eg, a ball, an automobile dashboard, or a fist). An orbital blowout fracture should be suspected in any patient who has received a periorbital blow forceful enough to cause ecchymosis. Physical examination typically reveals the following:

- *Eyelid signs.* Ecchymosis and edema of the eyelids may be present, but external signs of injury can be absent *(white-eyed blowout fracture).*
- *Diplopia with limitation of upgaze, downgaze, or both.* Limited vertical movement of the globe on attempted supraduction with vertical diplopia and pain in the inferior orbit can be consistent with entrapment of the inferior rectus muscle or its adjacent septa in the fracture, especially in cases of pediatric orbital trauma. However, orbital edema and/or hemorrhage is a more likely cause of diplopia in the acute posttraumatic period and can take weeks to months to completely resolve. Less commonly, damage to the extraocular muscles or their innervation can result in significant limitation of both horizontal and vertical eye movements. If entrapment is present, a *forced duction test (traction test)* will show restriction of passive movement of the eye. This test can be performed with the instillation of anesthetic eyedrops followed by a cotton pledget of topical anesthetic in the inferior cul-de-sac for several minutes. Using toothed forceps, the examiner engages the insertion of the inferior rectus muscle through the conjunctiva and attempts to rotate the globe gently up and down. This test may be uncomfortable for a conscious patient and may be deferred to the time of surgery, when the patient is under anesthesia. It can help determine appropriate release of incarcerated tissue during surgery. Another characteristic finding of inferior rectus entrapment is an increase in intraocular pressure (IOP) in upgaze in comparison to primary gaze.
- *Enophthalmos and ptosis of the globe.* These findings can occur with large fractures in which the orbital soft tissues prolapse into the maxillary sinus. If associated with the orbital floor fracture, a medial wall fracture may significantly contribute to enophthalmos because of the prolapse of orbital tissues into both the ethmoid and maxillary

sinuses. Enophthalmos may be masked by orbital edema immediately following injury and may become more apparent as edema subsides.

- *Hypoesthesia in the distribution of the infraorbital nerve.*
- *Emphysema of the orbit and eyelids.* Any fracture that extends into a sinus may allow air to escape into the subcutaneous tissues and is commonly associated with fractures of the medial orbital wall. Patients with fractures are advised to avoid nose blowing to prevent orbital emphysema.

In patients with orbital floor fractures, vision loss can result from globe trauma, injury to the optic nerve, or increased orbital pressure causing a *compartment syndrome* (discussed later in this chapter, in the section Orbital Compartment Syndrome). An orbital hemorrhage should be suspected if loss of vision is associated with proptosis and increased IOP. Injuries to the globe and ocular adnexa may also be present.

Management

Orbital CT with coronal, axial, and sagittal views enables evaluation of the fracture size and extraocular muscle relationships, providing information that may help predict enophthalmos and muscle entrapment. However, despite the publication of multiple studies suggesting neuroimaging criteria for extraocular muscle entrapment, restrictive strabismus related to blowout fracture remains a clinical diagnosis.

Most orbital floor fractures do not require surgical intervention. Patients may be observed from weeks to months to allow edema and orbital hemorrhage to subside. Oral steroids (1 mg/kg per day for the first 7 days) decrease edema and may help hasten the decision of whether surgery for diplopia is necessary.

An exception to observation is in pediatric patients (Fig 6-5) in which the inferior rectus muscle is more likely to become tightly ensnared within a trapdoor fracture. In these patients, vertical globe excursion is significantly limited, and CT reveals the inferior rectus muscle within the fracture site along the maxillary sinus. Eye movement may stimulate the oculocardiac reflex (Video 6-1), causing pain, nausea, and bradycardia. Urgent repair should be undertaken in these cases. Immediate release of the entrapped muscle may improve the final ocular motility by limiting fibrosis.

> ▶ **VIDEO 6-1** Orbital fracture associated with oculocardiac reflex.
> *Courtesy of David Kuo, MD and Bobby S. Korn, MD PhD.*
> Access all Section 7 videos at www.aao.org/bcscvideo_section07.

Otherwise, the indications and timing for surgery remain controversial. Presently, there are no prospective, randomized clinical trials to guide decision making, and recommendations are based on noncomparative, retrospective reports or case series. The following 3 criteria are suggested to define when surgery may be indicated:

- *Diplopia with limitation of upgaze and/or downgaze within 30° of the primary position; positive forced duction test; and radiologic confirmation of an orbital floor fracture.* These findings may indicate functional entrapment of tissues affecting the inferior rectus muscle. Diplopia will improve significantly over the course of the first several weeks to months as orbital edema and/or hemorrhage resolve and the entrapped tissues stretch. If the findings are still present after 2 weeks, some surgeons prefer

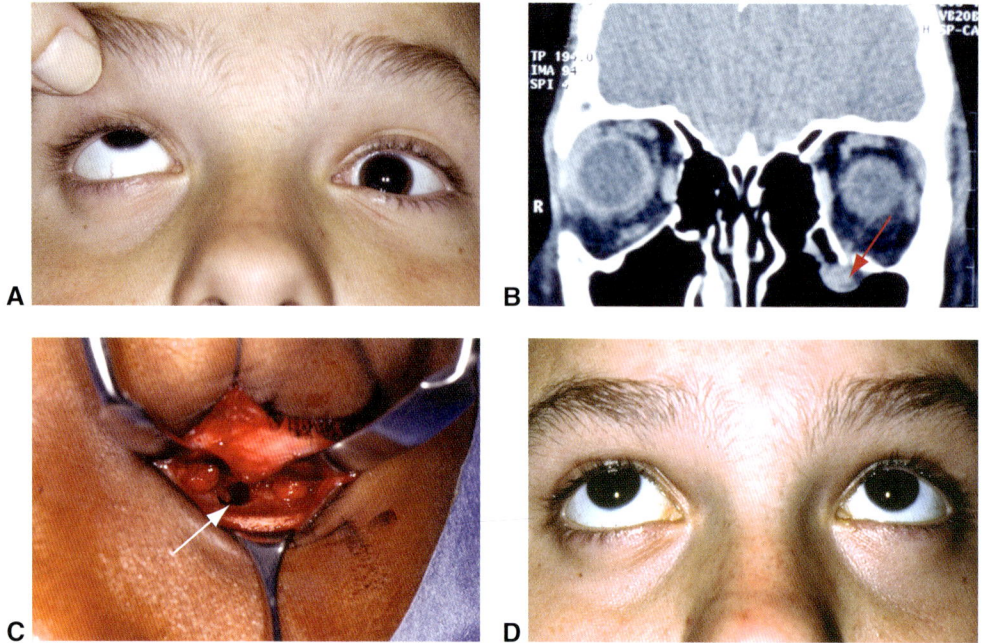

Figure 6-5 Orbital floor fracture. **A,** Teenaged patient following blunt trauma to the eye and orbit. With attempted gaze up, there is limited supraduction of the left eye. Note the lack of ecchymosis of the left side (white-eyed blowout fracture). **B,** Coronal CT scan of the orbit shows a small orbital floor fracture and inferior rectus muscle prolapsing into the maxillary sinus *(arrow)*. **C,** Intraoperative view of a similar case shows an orbital floor defect *(arrow)* enlarged surgically to release and extract inferior rectus muscle. **D,** In a photo taken 2 months postoperatively, the patient demonstrates resolution of upgaze limitation. *(Courtesy of John B. Holds, MD.)*

to repair the fracture whereas others prefer to continue observing until findings are no longer improving. As mentioned earlier, tight entrapment of the inferior rectus muscle with possible muscle ischemia is an indication for immediate repair.

- *Enophthalmos that exceeds 2 mm and is cosmetically unacceptable to the patient.* Enophthalmos can be masked by orbital edema immediately after the injury and may delay recognition of the enophthalmos for weeks to months. Exophthalmometry measurements are taken at the initial evaluation and at subsequent visits to monitor for enophthalmos. Some surgeons believe that when significant enophthalmos is present within the first 2 weeks of a large orbital floor fracture, greater enophthalmos may ensue, and thus intervention is indicated. Others believe that late enophthalmos is rare, even in the case of large fractures, and thus longer observation is appropriate, with the patient ultimately deciding whether the degree of enophthalmos is aesthetically unacceptable.

- *Large fractures involving at least half of the orbital floor, particularly when associated with large medial wall fractures as determined by CT.* Orbital fractures of this size may have a higher incidence of subsequent significant enophthalmos, and early repair may be sought. However, studies have shown that it can be difficult to predict who will proceed to develop significant enophthalmos based on imaging alone.

Burnstine MA. Clinical recommendations for repair of isolated orbital floor fractures: an evidence-based analysis. *Ophthalmology.* 2002;109(7):1207–1210.

Kersten RC, Vagefi MR, Bartley GB. Orbital "blowout" fractures: time for a new paradigm. *Ophthalmology.* 2018;125(6):796–798.

Surgical management of orbital fractures Some surgeons prefer to proceed with the repair within 2 weeks of the initial trauma, believing that scar tissue formation and contracture of the prolapsed tissue make later correction of diplopia and/or enophthalmos difficult. Other surgeons prefer to observe the fracture to allow complete resolution of the orbital edema and/or hemorrhage with a determination of whether residual diplopia and/or aesthetically significant enophthalmos merits repair. Satisfactory correction of diplopia and enophthalmos is obtainable even if surgery is delayed.

The surgical approach to blowout fractures of the orbital floor is ideally performed through an inferior transconjunctival incision either with or without a lateral canthotomy and inferior cantholysis. The approaches through the lower eyelid have the following steps in common: elevation of the periorbita from the orbital floor, release of the prolapsed tissues from the fracture, and, usually, placement of an implant over the fracture to prevent recurrent adhesions and prolapse of the orbital tissues.

Orbital implants can be alloplastic (porous polyethylene, nylon foil, polytetrafluoro-ethylene, silicone sheet, or titanium mesh) or autogenous (split cranial bone, iliac crest bone, or fascia). Alloplastic implants combined with both synthetic and metallic components enable microplating and are an option for the management of large orbital floor and/or combined medial wall fractures. The harvesting of autologous grafts requires an additional operative site, and bone grafts are rarely indicated.

Delayed treatment of blowout fractures to correct persistent restrictive diplopia or cosmetically unacceptable enophthalmos may include exploration of the orbital floor to free prolapsed tissue and reposition it in the orbit. In late surgery for enophthalmos, placement of an implant to reposition the globe anteriorly and/or superiorly may be necessary. Other treatment options include strabismus surgery and procedures to camouflage the narrowed palpebral fissure and deep superior sulcus associated with enophthalmos.

Complications of blowout fracture surgery include decreased vision or blindness, persistent or new diplopia, undercorrection or overcorrection of enophthalmos, retraction of the lower eyelid, hypoesthesia of the infraorbital nerve, infection, early or late extrusion of the implant, lymphedema, delayed orbital hemorrhage around the implant, and damage to the lacrimal drainage system.

Intraorbital Foreign Bodies

Orbital CT is the study of choice to localize an orbital foreign body (Fig 6-6). An inorganic foreign body may be difficult to visualize on CT and is better observed on magnetic resonance imaging (MRI). However, MRI should be avoided if there is a possibility that the foreign object is ferromagnetic. Orbital ultrasonography may be helpful for foreign bodies positioned more anteriorly. Treatment of orbital foreign bodies initially involves culturing the wound (or the foreign body if it is removed) and administering antibiotics. Foreign

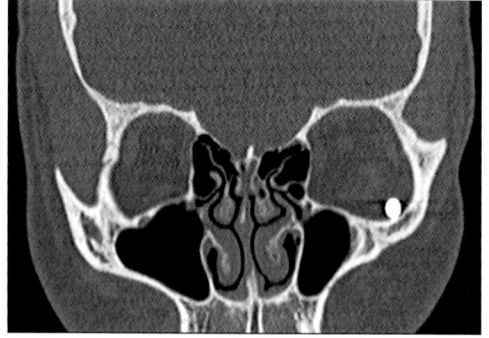

Figure 6-6 Intraorbital foreign body. Coronal CT demonstrates a metallic, extraconal foreign body of the left orbit resting along the zygomatic bone that is consistent with a pellet from a BB gun. This type of foreign body may be observed without surgery. *(Courtesy of M. Reza Vagefi, MD.)*

bodies should be removed if they are composed of vegetable matter or if they are easily accessible in the anterior orbit. If an embedded foreign body causes an orbital infection that drains to the skin surface, it is sometimes possible to locate the object by surgically following the fistulous tract posteriorly. In many cases, objects can be safely observed without surgery if they are inert and have smooth edges or are located in the posterior orbit. Pellets from BB guns are common intraorbital foreign bodies and are usually best left in place. MRI can be safely performed with a BB pellet present in the orbit.

Ho VH, Wilson MW, Fleming JC, Haik BG. Retained intraorbital metallic foreign bodies. *Ophthalmic Plast Reconstr Surg.* 2004;20(3):232–236.

Orbital Compartment Syndrome

Orbital compartment syndrome (OCS) occurs as a result of an acute rise in orbital pressure from hemorrhage (Fig 6-7) or introduction of air into the orbit. It most commonly occurs in association with trauma, surgery, retrobulbar or peribulbar injections, or preexisting orbital disease.

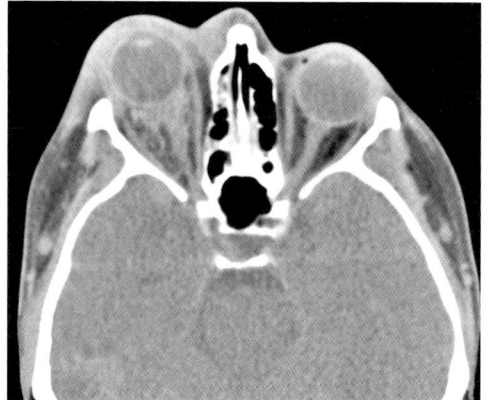

Figure 6-7 Orbital compartment syndrome (OCS). Axial CT image shows OCS on the right side secondary to a retrobulbar hemorrhage in a teenaged patient struck by a softball. Image demonstrates proptosis and the presence of intraconal blood. *(Courtesy of M. Reza Vagefi, MD.)*

Because the orbit has a fixed volume, there is limited room to accommodate any expansion of its contents. As orbital pressure increases, associated vision loss can be attributed to 1 of the 4 following mechanisms:

- central retinal artery occlusion
- direct compressive optic neuropathy
- compression of optic nerve vasculature
- ischemic optic neuropathy that results from stretching of nutrient vessels

Examination of a patient with OCS reveals decreased vision, afferent pupillary defect, and increased IOP. Elevated IOP in cases of OCS reflects the increased orbital pressure and is not indicative of glaucoma. In addition, a tight orbit with decreased extraocular movements and proptosis is often observed. Patients should undergo emergent decompression of the orbit, as described in Figure 6-8. Because vision loss can progress rapidly, this procedure should not be delayed for orbital imaging. If OCS is present in a patient with antecedent eyelid or orbital surgery, the wound should be opened and the hematoma evacuated, followed by exploration and cautery of active bleeding. Otherwise, decompression is most easily achieved by lateral canthotomy and cantholysis, in which the eyelids are disinserted from the lateral orbital rim, allowing the orbital volume to expand anteriorly. Lateral canthotomy alone does not sufficiently decrease orbital pressure; inferior cantholysis and sometimes superior cantholysis are also required. Careful monitoring and reassessment of the ophthalmic examination are necessary to determine whether further surgical intervention is needed.

Lima V, Burt B, Leibovitch I, Prabhakaran V, Goldberg RA, Selva D. Orbital compartment syndrome: the ophthalmic surgical emergency. *Surv Ophthalmol.* 2009;54(4):441–449.

Traumatic Vision Loss With Clear Media

Many patients report decreased vision following periocular trauma. It is imperative that a complete ophthalmic examination be performed to rule out direct globe injury or OCS. Reduction in visual acuity may be due to associated injuries of the cornea, lens, vitreous, retina, or orbit. In addition, eyelid edema may impede opening of the eyes to sufficiently clear the visual axis. However, a small percentage of patients have true vision loss without any evidence of globe injury. Vision loss in these cases suggests traumatic dysfunction of the optic nerve, also known as *traumatic optic neuropathy.* Such vision loss results from 1 of the 2 following mechanisms:

- direct injury to the optic nerve from a penetrating wound, bone fragment, or nerve avulsion
- indirect injury caused by force from a frontal blow transmitted to the intracanalicular portion of the optic nerve

The presence of an afferent pupillary defect in patients with an intact globe strongly suggests traumatic optic neuropathy. However, detection of an afferent defect may be difficult if the patient has received narcotics that cause pupillary constriction or if the traumatic optic nerve injury is bilateral and symmetric.

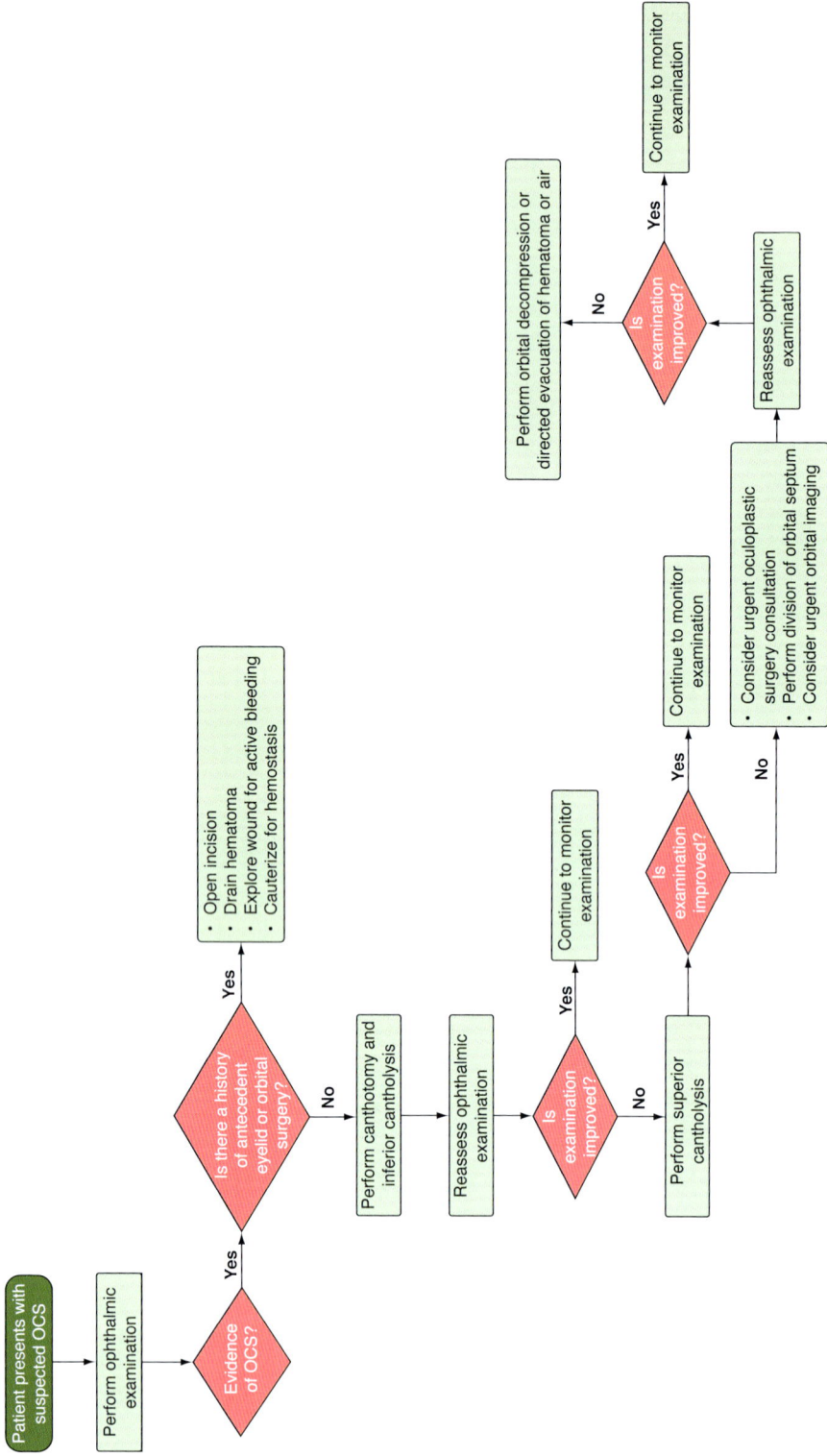

Figure 6-8 Orbital compartment syndrome treatment algorithm. The OCS treatment algorithm should be invoked in patients with decreased vision, afferent pupillary defect, and increased intraocular pressure in association with trauma, surgery, retrobulbar or peribulbar injections, or preexisting orbital disease. *(Courtesy of M. Reza Vagefi, MD.)*

The details of the injury and orbital imaging can help differentiate direct optic nerve injury from indirect. A penetrating wound likely indicates direct injury. History of blunt trauma to the frontal region or rapid deceleration of the cranium, often in patients who have experienced loss of consciousness, is suggestive of indirect injury. CT imaging of the orbits can demonstrate disruption of the optic nerve or fracture involving the orbital apex and/or optic canal in cases of direct injury but is often unremarkable in patients with indirect injury (Fig 6-9).

The proper management of neurogenic vision loss after blunt head trauma is controversial. Observation alone, high-dose corticosteroids, and surgical decompression of the optic canal have been considered as treatment options for indirect traumatic optic neuropathy. However, recent studies have shown that high-dose corticosteroid therapy may not provide any additional vision benefit over observation alone, and such treatment is contraindicated in patients with concomitant traumatic brain injury. In addition, other studies have shown that decompression of the optic nerve provides no additional benefit over observation alone while subjecting patients to the risks associated with surgery. The optimal management of indirect traumatic optic neuropathy remains unresolved. Future research focused on neuroprotection and regeneration is needed.

Ultimately, vision loss after trauma can have serious consequences relating to employment, education, driving, and/or other daily activities. Referral for a comprehensive vision rehabilitation assessment and intervention should be an integral part of the treatment plan for the patient. Significant psychosocial issues may also need to be addressed.

American Academy of Ophthalmology PPP Vision Rehabilitation Committee, Hoskins Center for Quality Eye Care. Preferred Practice Pattern® Guidelines. *Vision Rehabilitation*. San Francisco: American Academy of Ophthalmology; 2017. Available at www.aao.org/ppp.

Steinsapir KD, Goldberg RA. Traumatic optic neuropathy: an evolving understanding. *Am J Ophthalmol*. 2011;151(6):928–933.

Yu-Wai-Man P, Griffiths PG. Steroids for traumatic optic neuropathy. *Cochrane Database Syst Rev*. 2013;6:CD006032.

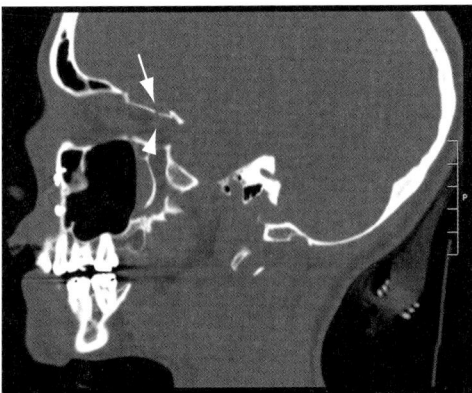

Figure 6-9 Direct traumatic optic neuropathy. A middle-aged woman presents with vision loss of the right eye after sustaining head trauma from a bicycle fall. Globe examination is normal; however, a sagittal CT image demonstrates a direct traumatic optic neuropathy with an inferiorly displaced roof fracture *(arrow)* compressing the optic nerve *(arrowhead)*. *(Courtesy of M. Reza Vagefi, MD.)*

Mass Casualty Incidents

A mass casualty incident (MCI) is defined as an event in which the need for emergency care exceeds the available medical resources, including personnel and equipment. With the rise of global and domestic terrorism, MCIs have unfortunately become more commonplace. Unless physicians have had prior experience treating battlefield injuries, they have undergone little training in the management of wounds arising from an MCI. An understanding of the mechanisms of injury, appropriate triage, and primary goals of initial surgery is needed to properly treat an MCI. These incidents often involve high-velocity weapons (eg, improvised explosive devices and assault rifles) that cause a pattern of injury different from the wounds resulting from low-velocity weapons that a trauma center would typically see. In addition, hospitals are seldom prepared for the large number of injured patients seeking treatment after an MCI occurs.

Lessons learned from physicians who have worked in combat zones have greatly improved the understanding of these types of injuries and enabled the application of these management principles in the civilian sector. On the battlefield, medics triage injured soldiers into 4 categories of urgency. The injured are stabilized accordingly and prepared for urgent medical evacuation to a combat-support hospital, where a team of specialists evaluate and surgically stabilize them. Once patients are hemodynamically stable, ophthalmic evaluation and primary surgical repair can be performed within hours of the injury. In the combat operations Iraqi Freedom and Enduring Freedom, ocular injuries were the fourth most common injury observed. Of the soldiers sustaining ocular trauma, 85% had other systemic injuries.

In the management of an MCI, similar principles of triage and identification of immediate life-threatening injuries, with a focus on airways, breathing, and circulation, are required. Following the 2013 Boston Marathon bombing, 62% of the casualties were transported to level I trauma centers, and 13.4% of those patients required ophthalmology consultation. These combat-medic principles allow physicians to provide the greatest benefit to the highest number of patients.

Majors JS, Brennan J, Holt GR. Management of high-velocity injuries of the head and neck. *Facial Plast Surg Clin North Am.* 2017;25(4):493–502.

Weichel ED, Colyer MH. Combat ocular trauma and systemic injury. *Curr Opin Ophthalmol.* 2008;19(6):519–525.

Yonekawa Y, Hacker HD, Lehman RE, et al. Ocular blast injuries in mass-casualty incidents: the marathon bombing in Boston, Massachusetts, and the fertilizer plant explosion in West, Texas. *Ophthalmology.* 2014;121(9):1670–1676.e1.

CHAPTER 7

Orbital Surgery

Highlights

- The orbit is divided into 5 surgical spaces: subperiosteal, extraconal, sub-Tenon, subarachnoid, and intraconal.
- The type of surgical approach to the orbit is based on the location of the pathology. A good understanding of orbital anatomy enables an appropriate surgical plan that minimizes morbidity.
- Orbital decompression surgery is performed in cases of thyroid eye disease to address compressive optic neuropathy, disfiguring proptosis, or corneal exposure.

Surgical Spaces

There are 5 surgical spaces within the orbit (Fig 7-1):

- the *subperiosteal surgical space,* which is the potential space between the bone and the periorbita (periosteum of the orbit)
- the *extraconal surgical space*, which lies between the periorbita and the muscle cone

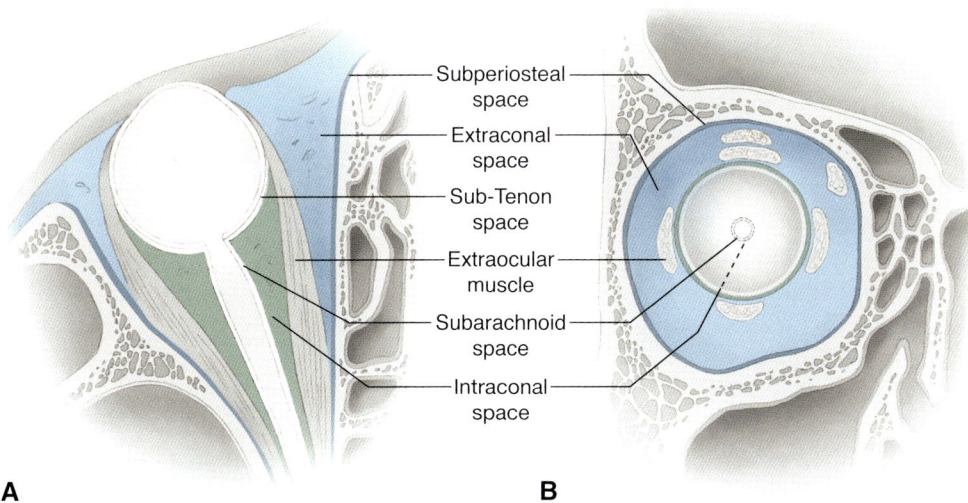

Figure 7-1   Surgical spaces of the orbit. **A,** Axial view. **B,** Coronal view. *(Illustration by Cyndie C. H. Wooley.)*

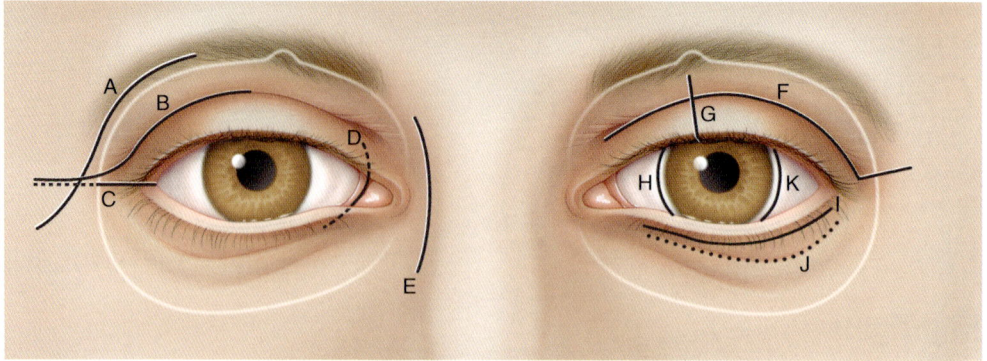

Figure 7-2 Sites of surgical entry into the orbit. *A,* Curvilinear lateral orbitotomy. *B,* Eyelid crease lateral orbitotomy. *C,* Lateral canthotomy/cantholysis orbitotomy. *D,* Retrocaruncular medial orbitotomy. *E,* Frontoethmoidal medial orbitotomy. *F,* Upper eyelid crease anterior orbitotomy. *G,* Vertical eyelid split superomedial orbitotomy. *H,* Medial bulbar conjunctival orbitotomy. *I,* Subciliary inferior orbitotomy. *J,* Transconjunctival inferior orbitotomy. *K,* Lateral bulbar conjunctival orbitotomy. *(Illustration by Christine Gralapp, after a drawing by Jennifer Clemens.)*

- the *sub-Tenon surgical space,* which lies between the Tenon capsule and the globe
- the *subarachnoid surgical space,* which lies between the optic nerve and the nerve sheath
- the *intraconal surgical space,* which lies within the muscle cone

A single orbital lesion may involve more than 1 surgical space, and a combination of approaches may be necessary for pathologic processes affecting the orbit. An operating microscope is sometimes used, particularly for dissection inside the muscle cone. The approaches to these spaces—superior, inferior, medial, and lateral—are discussed in the following sections. Incisions used to reach these surgical spaces are shown in Figure 7-2.

Orbitotomy

Superior Approach

More orbital lesions are found in the superoanterior part of the orbit than in any other location. Lesions in this area can usually be accessed through a transcutaneous incision. When this approach is used, care must be taken to avoid damaging the levator muscle, superior oblique muscle, trochlea, lacrimal gland, and sensory nerves and vessels entering or exiting the orbit along the superior orbital rim.

Transcutaneous incisions

A well-hidden incision in the upper eyelid crease provides access to the superior orbital space (Fig 7-3) and offers better cosmesis than an incision placed directly over the superior orbital rim. Both the subperiosteal space and the extraconal space may be approached through this incision. To reach the subperiosteal space, dissection is performed superiorly toward the orbital rim in a plane between the orbicularis oculi muscle and the orbital septum. An

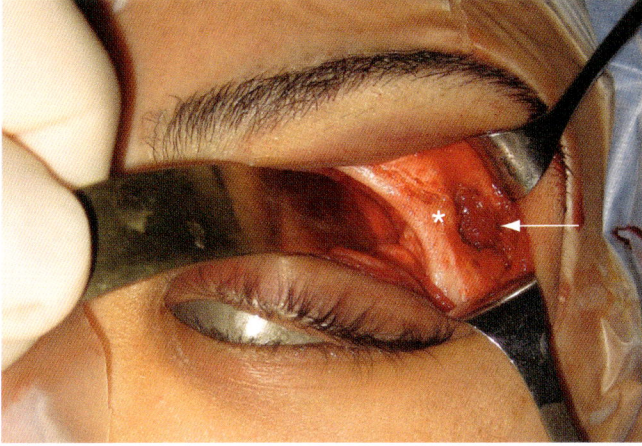

Figure 7-3 Transcutaneous upper eyelid incision for superior and lateral approach. The upper eyelid crease incision allows access to the superior and lateral orbit and anterior temporalis fossa, as demonstrated in this surgical excision of a dumbbell dermoid involving the lateral orbital wall *(asterisk)* and anterior temporal fossa *(arrow)* on the left side. *(Courtesy of Morris E. Hartstein, MD.)*

incision is then made at the arcus marginalis where the periosteum of the frontal bone reflects to become the orbital septum, thus entering the subperiosteal space. To access the superior extraconal space, the dissection is instead carried posteriorly through the orbital septum after the skin incision.

The upper eyelid crease incision may also be used for entry into the medial intraconal space. After opening the orbital septum, the surgeon identifies the medial edge of the levator muscle. Dissection is kept medial to this landmark and proceeds between the medial and central fat pads through the intermuscular septum that extends from the superior rectus muscle to the medial rectus muscle. This approach may be used for biopsy of the optic nerve, for optic nerve sheath fenestration in cases of idiopathic intracranial hypertension, or for accessing intraconal lesions medial to the optic nerve.

The coronal approach to the superior orbit is most often used for trauma or craniofacial surgery. This approach is also used for transcranial orbitotomies to provide better access to apical-based tumors, orbital tumors with intracranial extension, and skull-based tumors with orbital involvement.

Transconjunctival incisions

Incisions in the superior conjunctiva can be used to reach the superomedial, sub-Tenon, intraconal, or extraconal surgical spaces. Dissection must be performed medial to the levator muscle to prevent postoperative blepharoptosis. Care should also be taken in the superolateral fornix to avoid damage to the lacrimal ductules.

Vertical eyelid splitting

Vertical splitting of the upper eyelid via a full thickness incision allows an extended transconjunctival exposure for the removal of superomedial intraconal tumors. Careful realignment of the tarsal plate and levator aponeurosis prevents postoperative blepharoptosis, eyelid notching, and eyelid retraction.

Inferior Approach

The inferior approach is useful for accessing masses that are visible or palpable in the inferior conjunctival fornix of the lower eyelid, as well as for deeper inferior extraconal or intraconal orbital masses. This approach is also commonly used to approach the orbital floor for fracture repair or decompression.

Transcutaneous incisions

Visible scarring can be minimized by use of a subciliary blepharoplasty incision in the lower eyelid skin (Fig 7-4). The orbital septum is exposed through the preseptal orbicularis oculi muscle toward the inferior orbital rim. A cutaneous incision in the lower eyelid crease or directly over the inferior orbital rim can provide similar access but may leave a more noticeable scar and result in eyelid retraction. Once the skin–muscle flap is created, the surgeon can open the septum to expose the extraconal surgical space. Alternatively, for access to the inferior subperiosteal space, the periosteum is incised and elevated at the arcus marginalis to expose the orbital floor. Fractures of the orbital floor are reached by the subperiosteal route.

Transconjunctival incisions

For access to tumors and fractures of the inferior and medial orbit, the transconjunctival approach (Fig 7-5) has largely replaced the transcutaneous approach. An incision is made through the inferior conjunctiva and lower eyelid retractors to reach the extraconal surgical space and the orbital floor. This incision is placed either just below the inferior tarsal border or in the conjunctival fornix, and the conjunctiva is placed on superior traction. When using cutting cautery, care should be taken to avoid causing thermal damage to the conjunctiva and tarsus. Caution should also be taken to avoid injuring the inferior oblique muscle, inferior rectus muscle, and infraorbital neurovascular bundle (see Fig 7-5C). The optical cavity can be enlarged via a lateral canthotomy and inferior cantholysis. Dissection is performed in a similar fashion on a preseptal plane inferiorly toward the orbital rim. The extraconal space can be accessed by incising the orbital septum, and the subperiosteal space can be accessed by incising at the arcus marginalis and elevating the periosteum. Further dissection between the inferior rectus and lateral rectus muscles enables access to the intraconal space.

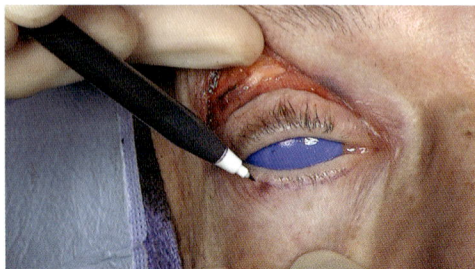

Figure 7-4 Transcutaneous lower eyelid incision for inferior approach. A well-hidden subciliary incision is made beneath the eyelashes and allows access to the inferior orbit. *(Courtesy of Bobby S. Korn, MD, PhD.)*

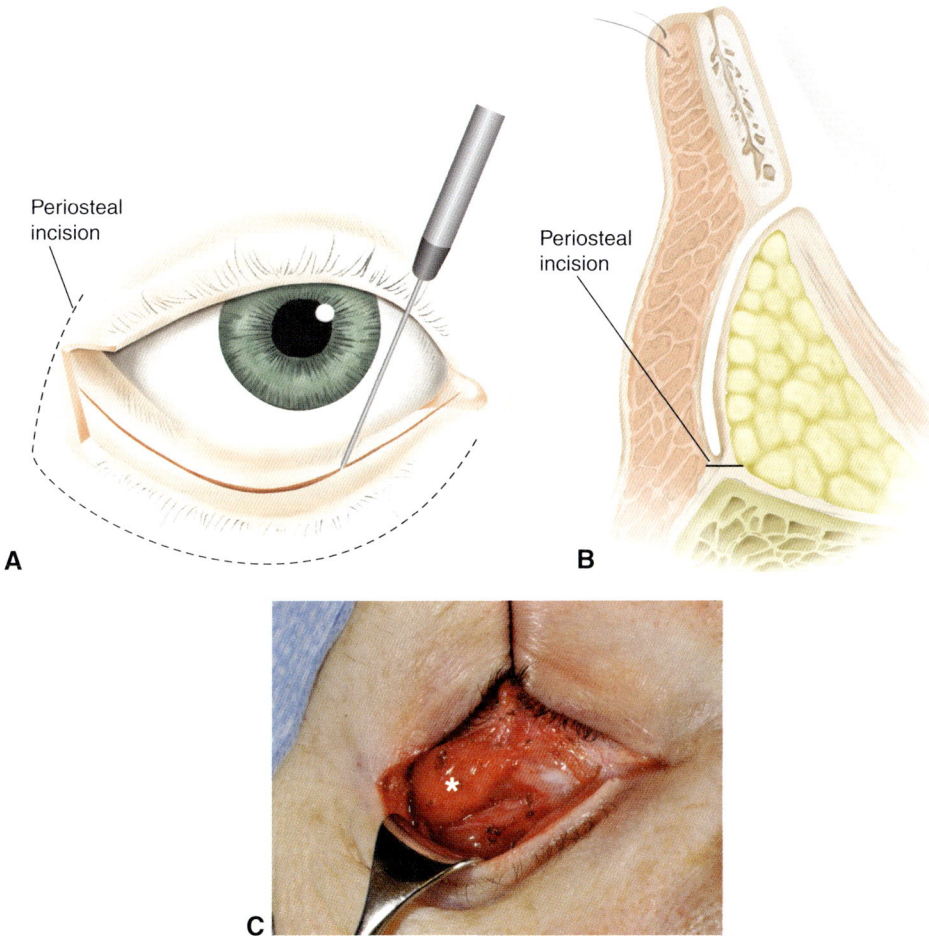

Figure 7-5 Transconjunctival approach to the inferior orbit. **A,** Conjunctival incision with or without canthotomy/cantholysis. **B,** Plane of dissection anterior to orbital septum. **C,** The conjunctiva is placed on superior traction and the orbital septum is opened to biopsy an inferior extraconal mass *(asterisk).* *(Parts A and B illustration by Cyndie C. H. Wooley; part C courtesy of M. Reza Vagefi, MD.)*

Alternatively, an incision of the bulbar conjunctiva and Tenon capsule allows entry to the sub-Tenon surgical space. This approach is also used to gain access to the intraconal surgical space by retracting or reflecting the inferior rectus muscle from the globe.

Medial Approach

Approach to the medial orbit is used in several circumstances, including repair of medial wall trauma, orbital decompression, and access to lacrimal sac or sino-nasal tumors with orbital involvement. When dissecting in the medial orbit, care should be taken to avoid damaging the medial canthal tendon, lacrimal canaliculi and sac, trochlea, superior oblique tendon and muscle, inferior oblique muscle, and the sensory nerves and vessels along the medial aspect of the superior orbital rim.

Transcutaneous incision

Tumors within or near the lacrimal sac or the frontal or ethmoid sinuses can be approached through a frontoethmoidal skin incision placed vertically just medial to the insertion of the medial canthal tendon. This route is generally used to enter the subperiosteal space by reflecting the medial canthal tendon in conjunction with the periosteum, thus preserving the lacrimal drainage apparatus.

Transconjunctival incision

An incision in the bulbar conjunctiva allows entry into the extraconal or sub-Tenon surgical space. If the medial rectus muscle is detached, the intraconal surgical space can be entered in the region of the anterior optic nerve for exploration or biopsy. If the posterior optic nerve or muscle cone needs to be accessed, a combined lateral/medial orbitotomy can be performed. A lateral orbitotomy with removal of the lateral orbital wall allows the globe to be displaced temporally, maximizing medial exposure to the deeper orbit.

Retrocaruncular incision

This incision may be used for repair of medial wall fractures, for medial orbital bone decompression, and for drainage of medial subperiosteal abscesses. An incision posterior to the caruncle allows excellent exposure of the medial orbit (Fig 7-6). Blunt dissection is carried medially, followed by incision and elevation of the periosteum to gain access to the subperiosteal space. In addition, by combining the retrocaruncular incision with an inferior transconjunctival incision, panoramic exposure of the inferior and medial orbit is possible. The inferior oblique muscle may be divided at its origin along the inferomedial orbit rim and reattached at the end of surgery (Fig 7-7). This approach also provides better cosmesis than the traditional frontoethmoidal incision. However, to protect the canaliculi, care must be taken to remain posterior to the lacrimal drainage apparatus during dissection.

Lateral Approach

A lateral approach to the orbit is used when a lesion is located within the lateral intraconal space, behind the equator of the globe, or in the fossa of the lacrimal gland. In addition, because the orbit is relatively shallower in children than in adults, extensive exposure may be achieved in pediatric patients without the need for bone removal.

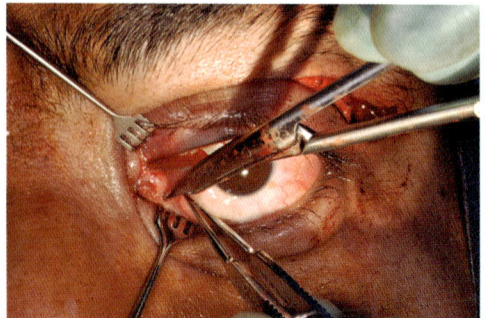

Figure 7-6 Retrocaruncular approach to the medial orbit. The retrocaruncular approach allows access to the medial orbit for surgeries such as orbital decompression, repair of orbital trauma, and orbital abscess drainage. *(Courtesy of M. Reza Vagefi, MD.)*

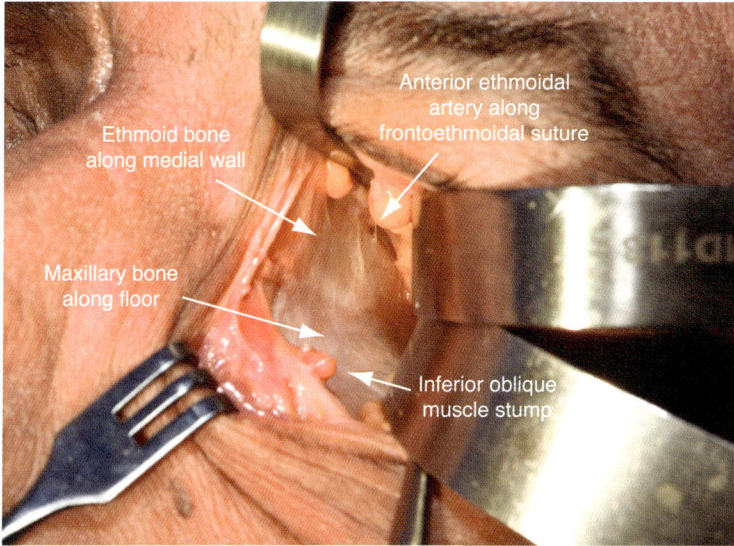

Figure 7-7 Combined retrocaruncular and inferior transconjunctival approach. Combined approach with division of the inferior oblique muscle provides wide exposure to the inferomedial orbit. *(Courtesy of Bobby S. Korn, MD, PhD.)*

The traditional curvilinear incision (see Fig 7-2), which extends from beneath the lateral eyebrow along the zygomatic arch, allows good exposure of the lateral rim but leaves a noticeable scar. It has largely been replaced by approaches through either an upper eyelid crease incision or an extended lateral canthotomy incision. After reflection of the temporalis muscle and the periosteum of the orbit, both approaches allow exposure of the lateral orbital rim and the anterior portion of the zygomatic arch. Dissecting through the periorbita and then the intermuscular septum, either above or below the lateral rectus muscle and posterior to the equator of the globe, provides access to the intraconal retrobulbar space. If a lesion cannot be adequately exposed through a soft tissue lateral incision, an oscillating saw is used to remove the bone of the lateral rim to provide further access (Fig 7-8). This procedure is also known as a marginotomy.

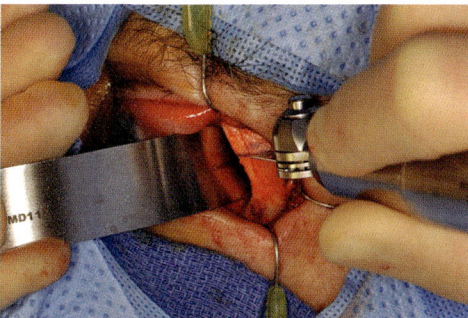

Figure 7-8 Lateral approach to the orbit. A lateral orbitotomy with removal of the lateral rim (marginotomy) provides improved access to the deep lateral orbit and intraconal space. *(Courtesy of M. Reza Vagefi, MD.)*

Complete hemostasis is achieved before closure. To help prevent postoperative intra-orbital hemorrhage, an external drain may be placed in the deep orbit. The lateral orbital rim is usually repositioned and sutured back into place through predrilled tunnels. Alternatively, rigid fixation with a microplating system can be employed.

Orbital Decompression

Orbital decompression is a surgical procedure used to improve the volume-to-space discrepancy that occurs primarily in patients with thyroid eye disease (TED). The goal of orbital decompression is to allow the enlarged muscles and orbital fat to expand into the additional space that is created during the surgery (Fig 7-9). This expansion relieves pressure on the optic nerve and its blood supply; it also reduces proptosis and orbital congestion.

Historically, decompression included removal of the medial orbital wall and much of the orbital floor, including the maxillo-ethmoidal strut, allowing the orbital tissues to expand into the ethmoid and maxillary sinuses. The approach was made through a maxillary vestibular or transcutaneous incision. However, globe ptosis and upper eyelid retraction could be exacerbated postoperatively, especially in patients with large, restricted inferior rectus muscles. This type of decompression could also disrupt globe excursion due to prolapse of the muscles into the sinus space and displacement of the orbital contents.

The approach currently used by many orbital surgeons combines 1 or more discrete incisions that allow access to the lateral, inferior, and/or medial walls. Entry to the lateral and inferior orbit is provided by an upper eyelid crease incision, an extended lateral canthotomy incision, or an inferior transconjunctival incision combined with a lateral canthotomy/inferior cantholysis. Decompression of the lateral wall can be achieved by using rongeurs and/or a drill to remove bone along the sphenoid wing (Fig 7-10). A retro-caruncular incision allows an excellent approach to the medial orbital wall; it can be

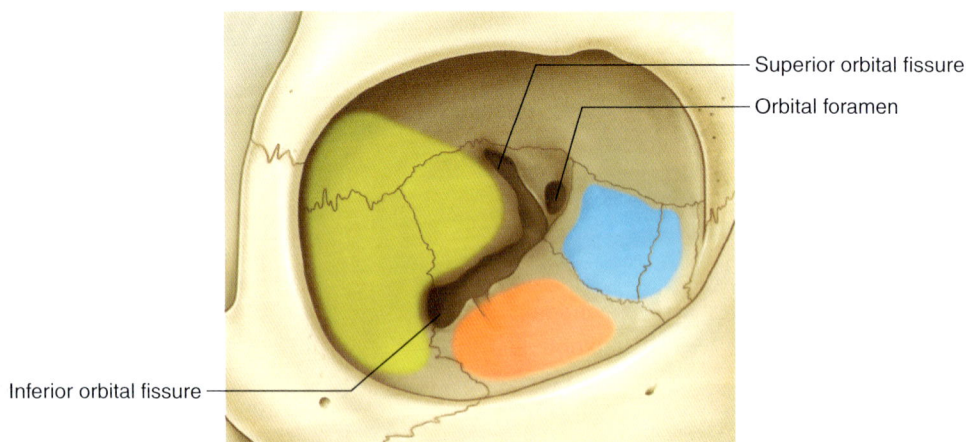

Figure 7-9 Bony anatomy of the right orbit. Potential sites for orbital decompression include the medial wall *(blue)*, lateral wall *(yellow)*, and floor of the orbit *(orange)*. *(Courtesy of Bobby S. Korn, MD, PhD.)*

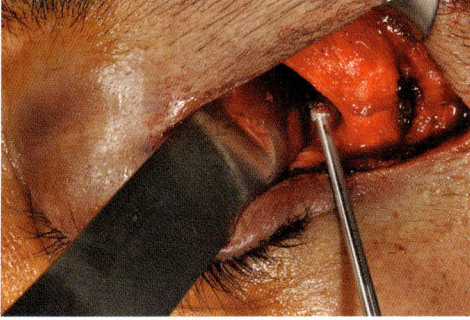

Figure 7-10 Orbital decompression of the lateral wall. A drill is introduced through a left lateral upper eyelid crease incision to remove bone along the greater sphenoid wing during orbital decompression in a patient with thyroid eye disease. *(Courtesy of M. Reza Vagefi, MD.)*

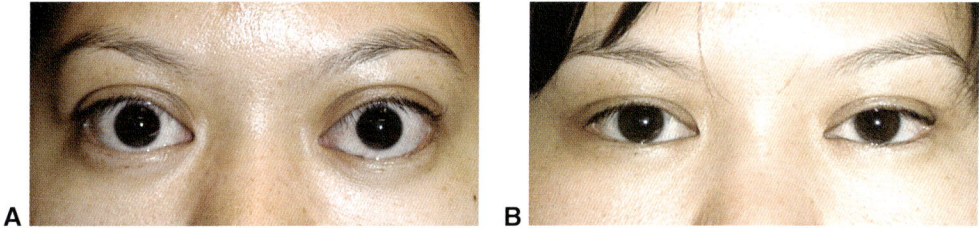

A   **B**

Figure 7-11 Orbital decompression for thyroid eye disease. Before **(A)** and after **(B)** bilateral, "balanced" orbital decompression of the medial and lateral orbital walls. *(Courtesy of Bobby S. Korn, MD, PhD.)*

used in conjunction with a transconjunctival incision for further access. Alternatively, a transnasal endoscopic approach to the medial orbit via the ethmoid sinus may be used to access the medial wall.

Some surgeons choose to decompress the orbit in a "balanced" manner by removing bone from the opposing walls, believing this will reduce the risk of worsened or new onset diplopia (Fig 7-11). For further decompression, occasionally some surgeons will remove the lateral orbital rim and/or reposition it anteriorly at the time of closure. Anterior displacement of the lateral canthus may also aid in the reduction of eyelid retraction.

Fat decompression with removal of retrobulbar fat further reduces proptosis and has also been shown to be beneficial in patients with compressive optic neuropathy. However, decompression through the orbital roof into the anterior cranial fossa is inadvisable.

Rootman DB. Orbital decompression for thyroid eye disease. *Surv Ophthalmol.* 2018;63(1):86–104.

Postoperative Care for Orbital Surgery

Measures used to reduce postoperative edema include elevation of the head, iced compresses on the eyelids, administration of systemic corticosteroids, and optional placement of a drain. Ice packs minimize swelling and allow for observation of the operative site and monitoring of visual acuity. The patient is instructed to promptly contact the surgeon with any change of vision. Prophylactic systemic antibiotics may also be given.

Special Surgical Techniques in the Orbit

Fine-needle aspiration biopsy (FNAB) may have value in selected cases, including lymphoid lesions, secondary tumors invading the orbit from the sinuses, suspected metastatic tumors, and blind eyes with optic nerve tumors (Fig 7-12). This technique is not very effective for obtaining tissue from fibrous inflammatory lesions because of the difficulty in successfully aspirating cells. Although historically FNAB has not been considered effective for biopsy in lymphoproliferative disorders, technological advances have improved its diagnostic yield when used in combination with flow cytometry and monoclonal antibodies or polymerase chain reaction analysis. If necessary, imaging techniques, such as ultrasonography or computed tomography, can be used to help guide the needle into the tumor. Cells (and occasionally a small block of tissue) are aspirated from the lesion. A skilled cytologist is required to study the specimen. See BCSC Section 4, *Ophthalmic Pathology and Intraocular Tumors,* for further discussion of FNAB.

Because of the anatomic relationship of the ethmoid and maxillary sinuses to the medial and inferior orbit, respectively, endoscopic transnasal surgery may be considered. Such an approach may permit biopsy and/or resection of some intraconal pathology. It may also be combined with open orbitotomy to allow improved access to apical processes. In addition, decompression of the orbit or optic canal may be considered for patients with TED or nontraumatic compressive optic neuropathy. Such an approach can also be used for drainage of medial subperiosteal orbital abscesses in patients with sinusitis or for debridement of necrotic tissue in patients with fungal orbital cellulitis.

Tumors and traumatic injuries of the skull base may involve the superior and posterior orbit. Advanced surgical techniques allow access to these areas via a frontal craniotomy or frontotemporal-orbitozygomatic (FTOZ) approach. Such procedures require a multidisciplinary team. The neurosurgeon provides the orbital surgeon with unparalleled access to the deep superior and lateral orbit by removing the frontal bar and the orbital roof. These techniques enable the decompression of the optic canal, as well as resection of tumors such as

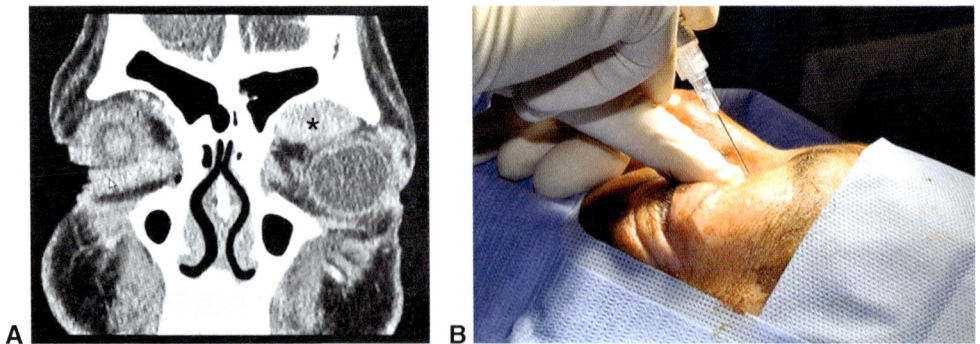

Figure 7-12 Fine-needle aspiration biopsy (FNAB). **A,** Coronal computed tomography image of a left extraconal superomedial orbital mass *(asterisk).* **B,** FNAB is performed to avoid significant blood loss from an open biopsy and reveals metastatic hepatocellular carcinoma. *(Courtesy of M. Reza Vagefi, MD.)*

meningiomas, fibrous dysplasia, cavernous venous malformations, solitary fibrous tumors, schwannomas, and gliomas.

Wiktorin ACH, Dafgård Kopp EME, Tani E, Söderén B, Allen RC. Fine-needle aspiration biopsy in orbital lesions: a retrospective study of 225 cases. *Am J Ophthalmol.* 2016;166:37–42.

Complications of Orbital Surgery

The surgeon can reduce complications from orbital surgery by performing a complete preoperative evaluation with orbital imaging when indicated, choosing the appropriate surgical approach, obtaining adequate exposure, manipulating the tissues carefully, employing proper instrumentation and illumination, maintaining excellent hemostasis, and using a team approach when appropriate.

Decreased or lost vision is a serious complication of surgery that may be caused by excessive traction on the globe and optic nerve, contusion of the optic nerve, postoperative infection, or hemorrhage, which leads to increased orbital pressure and consequent ischemic injury to the optic nerve. A patient who has severe orbital pain postoperatively should be evaluated immediately for possible orbital hemorrhage. If this pain is associated with decreased vision, proptosis, ecchymosis, increased intraocular pressure, and an afferent pupillary defect, the surgeon should consider opening the wound to minimize the effects of orbital compartment syndrome (see Chapter 6 in this volume), evacuating any hematoma, and controlling active bleeding.

In addition to vision loss, possible complications after orbital surgery include:

- blepharoptosis
- cerebrospinal fluid leak
- ciliary ganglion dysfunction with loss of accommodation
- cranial neuropathy resulting in extraocular muscle weakness or palsy
- hypoesthesia in the distribution of the trigeminal nerve (divisions V_1 and V_2)
- infraplacement of the globe after decompression
- keratitis sicca
- motility disturbance resulting in diplopia
- neuroparalytic keratopathy
- orbital cellulitis
- pupillary dysfunction
- retinal detachment
- vitreous hemorrhage

Ting DS, Perez-Lopez M, Chew NJ, Clarke L, Dickinson AJ, Neoh C. A 10-year review of orbital biopsy: the Newcastle Eye Centre Study. *Eye (Lond).* 2015;29(9):1162–1166.

CHAPTER 8

The Anophthalmic Socket

Highlights

- Enucleation is removal of the entire globe and a segment of the optic nerve after releasing the extraocular muscles from sclera.
- Evisceration is removal of the ocular contents, leaving the sclera and extraocular muscles intact.
- Exenteration is removal of the entire globe and either portions or all of the orbital components.
- The goals of anophthalmic socket surgery include maximizing orbital implant volume; achieving optimal eyelid contour, volume, and tone; establishing a socket lining with deep fornices; transmitting motility from the implant to the overlying prosthesis; and achieving comfort and symmetry.
- Orbital implants may be inert or biointegrated.
- Complications of the anophthalmic socket include superior sulcus defect, conjunctival surface changes, implant exposure, fornix/socket contraction, and eyelid malposition.

Introduction

Patients can present with conditions that lead to the removal of an eye or the orbital contents in order to safeguard life, to preserve vision in the fellow eye, or to enhance comfort and cosmesis.

The goals of anophthalmic socket surgery are

- maximizing orbital implant volume with good centration within the orbit
- achieving optimal eyelid contour, volume, and tone
- establishing a socket lining with deep fornices to retain the prosthesis
- transmitting motility from the implant to the overlying prosthesis
- achieving comfort and symmetry

The indications for anophthalmic surgery are diverse, and the procedure of choice varies. *Enucleation* involves removal of the entire globe while preserving remaining orbital tissues. *Evisceration* is the removal of the intraocular contents (lens, uvea, retina, and vitreous), leaving the sclera, extraocular muscles, and optic nerve intact. *Exenteration* refers to the removal of some or all of the orbital tissues, including the globe. The cosmetic goals in anophthalmic surgery are to minimize any condition that draws attention to the anophthalmia. Surgical efforts to produce orbital and eyelid symmetry and to promote good prosthetic position and motility enhance cosmesis.

Congenital anophthalmia (absence of the globe) and microphthalmia (globe diminished in size) and their management are discussed in Chapter 3 in this volume. Management of infants with these disorders differs from management of adults with anophthalmia because of the opportunity for orbital and tissue expansion in infants. However, the principles of socket surgery described in this chapter may also be applied to these children.

Loss of an eye may cause degraded self-image or depression. The ophthalmologist can assist patients both before and after surgery by providing reassurance and psychological support. Discussions of the procedure, the rehabilitation process, and expected functional changes can help patients with adjustment. With very few exceptions, monocular patients may resume the full range of home, vocational, and recreational activities. When resuming full activity, patients should take a cautious approach to allow adjustment to the loss of some depth perception and visual field. This loss may result in occupational limitations. One of the most important roles for the ophthalmologist is to help safeguard the remaining eye through regular follow-up examinations and the prescription of polycarbonate safety glasses for full-time wear.

Brady FB. *A Singular View: The Art of Seeing With One Eye*. 7th ed. Vienna, VA: Michael O. Hughes; 2011.

Enucleation and Evisceration

Enucleation

Enucleation involves first releasing the extraocular muscles from the sclera, then removing the globe. Enucleation allows for complete histologic examination of the eye and optic nerve. It reduces the concern that surgery might contribute to the risk of sympathetic ophthalmia (discussed below) in the fellow eye. Enucleation is the procedure of choice if the nature of the intraocular pathology is unknown or if an ocular tumor is suspected in an eye with no view of the posterior pole.

Enucleation is indicated for primary intraocular malignancies that are not amenable to alternative types of therapy. The ocular tumors most commonly requiring enucleation are retinoblastoma and choroidal melanoma. When enucleation is performed on an eye with an intraocular tumor, the surgeon must take care to avoid penetrating the globe during surgery and to handle the globe gently to minimize the theoretical risk of disseminating tumor cells. In cases of suspected retinoblastoma, removing a long segment of optic nerve with the enucleation specimen increases the chance of complete resection of the tumor. Blind eyes with opaque media should be suspected of harboring an occult neoplasm unless another cause of ocular disease can be surmised. Ultrasonography is useful in evaluating and planning proper management of these eyes.

In severely traumatized eyes, early enucleation may be considered if the risk of sympathetic ophthalmia and harm to the remaining eye is judged to be greater than the likelihood of recovering useful vision in the traumatized eye. Sympathetic ophthalmia is thought to be a delayed hypersensitivity immune response to the uveal antigens. Enucleation with complete removal of the uveal pigment may be beneficial in preventing this subsequent immune response. The yearly incidence of sympathetic ophthalmia is estimated to be 0.03 cases per 100,000. The condition has been reported to occur from 9 days to 50 years after corneoscleral perforation. The infrequency of sympathetic ophthalmia, coupled with improved medical therapy for uveitis, has made early enucleation strictly for prophylaxis a debatable practice. (See BCSC Section 9, *Uveitis and Ocular Inflammation,* for additional information.)

Painful eyes without useful vision can be managed with enucleation or evisceration. Patients with end-stage neovascular glaucoma, chronic uveitis, or previously traumatized blind eyes can obtain dramatic relief from discomfort and improved cosmesis with either procedure. Enucleation can be performed satisfactorily under local or general anesthesia; however, most patients prefer general or monitored anesthesia when an eye is removed. For debilitated patients unable to undergo surgery and rehabilitation, retrobulbar injection of ethanol may provide adequate pain relief. Serious complications associated with retrobulbar injections of ethanol include chronic orbital inflammation, fibrosis, and pain.

For nonpainful, disfigured eyes, it is generally advisable to consider a trial of a cosmetic scleral shell prior to removal of the eye. If tolerated, scleral shells can provide excellent cosmesis and motility.

Tan XL, Seen S, Dutta Majumder P, et al. Analysis of 130 cases of sympathetic ophthalmia—a retrospective multicenter case series. *Ocul Immunol Inflamm.* 2018:1–8.

Enucleation in childhood

Enucleation in early childhood, as well as congenital anophthalmia or microphthalmia, may lead to underdevelopment of the involved bony orbit with secondary facial and eyelid asymmetry. Orbital soft-tissue volume is a critical determinant of orbital bone growth. Thus, for an anophthalmic socket in a young child, the surgeon aims to select an implant that maximally replaces the lost orbital volume but exerts minimal tension on the wound.

In young children, autogenous dermis-fat grafts can be used successfully as primary anophthalmic implants. These grafts have been shown to grow along with the expanding orbit. The opposite effect has been observed in adults, in whom a loss of volume generally occurs when dermis-fat grafts are used as primary anophthalmic implants.

Quaranta-Leoni FM, Sposato S, Raglione P, Mastromarino A. Dermis-fat graft in children as primary and secondary orbital implant. *Ophthalmic Plast Reconstr Surg.* 2016;32(3):214–219.

Evisceration

Evisceration involves the removal of the contents of the globe, leaving the sclera, extraocular muscles, and optic nerve intact. Evisceration should be considered *only* if the presence of an intraocular malignancy has been ruled out.

Advantages of evisceration

The advantages of evisceration include the following:

- *Less disruption of orbital anatomy.* Because there is less dissection within the orbit, there is a lower chance of injury to the extraocular muscles and nerves and a lower chance of fat atrophy. The relationships between the muscles, globe, eyelids, and fornices remain undisturbed.
- *Better motility of the prosthesis.* The extraocular muscles remain attached to the sclera.
- *Treatment of endophthalmitis.* In cases of endophthalmitis, some surgeons prefer evisceration, because the ocular contents can be extirpated and drained without invasion of the orbit. The chance of contamination of the orbit and possible subsequent orbital cellulitis or intracranial extension is therefore theoretically reduced.
- *A technically simpler procedure.* Performing this less invasive procedure may be important when general anesthesia is contraindicated or when bleeding disorders increase the risk of orbital dissection. Because evisceration requires less manipulation of the orbital contents, less anesthetic sedation may be necessary.
- *Lower rate of migration or extrusion of the implant, and subsequent reoperation.*
- *Easier prosthesis fitting by the ocularist.*

Disadvantages of evisceration

The disadvantages of evisceration include the following:

- *Not every patient is a candidate.* Evisceration should never be performed if a malignant ocular tumor is suspected. Severe phthisis bulbi limits the size of the orbital implant that can be placed unless posterior sclerotomies are performed.
- *Theoretical increased risk of sympathetic ophthalmia.* Early reports, however, have not been confirmed.
- *Evisceration affords a less complete specimen for pathologic examinations.*

Intraoperative Complications of Enucleation and Evisceration

Removal of the wrong eye

Removal of the wrong eye is one of the most feared complications in ophthalmology. Taking a "time-out" immediately before enucleation or evisceration to reexamine the patient's medical record, the operative permit, and the patient with ophthalmoscopy in the operating room is of critical importance. Marking the skin near the eye to be enucleated or eviscerated after having the patient and family point to the involved eye gives further assurance.

AAO Wrong-Site Task Force, Hoskins Center for Quality Eye Care. Patient Safety Statements. *Recommendations of American Academy of Ophthalmology Wrong-Site Task Force—2014.* San Francisco: American Academy of Ophthalmology; 2014. www.aao.org/patient-safety-statement/recommendations-of-american-academy-ophthalmology-. Accessed February 20, 2019.

Ptosis and extraocular muscle damage

Avoiding excessive dissection, especially near the orbital roof and apex, reduces the chance of damaging the extraocular muscles, the levator muscle, and/or their innervation.

Orbital Implants

An orbital implant's function is to replace lost orbital volume, maintain the structure of the orbit, and impart motility to the overlying ocular prosthesis. Implants may be grouped according to the materials from which they are manufactured: *inert materials,* such as glass, silicone, or methylmethacrylate; and *biointegrated materials,* such as hydroxyapatite, porous polyethylene, and aluminum oxide (Fig 8-1). Biointegrated materials are designed to be incorporated by soft-tissue ingrowth from the socket.

Inert spherical implants provide comfort, have low extrusion rates, and are considered an appropriate cost-effective choice in patients not requiring implant integration. Disadvantages of nonporous implants include the possibilities of decreased motility and implant migration. Spheres of inert materials may be wrapped in sclera, polyglactin mesh, or autogenous materials (eg, fascia, dermis, or muscle) to provide a substrate for attachment of the extraocular muscles. Inert implants transfer motility to the prosthesis only through passive movement of the socket. Buried motility implants with anterior surface projections push the overlying prosthesis with direct force and can improve prosthetic motility.

Porous implants allow for direct attachment of the extraocular muscles as well as drilling and placement of a peg to integrate the prosthesis directly with the moving implant (see Fig 8-1B). Peg placement is usually carried out 6–12 months after enucleation to allow for complete vascular biointegration. Although pegged porous implants offer excellent motility, they also have a higher rate of postoperative complications, including inflammation and exposure. In fact, most porous implants are never pegged and are still able to achieve adequate motility.

After enucleation, implants are placed either within the Tenon capsule or in the muscle cone behind the posterior Tenon capsule. After evisceration, implants are placed either behind or within the sclera. Spheres may be covered with materials such as sclera (homologous or cadaveric), autogenous fascia, or polygalactin mesh, which serve as further barriers

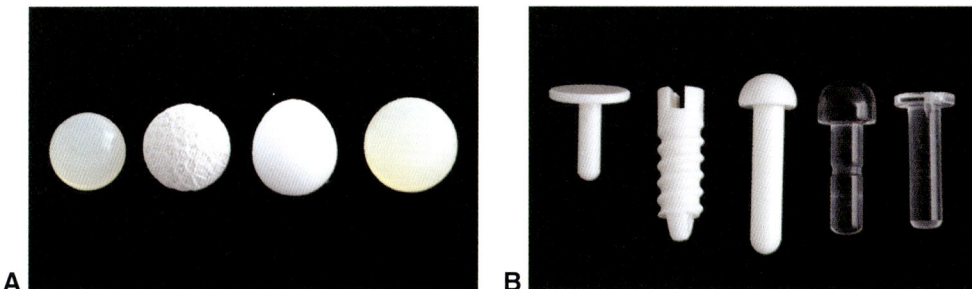

Figure 8-1 Orbital implants. **A,** Examples of various orbital implants *(from left to right)*: silicone, 18 mm; hydroxyapatite, 20 mm; porous polyethylene, 20 mm; silicone, 22 mm. **B,** Various pegs and rescue screws for integrated orbital implants. *(Courtesy of Christine C. Nelson, MD.)*

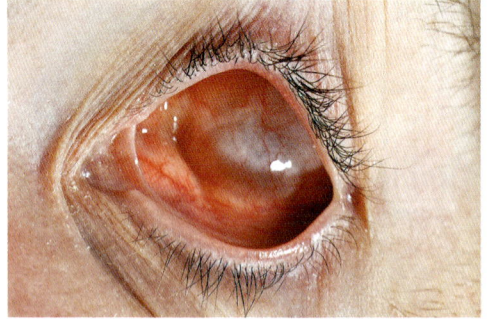

Figure 8-2 Superotemporal migration of an orbital implant secondary to displacement of the extraocular muscles. *(Courtesy of M. Reza Vagefi, MD.)*

to migration and extrusion. Secure closure of Tenon capsule over the anterior surface of an anophthalmic implant is an important barrier to potential later exposure. A dermis-fat graft may be placed instead of an implant or to increase the surface area of the conjunctiva. As the conjunctiva reepithelializes over the dermis, it adds to the socket surface area.

Extraocular muscles should not be crossed over the front surface of a spherical implant or purse-stringed anteriorly because the implant will migrate when the muscles slip off the anterior surface (Fig 8-2). Muscles sutured into the normal anatomical locations, either directly to the implant or to wrapping material (sclera, autogenous fascia, polygalactin mesh) surrounding the implant, allow superior motility and prevent implant migration.

Following enucleation or evisceration surgery, an acrylic or silicone conformer is placed in the conjunctival fornices to maintain the conjunctival space that will eventually accommodate the prosthesis.

Wladis EJ, Aakalu VK, Sobel RK, Yen MT, Bilyk JR, Mawn LA. Orbital implants in enucleation surgery: a report by the American Academy of Ophthalmology. *Ophthalmology*. 2018;125(2):311–317.

Prostheses

An ocular prosthesis is generally fitted 4 weeks after enucleation or evisceration. The ideal prosthesis is custom fitted to the exact dimensions of the patient's conjunctival fornices after postoperative edema has subsided (Fig 8-3). Eviscerations may be more amenable to prosthetic fitting. Premade or stock eyes are less satisfactory cosmetically, and they also limit prosthetic motility. In addition, they may trap secretions between the prosthesis and the socket. Typically, the patient might remove the prosthesis once a month for cleaning.

Figure 8-3 Right anophthalmic socket with an acceptable functional and cosmetic outcome. *(Courtesy of Keith D. Carter, MD.)*

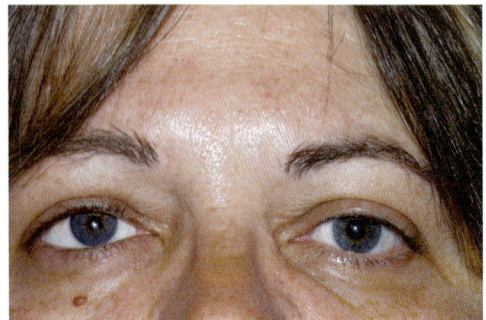

The American Society of Ocularists is an international nonprofit professional and educational organization founded by technicians specializing in the fabrication and fitting of custom ocular prosthetics. Its website includes information for both patients and physicians (www.ocularist.org).

Anophthalmic Socket Complications and Treatment

Deep Superior Sulcus

Deep superior sulcus deformity is caused by insufficient orbital volume (Fig 8-4). The surgeon can correct this deformity by increasing the orbital volume through placement of a subperiosteal secondary implant posteriorly along the orbital floor. This implant pushes the initial implant anteriorly and orbital fat upward to fill out the superior sulcus. Dermis-fat grafts may be implanted in the upper eyelid to fill out the sulcus; however, eyelid contour and function may be damaged, and the graft may undergo resorption. Superior sulcus deformity can also be corrected with replacement of the original implant with a larger secondary implant. Alternatively, modification of the ocular prosthesis may be used to correct a deep superior sulcus.

A related problem occurs when the superior conjunctival fornix is too deep. This leads to retention and buildup of mucus and debris, causing chronic discharge and infection. This condition, which is called *giant fornix syndrome*, is treated with a superior conjunctival resection.

> Farmer LD, Rajak SN, McNab AA, Hardy TG, Selva D. Surgical correction of giant fornix syndrome. *Ophthalmic Plast Reconstr Surg.* 2016;32(2):142–144.

Conjunctival Changes in Anophthalmic Socket

Conjunctival cyst

Conjunctival cysts form secondary to epithelial migration beneath the surface; poor wound closure during enucleation is typically the cause. These cysts may affect prosthetic function; however, treatment is typically not necessary unless the cyst size interferes with comfortable prosthesis wear (Fig 8-5).

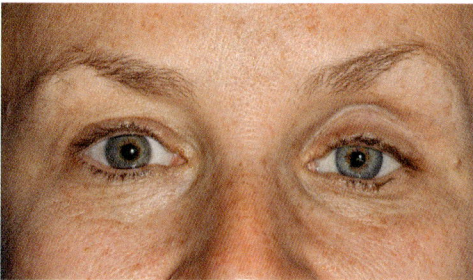

Figure 8-4 Superior sulcus deformity following enucleation of the left eye. *(Courtesy of Bobby S. Korn, MD, PhD.)*

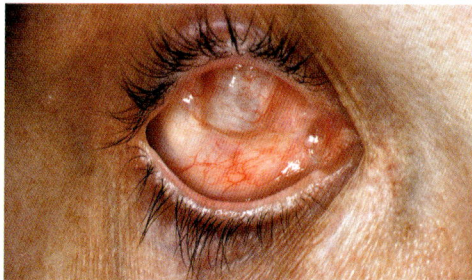

Figure 8-5 Subconjunctival cyst following enucleation of the right eye. *(Courtesy of M. Reza Vagefi, MD.)*

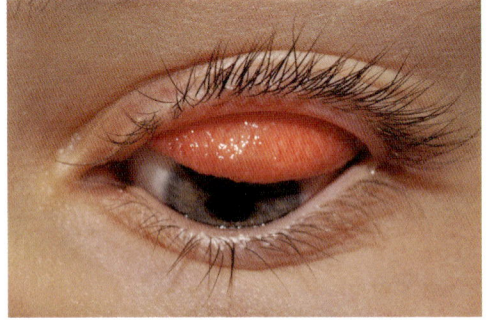

Figure 8-6 Giant papillary conjunctivitis of the left palpebral conjunctiva caused by friction against the prosthetic. *(Courtesy of M. Reza Vagefi, MD.)*

Giant papillary conjunctivitis

Giant papillary conjunctivitis (GPC) commonly develops with prosthesis wear, due to the mechanical friction between the palpebral conjunctival surface and the prosthesis. Everting the upper eyelid will demonstrate the papilla (Fig 8-6). Patients typically present with constant mucus discharge; the discharge has a stringy consistency. Treatment consists of topical corticosteroids and occasionally prosthetic modification.

Exposure and Extrusion of the Implant

Implants may extrude if placed too far forward, if closure of anterior Tenon capsule is not meticulous, or if the irregular surface of the implant mechanically erodes through the conjunctiva (Fig 8-7). Postoperative infection, poor wound healing, poorly fitting prostheses or conformers, pressure points between the implant and prosthesis, and compromised vascularity may also contribute to exposure of the implant. The formation of a pyogenic granuloma is suggestive of an implant exposure (Fig 8-8).

Exposed implants are subject to infection. Although small defects over porous implants may, in rare instances, close spontaneously, most exposures should be covered with scleral patch grafts or autogenous tissue grafts with a sufficient vascular bed to promote conjunctival healing. When implants are deeply seeded with infection, removal of the implant is usually required, followed by an autogenous dermis-fat graft (Fig 8-9).

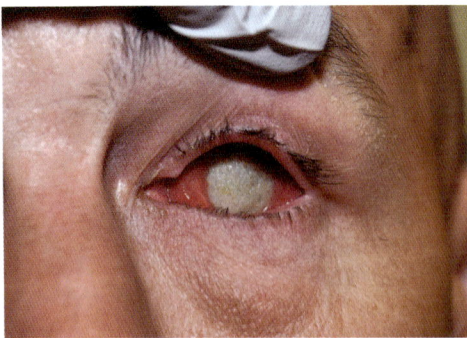

Figure 8-7 Exposure of a porous polyethylene implant in the left socket. *(Courtesy of Audrey C. Ko, MD.)*

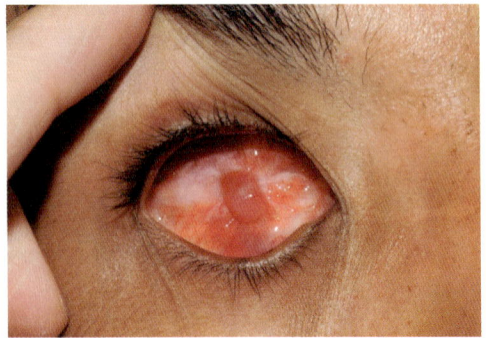

Figure 8-8 Pyogenic granuloma of the right socket following enucleation. *(Courtesy of Bobby S. Korn, MD, PhD.)*

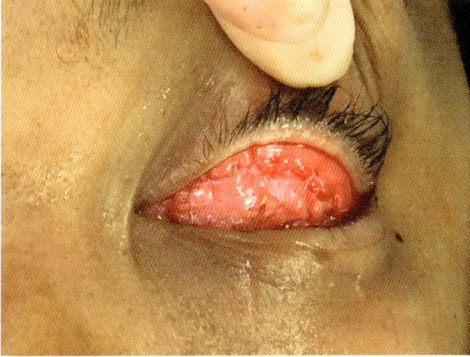

Figure 8-9 Dermis-fat graft placement in the left anophthalmic socket. *(Courtesy of Cat N. Burkat, MD.)*

Dermis-fat grafts may be used when a limited amount of conjunctiva remains in the socket. This graft increases the net amount of conjunctiva available as the conjunctiva re-epithelializes over the front surface of the dermis. Dermis-fat grafts should also be used in patients with a vascularized bed of tissue or vascularized implant. Unpredictable fat resorption is a drawback to the dermis-fat graft technique in adults. However, as stated earlier, dermis-fat grafts in children appear to grow along with the surrounding orbit and may help stimulate orbital development if enucleation is required during infancy or childhood.

Contracture of Fornices

Preventing contracted fornices includes preserving as much conjunctiva as possible and limiting dissection in the fornices. Placing extraocular muscles in their normal anatomical positions also minimizes shortening of the fornices. It is recommended that the patient wear a conformer in the immediate postoperative period to maintain soft-tissue anatomy and minimize conjunctival shortening. Conformers and prostheses should not be removed for periods greater than 24 hours. The prosthesis can be removed and cleaned, especially in the presence of infection, but should be replaced promptly after irrigation of the socket.

Contracted Sockets

Causes of contracted sockets include

- radiation treatment (usually as treatment of a tumor that necessitated removal of the eye)
- extrusion of an orbital implant
- severe initial injury (alkali burns or extensive lacerations)
- poor surgical techniques (excessive sacrifice or destruction of conjunctiva and Tenon capsule; traumatic dissection within the socket causing excessive scar tissue formation)
- multiple ocular and/or socket operations
- removal of the conformer or prosthesis for prolonged periods

Sockets are considered contracted when the fornices are too small to retain a prosthesis (Fig 8-10). Socket reconstruction procedures involve incision or excision of the

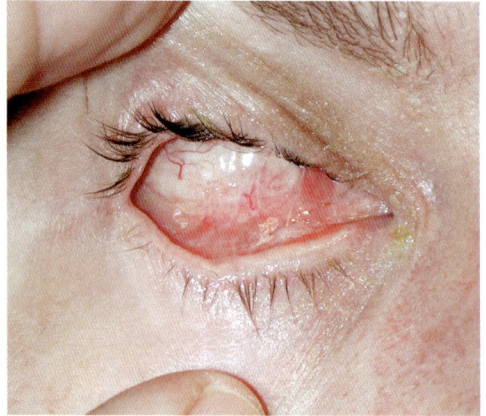

Figure 8-10 Contraction of the right anophthalmic socket. *(Courtesy of Keith D. Carter, MD.)*

scarred tissues and placement of a graft to enlarge the fornices. Full-thickness mucous membrane grafting is preferred as it allows the grafted tissue to match conjunctiva histologically. Amniotic membrane may also be used. Buccal mucosal grafts may be taken from the cheeks (avoid the duct from the parotid gland), the lower lip, or the upper lip, or from the hard palate for rigid tissue. Goblet cells and mucus production are preserved.

Contracture of the fornices alone (more common with the inferior fornix) is usually associated with milder degrees of socket contracture. In these cases, the buccal mucosal graft is placed in the defect, and a silicone sheet is attached by sutures to the superior or inferior orbital rim, depending on which fornix is involved. In 2 weeks, the sheet may be removed, and the prosthesis placed.

Anophthalmic Ectropion

Lower eyelid ectropion may result from the loosening of lower eyelid support under the weight of the prosthesis. Frequent removal of the prosthesis or use of a larger prosthesis accelerates the development of eyelid laxity (Fig 8-11). Tightening the lateral or medial canthal tendon may correct the ectropion. Surgeons may combine ectropion repair with deepening of the inferior fornix by recessing the inferior retractor muscle and grafting mucous membrane tissue.

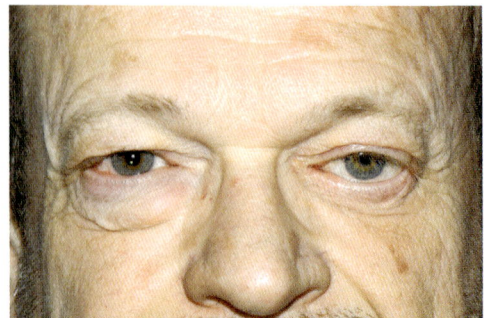

Figure 8-11 Anophthalmic ectropion of the left lower eyelid. *(Courtesy of Keith D. Carter, MD.)*

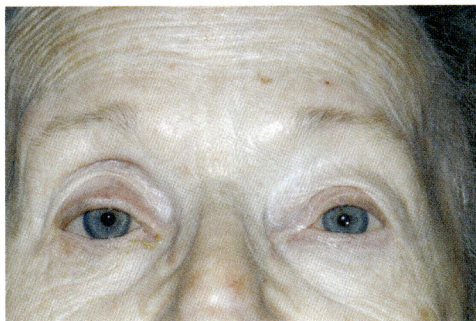

Figure 8-12 Anophthalmic ptosis of the right upper eyelid. *(Courtesy of Keith D. Carter, MD.)*

Anophthalmic Ptosis

Ptosis of the anophthalmic socket results from superotemporal migration of sphere implants, cicatricial tissue in the upper fornix, or damage to the levator muscle or nerve (Fig 8-12). Small amounts of ptosis may be managed by prosthesis modification. Greater amounts require advancement of the levator aponeurosis. This procedure is best done under local anesthesia with intraoperative adjustment of eyelid height and contour, because mechanical forces may cause the surgeon to underestimate true levator function. Ptosis surgery usually improves a deep sulcus by bringing the preaponeurotic fat forward. Mild ptosis may be corrected with Müller muscle–conjunctival resection; however, this may shorten the superior fornix. Frontalis suspension is usually a less useful procedure because there is no visual drive to stimulate contracture of the frontalis muscle to elevate the eyelid.

Lash Margin Entropion

Lash margin entropion, trichiasis, and ptosis of the eyelashes (Fig 8-13) are common in patients with an anophthalmic socket. Contracture of fornices or cicatricial tissue near the lash margin contributes to these abnormalities. Horizontal tarsal incisions and rotation of the lash margin may correct the problem. In more severe cases, splitting of the eyelid margins at the gray line with mucous membrane grafting to the eyelid margin may correct the entropic lash margin.

Cosmetic Optics

Spectacles with particular frame styles and tinted lenses can be used to help camouflage residual defects in reconstructed sockets, in addition to protecting the contralateral eye.

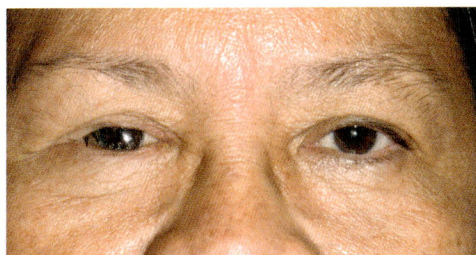

Figure 8-13 Lash ptosis of the right upper eyelid after enucleation. *(Courtesy of Bobby S. Korn, MD, PhD.)*

Plus (convex) lenses or minus (concave) lenses may be placed in the glasses in front of the prosthesis to alter the apparent size of the prosthesis. Prisms in the glasses may be used to change the apparent vertical position of the prosthesis.

Exenteration

In exenteration, some or all of the soft tissues of the orbit are removed, including the globe.

Considerations for Exenteration

Exenteration should be considered in the following circumstances:

- *Destructive tumors extending into the orbit from the sinuses, face, eyelids, conjunctiva, or intracranial space.* However, exenteration is not indicated for all such tumors; some are responsive to radiation, and some have extended too far to be completely removed by surgical excision.
- *Intraocular melanomas or retinoblastomas that have extended outside the globe (if evidence of distant metastases is excluded).* When local control of the tumor would benefit the nursing care of the patient, exenteration is indicated.
- *Malignant epithelial tumors of the lacrimal gland.* Although the procedure is somewhat controversial, these tumors may require extended exenteration with radical bone removal of the roof, lateral wall, and floor.
- *Fungal infection.* Subtotal or total exenteration (discussed in the next section) can be considered for the management of orbital mucormycosis.
- *Primary orbital malignancies that do not respond to nonsurgical therapy.*

Types of Exenteration

Exenterations can be categorized according to the amount of tissue that is removed. Following are the types of exenteration:

- *Subtotal.* The eye and adjacent intraorbital tissues are removed so that the lesion is locally excised (leaving part of the periorbita and eyelids). This technique is used for some locally invasive tumors, for debulking of disseminated tumors, or for partial treatment in selected patients.
- *Total.* All intraorbital soft tissues, including periorbita, are removed, with or without the skin of the eyelids (Fig 8-14A).
- *Extended.* All intraorbital soft tissues are removed, together with adjacent structures (usually bony walls and sinuses).

The technique selected depends on the pathologic process. The goal is to remove all lesions along with appropriate margins of adjacent tissue while retaining as much healthy tissue as possible. Following removal of the orbital contents, the bony socket may be allowed to spontaneously granulate and epithelialize, or it may be covered by a split-thickness skin graft (Fig 8-14B) or collagen skin replacement. The graft or skin replacement may be placed onto bare bone or over a temporalis muscle or temporoparietal fascial flap. Rehabilitation after exenteration may include a prosthesis attached to an eyeglasses frame, to the periorbital area (with adhesive), or to an osseointegrated implant, which may be facilitated with magnetic posts (Fig 8-15). The exenteration prosthesis restores the tissues that have been removed, including eyelids and an eye, but it does not blink or move.

Wei LA, Brown JJ, Hosek DK, Burkat CN. Osseointegrated implants for orbito-facial prostheses: preoperative planning tips and intraoperative pearls. *Orbit.* 2016;35(2):55–61.

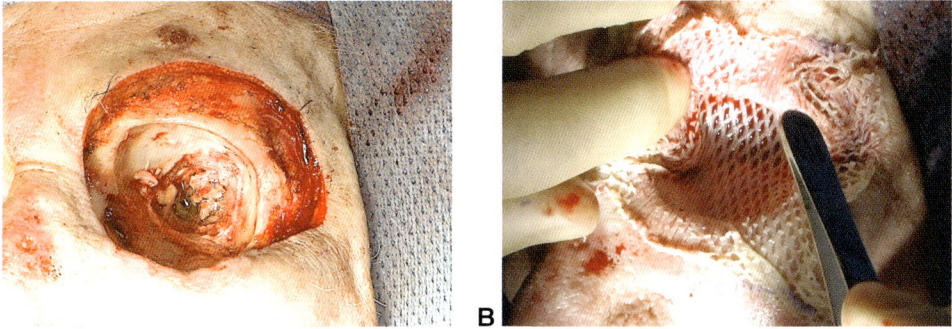

Figure 8-14 Total exenteration and reconstruction. **A,** Total exenteration of the left orbit for invasive squamous cell carcinoma. **B,** Socket reconstruction using a split-thickness skin graft. *(Courtesy of Bobby S. Korn, MD, PhD.)*

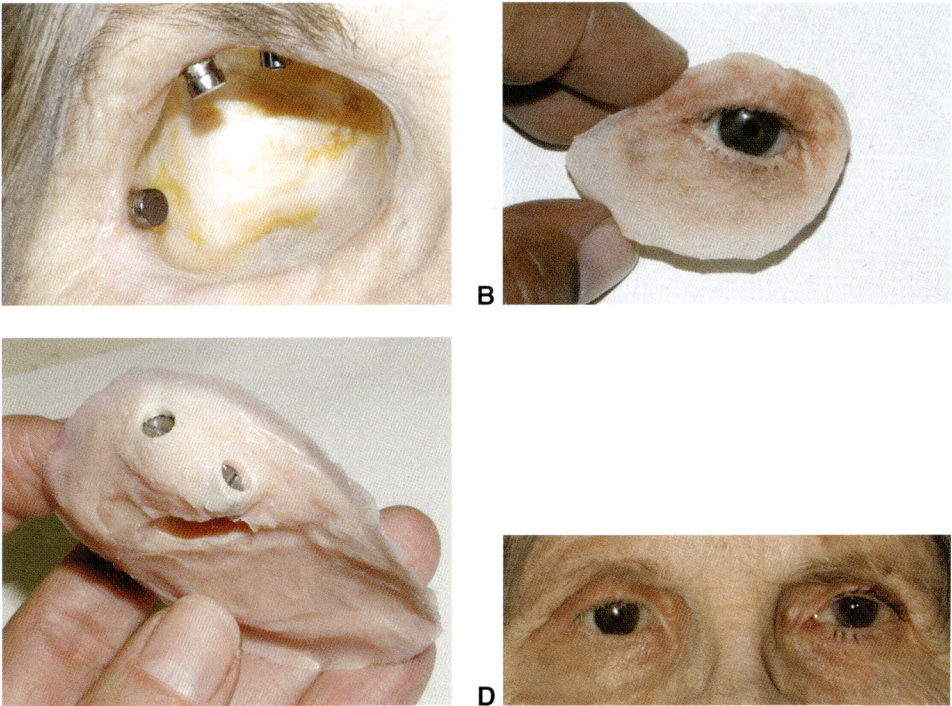

Figure 8-15 Osseointegrated prosthesis placement after exenteration. **A,** Osseointegrated magnetic coupling implants in the right orbit after exenteration. **B,** Front view of orbitofacial prosthetic. **C,** Back view of orbitofacial prosthetic with ferromagnetic posts. **D,** Orbitofacial prosthetic in place using magnetic fixation showing excellent contour to the skin. *(Parts A, B, D courtesy of Keith D. Carter, MD; part C courtesy of Cat N. Burkat, MD.)*

PART II

Periocular Soft Tissues

CHAPTER 9

Facial and Eyelid Anatomy

🖐 *This chapter includes related activities, which can be accessed by scanning the QR codes provided in the text or going to www.aao.org/bcscactivity_section07.*

Highlights

- A detailed understanding of the eyelid and facial anatomy is critical to safe and successful surgical outcomes.
- The temporal branch of the facial nerve becomes superficial as it crosses over the zygomatic arch, and it passes inferior to the superficial temporal artery in the temporoparietal fascial plane.
- Knowledge of the vascular network of the face is important when creating reconstructive flaps and helps minimize the risk of intravascular injection of dermal fillers.
- Maintaining the attachment of the medial canthal tendon to the posterior lacrimal crest is most critical in maintaining apposition of the eyelids to the globe.
- The inferior oblique muscle runs between the medial and central fat pads of the lower eyelid.

Face

The structural planes of the face include skin; subcutaneous tissue; *superficial musculo-aponeurotic system (SMAS)*; mimetic muscles; the deep facial fascia; and the plane containing the facial nerve, parotid duct, and buccal fat pad.

Superficial Musculoaponeurotic System and Temporoparietal Fascia

The superficial facial fascia, which is an extension of the superficial cervical fascia in the neck, invests the facial mimetic muscles to create the SMAS (Fig 9-1A, B). The SMAS distributes facial muscle contractions, facilitating facial expression. These muscle actions are transmitted to the skin by ligamentous attachments located between the SMAS and the dermis. The SMAS is also connected to the underlying bone by a network of fibrous septa and ligaments. Thus, facial support is transmitted from the deep fixed structures of the face to the overlying dermis. There are 2 major components of this system:

- the osteocutaneous ligaments (orbitomalar, zygomatic, and mandibular), which are thick fibrous attachments that originate from the bony periosteum

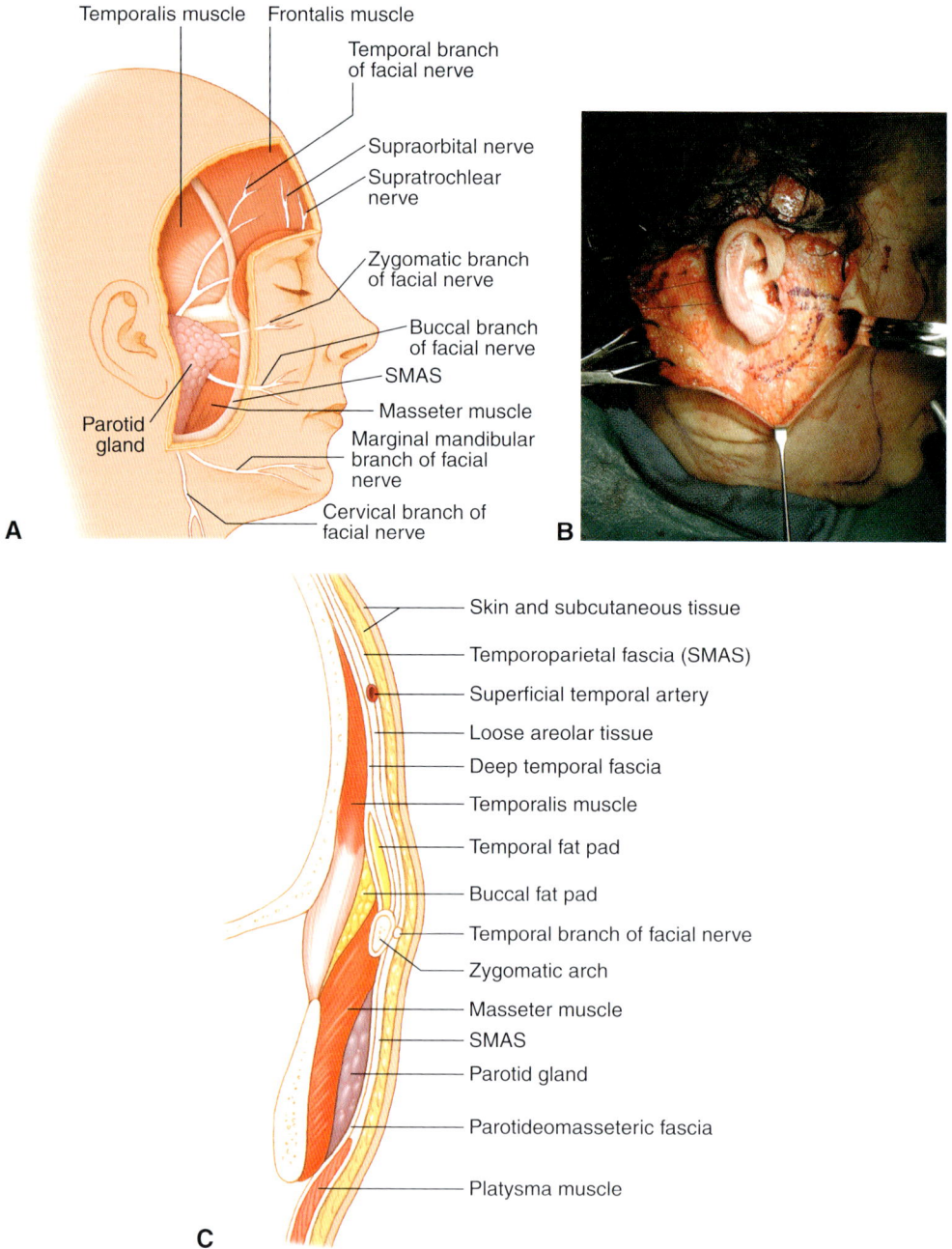

Figure 9-1 Superficial musculoaponeurotic system (SMAS). **A,** Illustration shows the SMAS; note that the facial nerve branches inferior to the zygomatic arch are deep to the SMAS. **B,** The SMAS exposed during a face-lift procedure. The horizontal surgical markings indicate the border of the zygomatic arch, and the oblique lines mark the area of planned excision of the SMAS during the procedure. **C,** Coronal section of the face. The temporal branch of the facial nerve is found within the superficial portion of the temporoparietal fascia (extension of the SMAS). *(Illustrations by Christine Gralapp. Clinical photo courtesy of Jill Foster, MD.)*

- the fascial cutaneous ligaments (parotidocutaneous and masseteric), which are formed by a condensation of superficial and deep facial fasciae

As these ligaments become attenuated in conjunction with facial dermal elastosis, facial aging becomes apparent. Dissection and repositioning of the SMAS have important implications for facial cosmetic surgery.

As the SMAS continues superiorly over the zygomatic arch, it becomes continuous with the *temporoparietal fascia* (also called the *superficial temporal fascia*). More superiorly, the SMAS becomes continuous with the galea aponeurotica. Beneath the loose areolar tissue and the temporoparietal fascia, the deep temporal fascia of the temporal muscle splits and envelops the temporal fat pad, creating deep and superficial layers of the deep temporal fascia (Fig 9-1C).

Mimetic Muscles

The mimetic muscles (Fig 9-2) can be grouped into upper face muscles and lower face muscles.

The upper face muscles include

- the corrugator supercilii (oblique and transverse heads) (Fig 9-3), depressor supercilii, and procerus muscles, which animate the glabella and medial eyebrow and cause vertical and oblique rhytids
- the orbicularis oculi muscle, which depresses the eyebrows and closes the eyelids
- the frontalis, which is the sole elevator of the eyebrows; contraction of this muscle causes transverse forehead rhytids

The lower face muscles include

- the *superficial mimetic muscles,* which receive their neurovascular supply on the posterior surfaces and include the platysma, zygomaticus major, zygomaticus minor, and risorius
- the *deep mimetic muscles,* which receive their neurovascular supply anteriorly and include the buccinator, mentalis, and levator anguli oris

Other facial muscles include the orbicularis oris, the levator labii superioris, the levator labii superioris alaeque nasi, the depressor anguli oris, the depressor labii inferioris, the masseter, the nasalis, and the temporalis.

Facial Nerve

In the neck, the superficial cervical fascia and platysma are continuous with the SMAS, and the deep cervical fascia is found on the superficial surface of the strap muscles, superior to the hyoid bone. The deep cervical fascia overlies the myelohyoid muscle and extends superiorly over the body of the mandible, continuing as the parotideomasseteric fascia. The facial nerve lies deep to this thin layer in the lower face. Above the zygomatic arch in the temporal region, the parotideomasseteric fascia is continuous with the deep temporal fascia, and the temporal (frontal) branch of the facial nerve lies superficial to this fascial layer. The transition of the temporal branch of the facial nerve from deep to superficial occurs as the

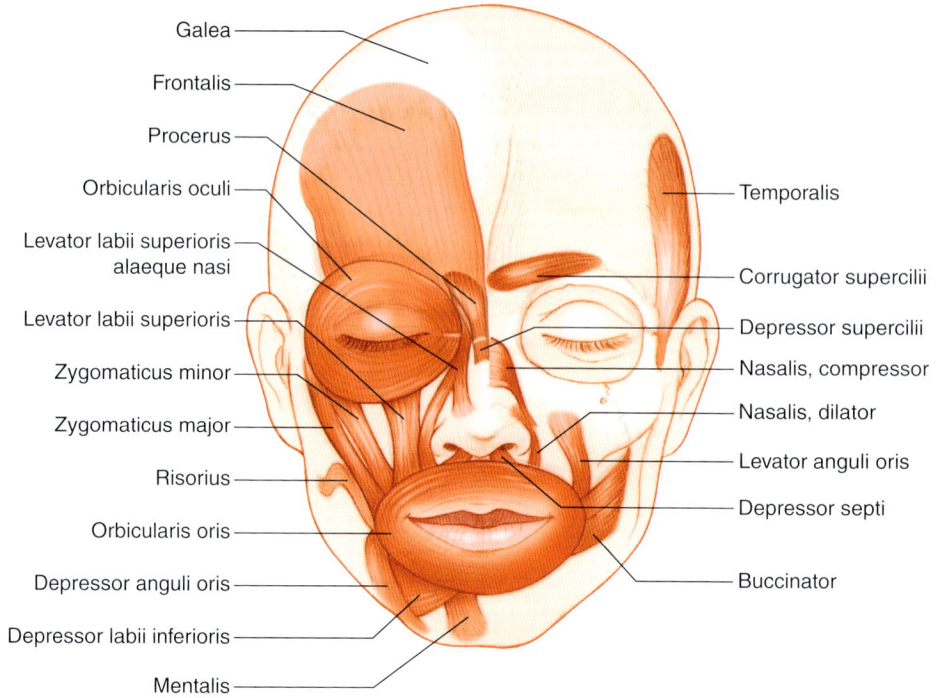

Figure 9-2 Facial mimetic muscles. *(Illustration by Christine Gralapp.)*

Figure 9-3 Oblique and transverse heads of the corrugator supercilii muscle. *(Courtesy of Cat N. Burkat, MD.)*

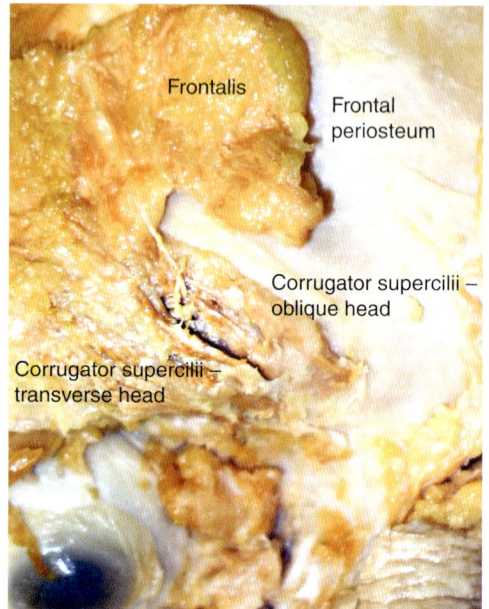

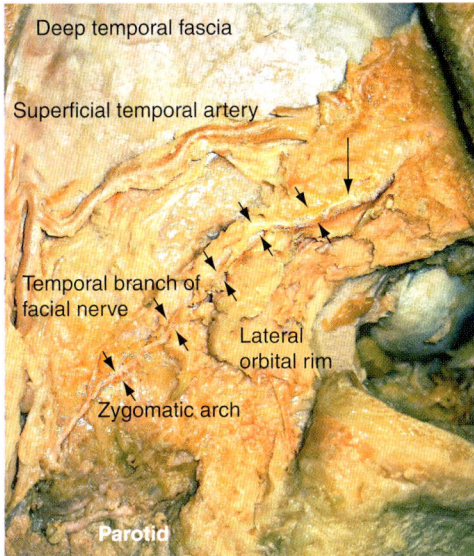

Figure 9-4 Temporal branch of the facial nerve below the superficial temporal artery. *(Courtesy of Cat N. Burkat, MD.)*

nerve crosses over the zygomatic arch. When biopsy of the superficial temporal artery is performed, care is taken to avoid injury to the temporal branch of the facial nerve passing just inferior to the artery, both of which lie in the temporoparietal fascial plane (Fig 9-4).

The facial nerve, cranial nerve VII (CN VII), innervates the mimetic muscles and divides into 5 major branches within or deep to the parotid gland (Fig 9-5): temporal (frontal), zygomatic, buccal, marginal mandibular, and cervical (Fig 9-6). Two surgical planes help surgeons avoid CN VII when operating: dissection on top of the deep temporal fascia (see Fig 9-4), which is deep to the SMAS and deep to CN VII, in the upper face and temporal region; and dissection superficial to the SMAS and CN VII branches in the lower face.

In the temporal area, the temporal branch of CN VII (see Figs 9-5, 9-6) crosses the zygomatic arch and courses superomedially in the deep layers of the temporoparietal fascia. The temporoparietal fascia is continuous with the SMAS of the lower face and the galea aponeurosis of the upper face. Deep to the temporoparietal fascia is the previously mentioned *deep temporal fascia*, a dense, immobile fascia that overlies the temporalis muscle and is continuous with the frontal periosteum (see Fig 9-1C). Dissection along this fascia allows mobilization of the temporal forehead while avoiding the overlying temporal branch of the facial nerve. This anatomic principle is important when performing brow-lifting and forehead-lifting procedures. When performing a rotation flap in the lateral canthus and temporal region, the safety zone is within 2 cm (on average) from the lateral canthal angle to avoid the frontal branch of the facial nerve as it crosses over the zygomatic arch (Fig 9-7).

In the lower face, the facial nerve branches, sensory nerves, vascular networks, and parotid gland and duct are deep to the SMAS (see Figs 9-1A, 9-6). Dissection just superficial to the SMAS, parotid gland, and parotideomasseteric fascia in the lower face avoids injury to these structures. The face receives sensory innervation from the 3 branches of CN V: V_1, ophthalmic; V_2, maxillary; and V_3, mandibular (Fig 9-8). Damage to these nerves causes

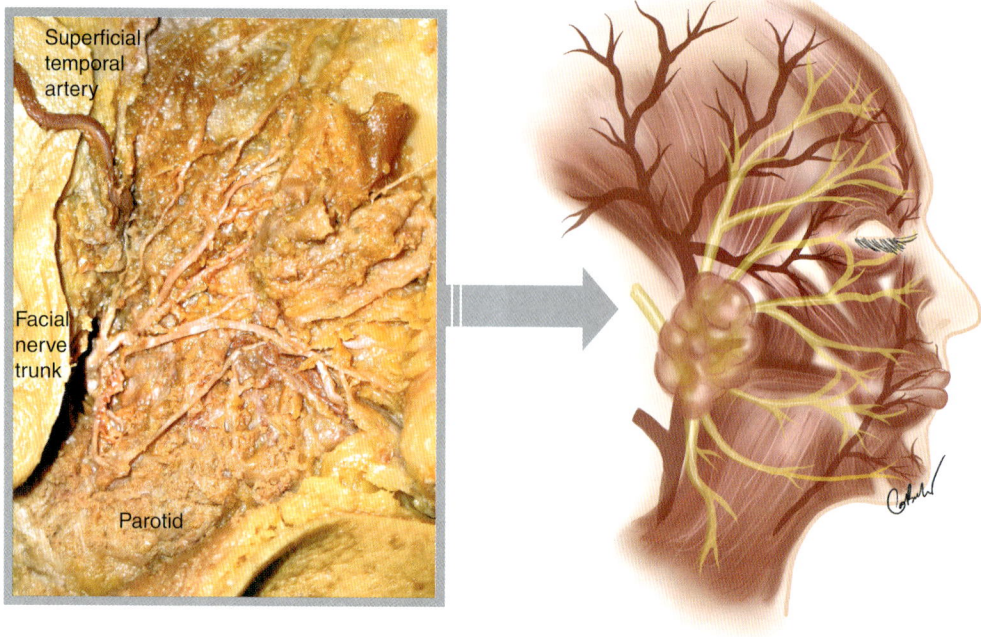

Figure 9-5   Facial nerve branching within the parotid gland. *(Courtesy of Cat N. Burkat, MD.)*

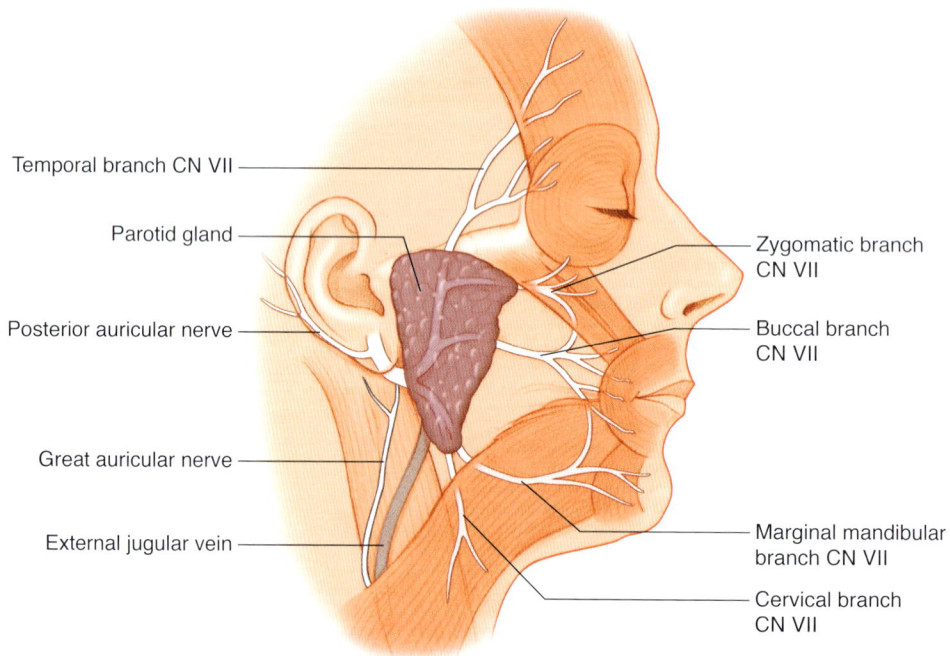

Figure 9-6   The 5 major branches of the facial nerve, cranial nerve (CN) VII. Note that the branches progress from deep beneath the parotid gland to more superficial layers as they cross the zygomatic arch or reach the anterior edge of the SMAS. *(Illustration by Christine Gralapp.)*

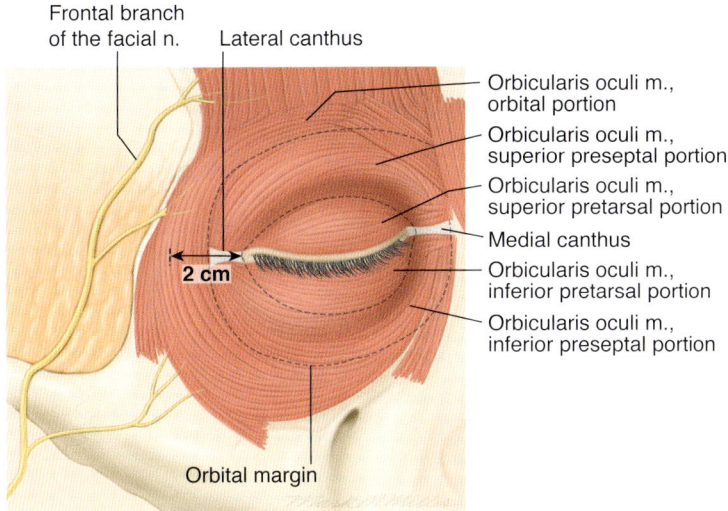

Figure 9-7 Orbicularis oculi muscle and the frontal branch of the facial nerve passing lateral to the canthal angle. *(Illustration by Mark Miller, based on a sketch by Cat N. Burkat, MD.)*

facial numbness and paresthesia. Fortunately, overlap of the distal branches makes permanent sensation loss unusual, unless injury occurs at the proximal neurovascular bundles or with extensive distal disruption, as can be seen with a coronal incision.

Arterial Network

An understanding of the vascular supply of the eyelids and face is crucial during facial surgery, as well as when performing nonsurgical facial procedures such as soft-tissue filler augmentation and neurotoxin chemodenervation. Although very rare (<0.001–0.5%), direct injection into a facial artery can result in skin necrosis; this has been reported for every filler type. The risk is highest for procedures performed in the glabella due to its limited collateral circulation; the supraorbital, supratrochlear, infraorbital, and angular arteries are the most vulnerable. Early signs of arterial vascular compromise are pain and skin pallor; signs of venous occlusion often have a delayed onset, presenting as dull pain and skin discoloration.

The most devastating adverse outcome associated with soft-tissue fillers is blindness resulting from occlusion of the ophthalmic artery and its branches. An intravascular bolus of filler can reach the ophthalmic artery via retrograde flow from any number of facial arteries, in particular, the dorsal nasal, angular, supratrochlear, or supraorbital vessels (Activity 9-1; Fig 9-9). Vision loss is often profound (no light perception) and permanent. Dissemination of filler in a facial artery can also result in focal brain infarctions, leading to hemiplegia and dysarthria. In rare instances, vascular occlusions in the periorbital area can also result in ophthalmoplegia and ptosis.

ACTIVITY 9-1 Arterial danger zones of the face during filler injection.
Illustration courtesy of Mark Miller, based on a sketch by Cat N. Burkat, MD.
Access all Section 7 activities at www.aao.org/bcscactivity_section07.

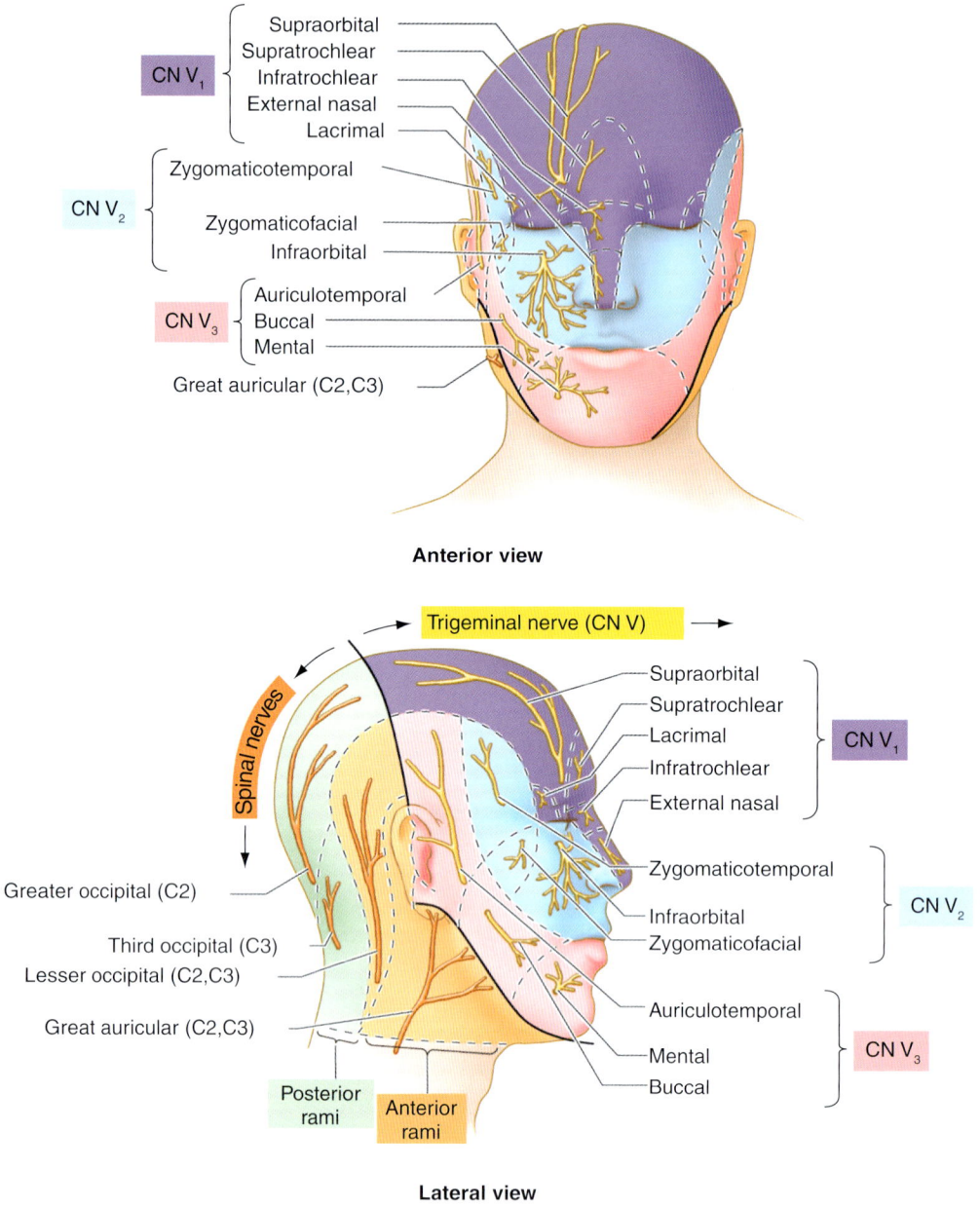

Figure 9-8 The face receives its sensory innervation from the 3 branches of CN V: V_1, ophthalmic; V_2, maxillary; and V_3, mandibular. *(Modified with permission from Moore KL, Dalley AF, Agur AMR. Clinically Oriented Anatomy. 7th ed. Baltimore: Lippincott Williams & Wilkins; 2013:851.)*

Park KH, Kim YK, Woo SJ, et al; Korean Retina Society. Iatrogenic occlusion of the ophthalmic artery after cosmetic facial filler injections: a national survey by the Korean Retina Society. *JAMA Ophthalmol.* 2014;132(6):714–723.

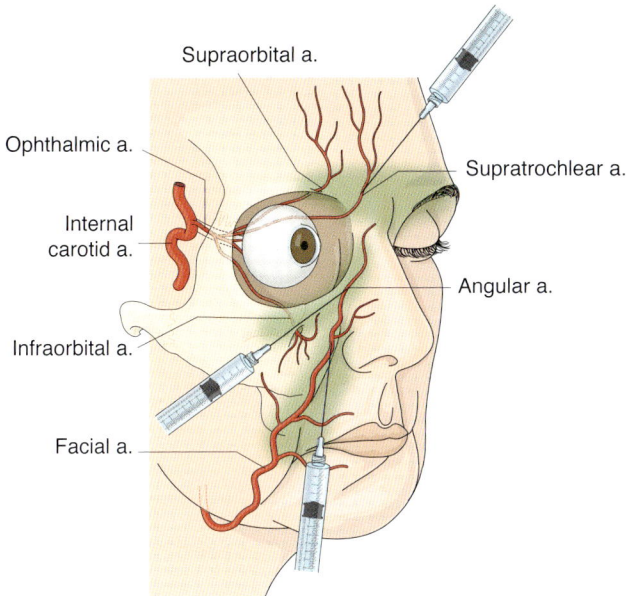

Figure 9-9 Arterial danger zones of the face. *Shading* denotes areas to inject with caution. *(Illustration courtesy of Mark Miller, based on a sketch by Cat N. Burkat, MD.)*

Eyelids

The eyelids can be divided into the following 7 structural layers:

- skin and subcutaneous connective tissue
- muscles of protraction
- orbital septum
- orbital fat
- muscles of retraction
- tarsus
- conjunctiva

Figure 9-10 details the anatomy of the eyelids; Activity 9-2 is an online interactive tool for self-testing knowledge of eyelid anatomy. See also BCSC Section 2, *Fundamentals and Principles of Ophthalmology,* for additional discussion and numerous illustrations.

ACTIVITY 9-2 Upper and lower eyelid anatomy. *Illustration modified from Stewart WB. Surgery of the Eyelid, Orbit, and Lacrimal System. Ophthalmology Monograph 8, vol 2. San Francisco: American Academy of Ophthalmology; 1994:23, 85. Illustration by Cyndie C. H. Wooley.*

Skin and Subcutaneous Connective Tissue

Eyelid skin is the thinnest skin of the body and is unique in having no subcutaneous fat layer. Because the thin skin of the eyelids is subjected to constant movement with each blink, the

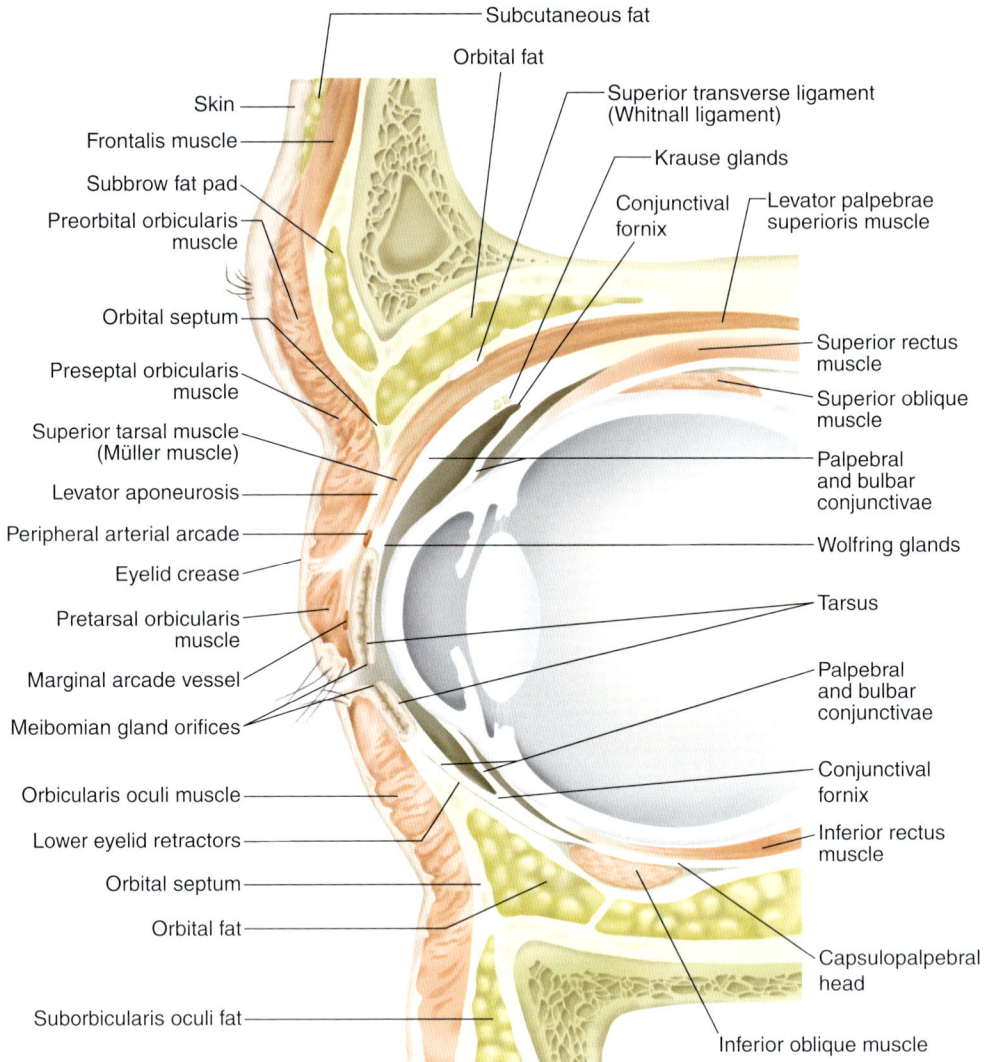

Figure 9-10 Upper and lower eyelid anatomy. *(Modified from Stewart WB. Surgery of the Eyelid, Orbit, and Lacrimal System. Ophthalmology Monograph 8, vol 2. San Francisco: American Academy of Ophthalmology; 1994:23, 85. Illustration by Cyndie C. H. Wooley.)*

laxity that often occurs with age is not surprising. In both the upper and the lower eyelids, the pretarsal tissues are normally firmly attached to the underlying tissues, whereas the preseptal tissues are more loosely attached, creating potential spaces for fluid accumulation. The contours of the eyelid skin are defined by the *eyelid crease* and the *eyelid fold:*

- The upper eyelid crease represents the attachments of the levator aponeurosis to the pretarsal orbicularis muscle and skin. In the non-Asian eyelid, this site is near or at the level of the superior tarsal border.

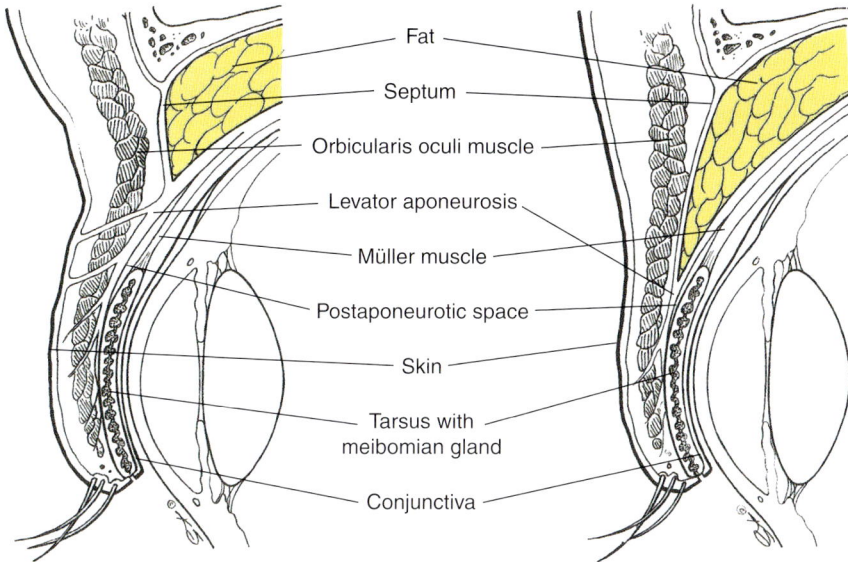

Fat

Septum

Orbicularis oculi muscle

Levator aponeurosis

Müller muscle

Postaponeurotic space

Skin

Tarsus with
meibomian gland

Conjunctiva

Figure 9-11 Racial variations in eyelid anatomy. Variant I *(left)*: the orbital septum fuses with the levator aponeurosis above the tarsus. Variant II (Asian, *right*): the orbital septum fuses with the levator aponeurosis between the eyelid margin and the superior border of the tarsus, and there are fewer aponeurotic attachments to the skin. *(Reproduced with permission from Katowitz JA, ed.* Pediatric Oculoplastic Surgery. *Philadelphia: Springer-Verlag; 2002.)*

- The upper eyelid fold consists of the loose preseptal skin and subcutaneous tissues resting above the confluence of the levator aponeurosis and orbital septum.

Racial variation can be seen in the location of the eyelid crease and eyelid fold. The eyelid of an Asian individual normally has a relatively low upper eyelid crease because the orbital septum fuses with the levator aponeurosis between the eyelid margin and the superior border of tarsus, in contrast to a supratarsal fusion (Fig 9-11). This also allows preaponeurotic fat to occupy a position more inferior and anterior in the eyelid. Although the lower eyelid crease is less well defined than the upper eyelid crease, these differences are apparent in the lower eyelid as well.

Muscles of Protraction

The orbicularis oculi muscle is the main protractor of the eyelid. Innervated by CN VII, contraction of this muscle narrows the palpebral fissure. Specific portions of this muscle also constitute the lacrimal pump. The orbicularis oculi muscle is divided into *pretarsal, preseptal,* and *orbital* parts (Fig 9-12; see also Fig 9-7). The palpebral (pretarsal and preseptal) parts are integral to involuntary eyelid movements (blinking), whereas the orbital portion is primarily involved in forced eyelid closure.

The pretarsal orbicularis muscle arises from deep origins at the posterior lacrimal crest and superficial origins at the anterior limb of the medial canthal tendon (Fig 9-13). Near the

Frontalis m.   Orbicularis oculi m.,
                    orbital portion
Lateral canthus

Corrugator m.

Procerus m.

Orbicularis oculi m.,
superior preseptal portion

Orbicularis oculi m.,
superior pretarsal portion

Medial canthus

Orbicularis oculi m.,
inferior pretarsal portion

Orbicularis oculi m.,
inferior preseptal portion

Orbital margin

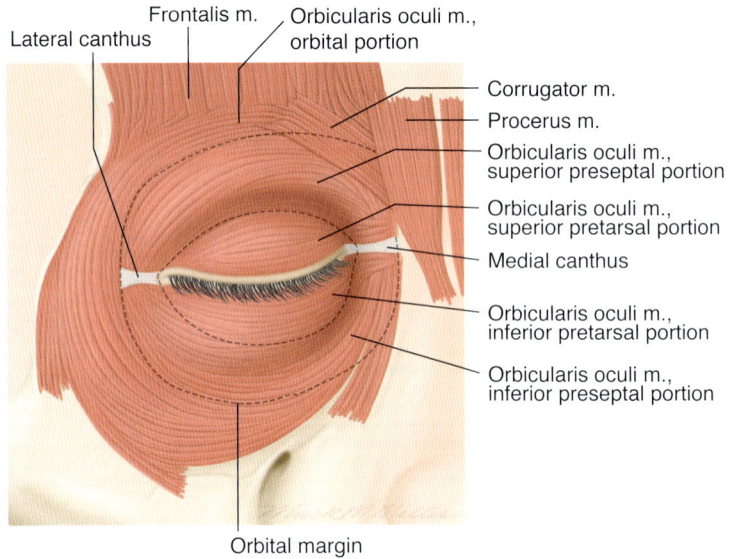

Figure 9-12   Segments of the orbicularis oculi muscle. *(Illustration courtesy of Mark Miller.)*

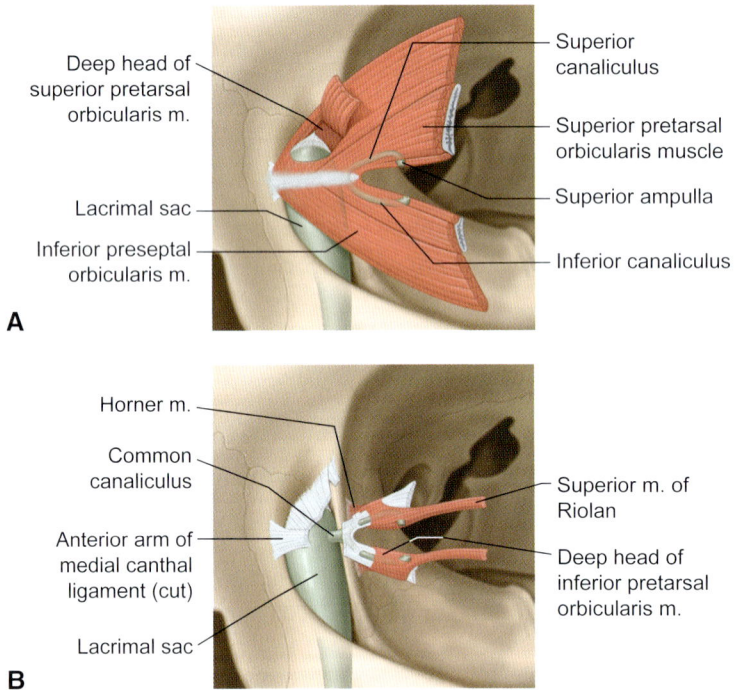

Deep head of
superior pretarsal
orbicularis m.

Superior
canaliculus

Superior pretarsal
orbicularis muscle

Superior ampulla

Lacrimal sac

Inferior preseptal
orbicularis m.

Inferior canaliculus

A

Horner m.

Common
canaliculus

Superior m. of
Riolan

Anterior arm of
medial canthal
ligament (cut)

Deep head of
inferior pretarsal
orbicularis m.

Lacrimal sac

B

Figure 9-13   Lacrimal drainage system. **A,** Medial attachments of the orbicularis oculi muscle. **B,** Deep head of the orbicularis oculi muscle. *(Illustrations courtesy of Mark Miller.)*

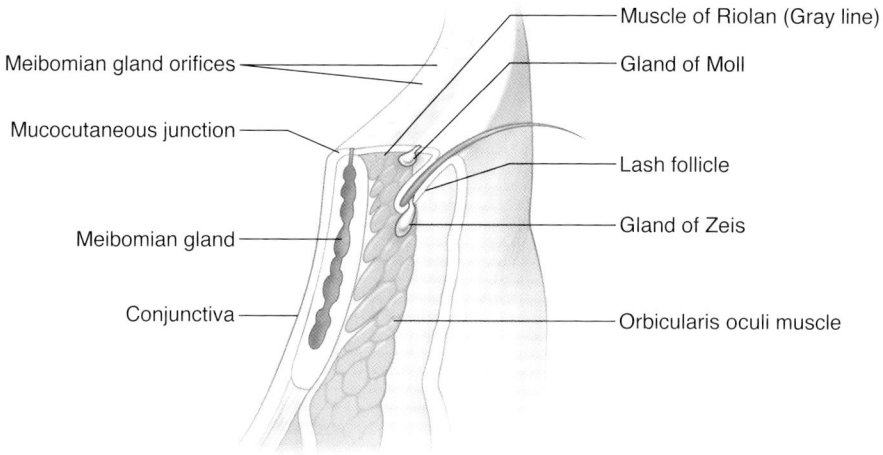

Figure 9-14 Eyelid margin anatomy. *(Illustration by Christine Gralapp.)*

common canaliculus, the deep heads of the pretarsal orbicularis fuse to form a prominent bundle of fibers known as the *Horner muscle,* which continues just behind the posterior arm of the medial canthal tendon to insert onto the posterior lacrimal crest. The upper and lower eyelid segments of the pretarsal orbicularis fuse in the lateral canthal area to become the lateral canthal tendon.

The preseptal orbicularis arises from the upper and lower borders of the medial canthal tendon, or as a single head from the common tendon. In the upper eyelid, the preseptal muscle has an anterior head from the common tendon and a posterior head from both the superior and posterior arms of the tendon. Laterally, the preseptal muscles form the lateral palpebral raphe.

The orbital portions of the orbicularis muscle arise from the anterior limb of the medial canthal tendon, the orbital process of the frontal bone, and the frontal process of the maxillary bone in front of the anterior lacrimal crest. Its fibers form a continuous ellipse and insert just below the point of origin. At the eyelid margin, a specialized bundle of striated muscle fibers, the *muscle of Riolan,* lies more posterior than the main portion of the orbicularis and creates the gray line (Fig 9-14). The muscle of Riolan may play a role in meibomian glandular discharge, blinking, and eyelash position.

Orbital Septum

The orbital septum, a thin, multilayered sheet of fibrous tissue, arises from the periosteum over the superior and inferior orbital rims at the arcus marginalis. In the upper eyelid, the orbital septum typically fuses with the levator aponeurosis 2–5 mm above the superior tarsal border, and below the superior tarsus in eyelids of Asian individuals (see Figs 9-10, 9-11). In the lower eyelid, the orbital septum fuses with the capsulopalpebral fascia at or just below the inferior tarsal border. Along with a small contribution from the inferior tarsal smooth muscle, the fused capsulopalpebral–orbital septum complex inserts on the posterior and anterior tarsal surfaces as well as the inferior border of the tarsus. Over time, thinning and attenuation of the septum and laxity of the orbicularis muscle contribute to anterior herniation of the orbital fat pads.

Orbital Fat

Orbital fat lies posterior to the orbital septum and anterior to the levator aponeurosis (upper eyelid) or the capsulopalpebral fascia (lower eyelid). In the upper eyelid, there are 2 fat pads: medial and central (preaponeurotic). In the lower eyelid, there are 3 fat pads: medial, central, and lateral (Fig 9-15). The inferior oblique muscle runs between the medial and central fat pads (Fig 9-16). These pockets are surrounded by thin fibrous capsules that are continuations of the anterior orbitoseptal system. The central orbital fat pad is an important landmark in both elective eyelid surgery and eyelid laceration repair because it lies directly behind the orbital septum and in front of the levator aponeurosis.

Muscles of Retraction

The upper eyelid retractors are the levator palpebrae superioris muscle with its aponeurosis and the superior tarsal muscle *(Müller muscle)*. In the lower eyelid, the retractors are the capsulopalpebral fascia and the inferior tarsal muscle.

Upper eyelid retractors

The levator muscle originates in the apex of the orbit, arising from the periorbita of the lesser wing of the sphenoid, just above the annulus of Zinn. The muscular portion of the levator is approximately 40 mm long; the aponeurosis is 14–20 mm in length (Fig 9-17). The superior transverse ligament *(Whitnall ligament)* is a sleeve of elastic fibers around

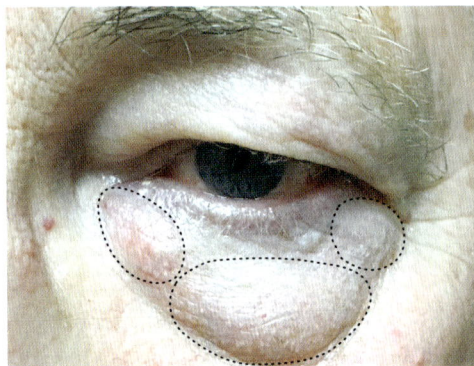

Figure 9-15 Clinical photo of the fat pads of the left lower eyelid. *(Courtesy of Cat N. Burkat, MD.)*

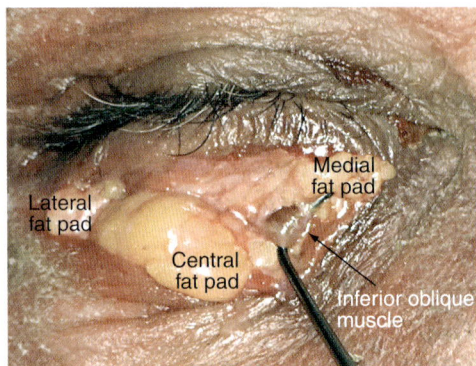

Figure 9-16 Photo of the right lower eyelid fat pads, demonstrating the inferior oblique muscle between the medial and central fat pads. *(Courtesy of Cat N. Burkat, MD.)*

the levator muscle. It is located near or above the area where the levator muscle transitions into the levator aponeurosis (Figs 9-18, 9-19).

The Whitnall ligament functions primarily as a suspensory support for the upper eyelid and the superior orbital tissues. The ligament also acts as a fulcrum for the levator, transferring its vector force from an anterior–posterior to a superior–inferior direction. Its analogue in the lower eyelid is the *Lockwood ligament.* Medially, the Whitnall ligament attaches to connective tissue around the trochlea and superior oblique tendon. Laterally, it forms septa through the lacrimal gland stroma, then arches upward to attach inside the lateral orbital wall several millimeters above the lateral orbital tubercle via attachments to the lacrimal gland fascia, with a small group of fibers extending inferiorly to insert onto the lateral retinaculum. The Whitnall ligament should not be confused with the horns of the levator aponeurosis, which lie more inferior and more toward the canthi (see Fig 9-18). The lateral horn inserts onto the lateral orbital tubercle; the medial horn inserts onto the posterior lacrimal crest. The lateral horn of the levator aponeurosis is robust and divides the lacrimal gland into the orbital and palpebral lobes, attaching firmly to

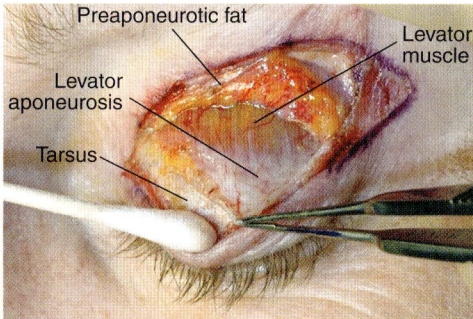

Figure 9-17   Levator muscle and aponeurosis. *(Courtesy of Cat N. Burkat, MD.)*

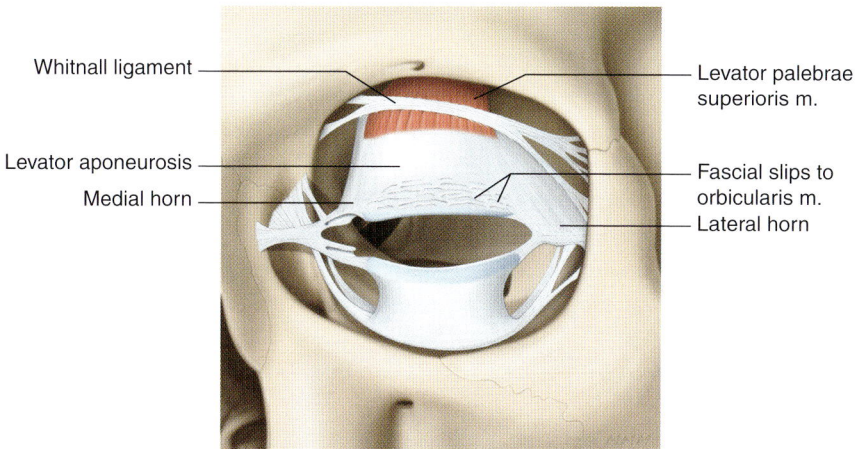

Figure 9-18   The suspensory and fibrous anatomy of the eyelid. *(Illustration courtesy of Mark Miller.)*

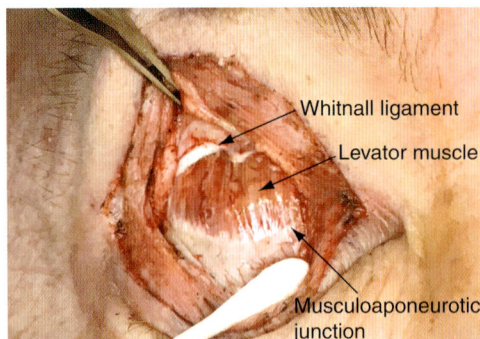

Figure 9-19 Whitnall ligament and levator complex. *(Courtesy of Cat N. Burkat, MD.)*

the orbital tubercle. The medial horn of the aponeurosis is more delicate and forms loose connective attachments to the posterior aspect of the medial canthal tendon and to the posterior lacrimal crest.

As the levator aponeurosis continues toward the tarsus, it divides into an anterior portion and a posterior portion a variable distance above the superior tarsal border. The anterior portion is composed of fine strands of aponeurosis that insert into the septa between the pretarsal orbicularis muscle bundles and skin. These fine attachments are responsible for the close apposition of the pretarsal skin and orbicularis muscle to the underlying tarsus. The upper eyelid crease is formed by the most superior of these attachments and by contraction of the underlying levator complex (see Fig 9-10). The upper eyelid fold is created by the overhanging skin, fat, and orbicularis muscle superior to the crease.

The posterior portion of the levator aponeurosis inserts firmly onto the anterior surface of the inferior half of the tarsus. It is most firmly attached approximately 3 mm above the eyelid margin and is only loosely attached to the superior 2–3 mm of tarsus. Disinsertion, dehiscence, or rarefaction of the aponeurosis following ocular surgery or due to intraocular inflammation, eyelid trauma, or senescence may give rise to ptosis. The levator muscle is innervated by the superior division of CN III, which also supplies the superior rectus muscle. A superior division palsy, resulting in ptosis and decreased upgaze, implies an intraorbital disruption of CN III.

The Müller muscle originates from the undersurface of the levator palpebrae superioris muscle approximately at the level of the Whitnall ligament, 12–14 mm above the upper tarsal border (Fig 9-20). The levator muscle divides into an anterior branch, which becomes the aponeurosis, and a posterior branch, which becomes the Müller muscle. This sympathetically innervated smooth muscle extends inferiorly to insert along the superior tarsal border. The muscle provides approximately 2–3 mm of elevation of the upper eyelid; if it is interrupted (as in Horner syndrome), mild ptosis results. The Müller muscle is firmly attached to the conjunctiva posteriorly, especially just above the superior tarsal border. The peripheral arterial arcade is found between the levator aponeurosis and the Müller muscle, just above the superior tarsal border (see Fig 9-20). This vascular arcade serves as a useful surgical landmark to identify the Müller muscle.

Ng SK, Chan W, Marcet MM, Kakizaki H, Selva D. Levator palpebrae superioris: an anatomical update. *Orbit.* 2013;32(1):76–84.

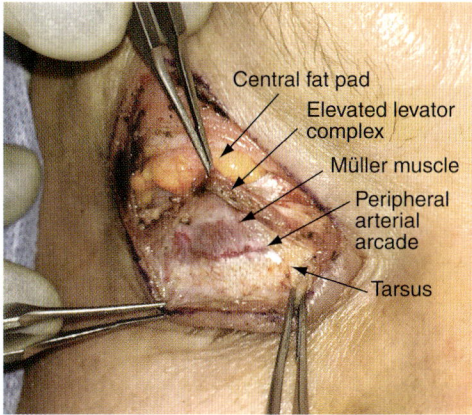

Figure 9-20 Müller muscle and peripheral arterial arcade superior to the upper tarsal border (levator complex reflected superiorly). *(Courtesy of Cat N. Burkat, MD.)*

Lower eyelid retractors

The capsulopalpebral fascia in the lower eyelid is analogous to the levator aponeurosis in the upper eyelid (Fig 9-21). The fascia originates as the capsulopalpebral head from attachments to the terminal muscle fibers of the inferior rectus muscle. The capsulopalpebral head divides as it encircles the inferior oblique muscle and fuses with the sheath of the inferior oblique muscle. Anterior to the inferior oblique muscle, the 2 portions of the capsulopalpebral head join to form the Lockwood suspensory ligament. The capsulopalpebral fascia extends anteriorly from this point, sending strands to the inferior conjunctival fornix, to the inferior tarsal border after fusing with the orbital septum, and to the skin to create the eyelid crease.

The inferior tarsal muscle in the lower eyelid is analogous to the Müller muscle, although it is less well developed structurally. It runs posterior to the capsulopalpebral fascia, with smooth muscle fibers most abundant in the area of the inferior fornix.

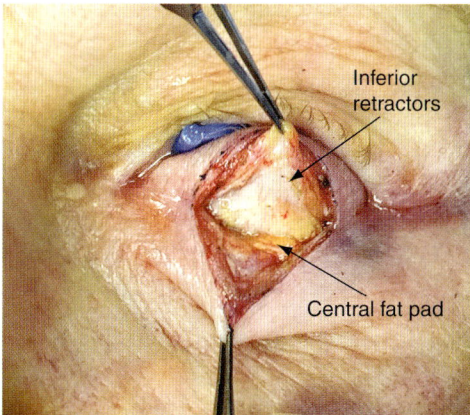

Figure 9-21 Inferior retractors of the lower eyelid. *(Courtesy of Cat N. Burkat, MD.)*

Tarsus

The tarsi are firm, dense plates of connective tissue that serve as the structural support of the eyelids (Fig 9-22). The upper eyelid tarsal plate measures 10–12 mm vertically in the central eyelid; the lower eyelid tarsal plate measures 3–4 mm. The tarsal plates are typically 1 mm thick and taper at the ends to form rigid attachments to the periosteum through the medial and lateral canthal tendons. They may become horizontally displaced with age as a result of stretching of the medial and lateral supporting tendons. The meibomian glands within the tarsus are modified holocrine sebaceous glands.

Conjunctiva

The conjunctiva is composed of nonkeratinized stratified squamous epithelium. It forms the posterior layer of the eyelids and contains the mucin-secreting goblet cells and the accessory lacrimal *glands of Wolfring* and *Krause*. The accessory lacrimal glands are found in the subconjunctival tissue mainly in the upper and lower eyelids. The glands of Wolfring are found primarily along the nonmarginal tarsal borders, and the glands of Krause are found in the fornices.

Additional Anatomical Considerations

Connective tissue

Suborbicularis fat pads Deep to the orbicularis muscle overlying the maxillary and zygomatic periosteum is a plane of nonseptate fat called the *suborbicularis oculi fat (SOOF)*. This fat is analogous to the superiorly located *retro-orbicularis oculi fat (ROOF),* which is situated deep to the eyebrow and extends into the eyelid, where it merges with postorbicularis fascia in the upper eyelid (see Fig 9-10).

The SOOF plays an important role in the gradual gravitational descent of the midfacial soft tissues with age. Repositioning of the SOOF can support involutional and cicatricial retraction of the lower eyelid. In aesthetic procedures, elevation of the SOOF restores more youthful contours in the lower eyelid and midfacial soft tissues.

Similarly, the ROOF undergoes gravitational descent, compounding redundant dermatochalasis and fullness. The descended ROOF, which is whiter and more fibrous, should not be confused with prominent prolapsed yellow preaponeurotic fat in the upper eyelid. In some patients, it is necessary to reposition the descended ROOF to the frontal periosteum during blepharoplasty to achieve an adequate functional and aesthetic result.

Lucarelli MJ, Khwarg SI, Lemke BN, Kozel JS, Dortzbach RK. The anatomy of midfacial ptosis. *Ophthalmic Plast Reconstr Surg.* 2000;16(1):7–22.
Mendelson BC, Muzaffar AR, Adams WP Jr. Surgical anatomy of the midcheek and malar mounds. *Plast Reconstr Surg.* 2002;110(3):885–896; discussion 897–911.

Canthal tendons The configuration of the palpebral fissure is maintained by the medial and lateral canthal tendons in conjunction with the attached tarsal plates (see Figs 9-18, 9-22). The 2 origins of the medial canthal tendon from the anterior and posterior lacrimal crests fuse just temporal to the lacrimal sac; they then split again into an upper limb and a

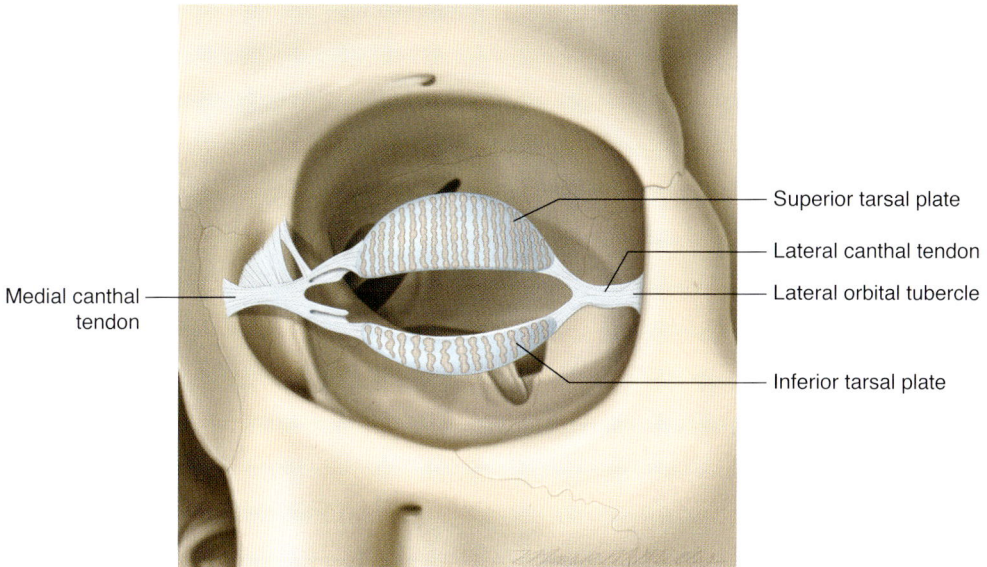

Figure 9-22 Tarsal plates and suspensory tendons of the eyelid. *(Illustration courtesy of Mark Miller.)*

lower limb that attach to the upper superior and lower inferior tarsal plates. The attachment of the tendon to the periosteum overlying the anterior lacrimal crest is diffuse and strong. The attachment to the posterior lacrimal crest is more delicate but is important in maintaining apposition of the eyelids to the globe, allowing the puncta to lie in the tear lake.

The lateral canthal tendon attaches at the lateral orbital tubercle 2–5 mm inside the lateral orbital rim. It splits into superior and inferior limbs that attach to the respective tarsal plates. Stretching or disinsertion of the medial canthal tendon may cause cosmetic or functional problems such as telecanthus (Fig 9-23). Horizontal eyelid instability is frequently the result of lateral canthal tendon lengthening. The lateral canthal tendon usually inserts 2 mm higher than the medial canthal tendon, giving the horizontal palpebral fissure a natural upward slope from medial to lateral. Insertion of the lateral canthal tendon inferior to the medial canthal tendon causes the horizontal palpebral fissure to slant downward.

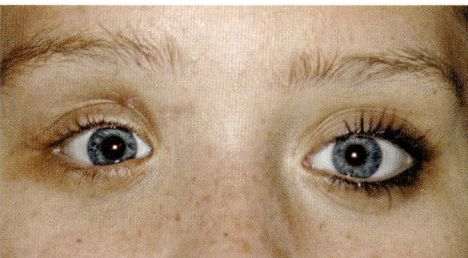

Figure 9-23 Traumatic telecanthus, right side. *(Courtesy of Cat N. Burkat, MD.)*

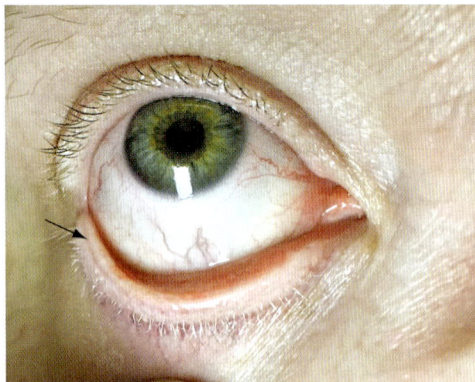

Figure 9-24 Eyelid margin gray line *(arrow)*. *(Courtesy of Cat N. Burkat, MD.)*

Eyelid margin

The eyelid margin is the confluence of the mucosal surface of the conjunctiva, the edge of the orbicularis, and the cutaneous epithelium. Along the margin are eyelashes and glands, which provide protection for the ocular surface. The *gray line* is an isolated section of pretarsal orbicularis muscle (Riolan) just anterior to the tarsus (Fig 9-24; also see Fig 9-14). The mucocutaneous junction is located posterior to the meibomian gland orifices on the eyelid margin. The horizontal palpebral fissure is approximately 30 mm long. The main portion of the margin, called the *ciliary margin,* has a rather well-defined anterior and posterior edge. Medial to the punctum and in the lateral quarter of the eyelid, the eyelid margin is thinner.

Eyelashes

There are approximately 100 eyelashes, or cilia, on the upper eyelid and 50 on the lower eyelid. The lashes originate in the anterior lamella of the eyelid margin just anterior to the tarsal plate, forming 2 or 3 irregular rows. A few cilia may be found in the caruncle.

Meibomian glands

The meibomian glands are sebaceous glands that contribute to the lipid layer of the tear film via modified holocrine secretion. They originate in the tarsus, numbering approximately 30–40 in the upper eyelid and 20 in the lower eyelid. During the second month of gestation, both the eyelashes and meibomian glands differentiate from a common pilosebaceous unit. This dual potentiality explains why, following trauma or chronic irritation, an eyelash follicle may develop from a meibomian gland *(acquired distichiasis)*. Similarly, an extra row of eyelashes arising from the meibomian orifices may be present from birth *(congenital distichiasis)*.

Vascular and lymphatic supply

The extensive vascularity of the eyelids promotes healing and helps defend against infection. The arterial supply of the eyelids comes from 2 main sources: (1) the internal carotid artery by way of the ophthalmic artery and its branches (supraorbital and lacrimal) and (2) the external carotid artery by way of the arteries of the face (angular and temporal). Collateral circulation between these 2 systems is extensive, anastomosing throughout the upper and lower eyelids and forming the marginal and peripheral arcades.

The *marginal arterial arcade* should not be confused with the peripheral arterial arcade. In the upper eyelid, the marginal arcade lies 2 mm superior to the margin, near the follicles of the cilia and anterior to the tarsal plate. The *peripheral arcade* lies superior to the tarsus, between the levator aponeurosis and the Müller muscle (see Figs 9-10, 9-20). The lower eyelid often has only 1 arterial arcade, located at the inferior tarsal border.

Eyelid venous drainage may be divided into a *preseptal* system, in which the preseptal tissues drain into the angular vein medially and into the superficial temporal vein laterally, and a *postseptal* system, in which drainage flows into the orbital veins and the deeper branches of the anterior facial vein and pterygoid plexus. Lymphatic vessels serving the medial portion of the eyelids typically drain into the submandibular lymph nodes. Lymphatic channels serving the lateral eyelids drain first into the superficial preauricular nodes and then into the deeper cervical nodes.

CHAPTER 10

Classification of Eyelid Disorders

Highlights

- The eyelids can be affected by congenital, acquired, infectious, inflammatory, and neoplastic conditions.
- The congenital ptosis seen in blepharophimosis syndrome typically requires frontalis suspension for adequate elevation.
- Epithelial hyperplasias, or papillomas, are the most common type of benign eyelid lesions.
- Targeted immune therapies for various cutaneous malignancies continue to evolve.
- Radiation therapy is not an acceptable primary treatment modality for sebaceous carcinoma.

Congenital Anomalies

Congenital anomalies of the eyelid may be isolated or associated with other eyelid, facial, or systemic anomalies. Careful evaluation of patients with hereditary syndromes is helpful before proceeding with treatment. Most congenital anomalies of the eyelids are rare and occur during the second month of gestation as a result of developmental arrest or failure of fusion. (See also BCSC Section 6, *Pediatric Ophthalmology and Strabismus.*)

Blepharophimosis–Ptosis–Epicanthus Inversus Syndrome

Blepharophimosis–ptosis–epicanthus inversus syndrome (BPES), also called *blepharophimosis syndrome,* is typically autosomal dominant in inheritance, although sporadic mutations can occur. Classic findings include

- blepharophimosis (profound shortening of the horizontal, and narrowing of the vertical, palpebral fissures)
- telecanthus (increased soft-tissue distance between the medial canthi)
- epicanthus inversus (fold of skin extending from the lower eyelid to the medial canthus)
- severe bilateral ptosis, often with poor levator function

The syndrome is caused by mutations in the *FOXL2* gene, located on chromosome 3. There are 2 types of BPES (types I and II), and both involve abnormalities of the eyelids.

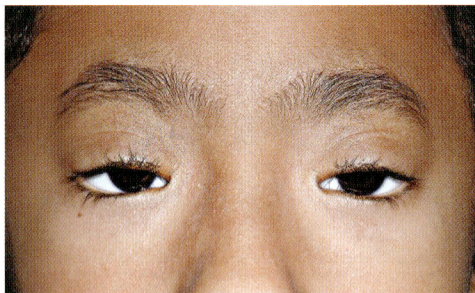

Figure 10-1 Patient with blepharophimosis–ptosis–epicanthus inversus syndrome (blepharophimosis syndrome). *(Courtesy of Cat N. Burkat, MD.)*

In addition to the characteristics listed above, findings may include lateral lower eyelid ectropion secondary to vertical eyelid deficiency, flat nasal bridge, superior orbital rim hypoplasia, ear deformities, high-arched eyebrows, and hypertelorism (Fig 10-1). Type I is also associated with premature ovarian failure, and infertility or reduced fertility in women.

Multiple surgeries may be required and are often performed in staged fashion. Medial canthal repositioning is typically addressed first with multiple Z-plasties (Fig 10-2) or with Y–V-plasties, sometimes combined with repositioning of the medial canthal tendons via transnasal wiring or suture fixation to a plate; however, horizontal traction on the upper eyelid may exacerbate the ptosis. Visually obstructive ptosis should be corrected promptly to avoid amblyopia; this procedure can be performed simultaneously with repair of the telecanthus. Additional surgeries may be necessary to address ectropion or orbital rim hypoplasia.

Congenital Ptosis of the Upper Eyelid

Congenital ptosis of the upper eyelid is discussed in Chapter 12.

Congenital Ectropion

Congenital ectropion rarely occurs as an isolated finding. It is more often associated with BPES, Down syndrome, or ichthyosis. Congenital ectropion is caused by a vertical insufficiency of the anterior lamella of the eyelid and may give rise to chronic epiphora and exposure keratitis. Mild congenital ectropion usually requires no treatment. If the condition is severe and symptomatic, surgical correction is similar to that used for cicatricial ectropion, with vertical lengthening of the anterior lamella with full-thickness skin grafting, and, frequently, horizontal tightening of the lateral canthal tendon.

Complete eversion of the upper eyelids occasionally occurs in newborns (Fig 10-3). Possible causes include anterior lamellar inflammation or shortage, inclusion conjunctivitis, and Down syndrome. Topical lubrication and short-term patching of both eyes may be curative. Full-thickness sutures or a temporary tarsorrhaphy is used when necessary, followed by definitive repair.

Euryblepharon

Euryblepharon is associated with both vertical shortening and horizontal lengthening of the lower eyelids and may be associated with BPES (Figs 10-4, 10-5). The lateral portion of the

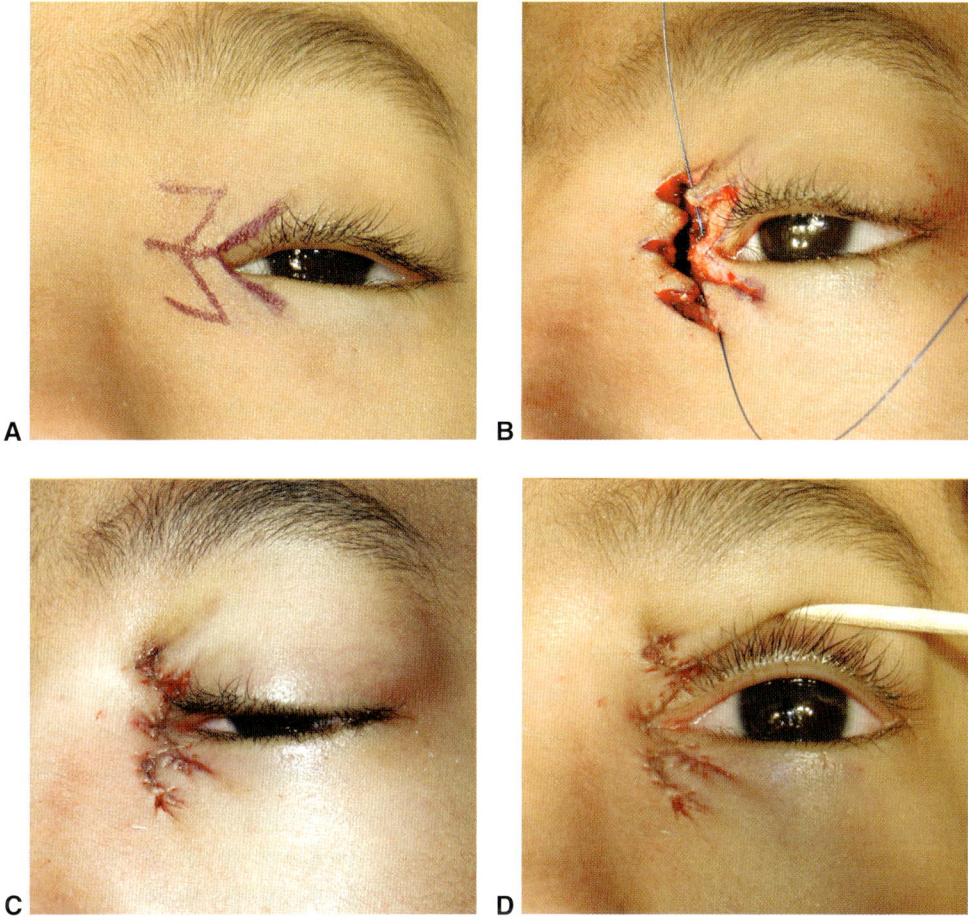

Figure 10-2 The 5-flap technique for blepharophimosis syndrome. **A,** The telecanthus is addressed with multiple Z-plasties or Y–V-plasties, marked along the epicanthal folds. **B,** After the flaps are elevated, the medial canthal tendon is repositioned with suture or transnasal wiring. **C,** The transposed flaps are sutured. **D,** Elevation of the upper eyelid demonstrates the improved medial canthal position and increased visibility of the medial sclera. *(Courtesy of Cat N. Burkat, MD.)*

eyelid is typically more involved than the medial aspect, and the palpebral fissure often has a downward slant due to an inferiorly displaced lateral canthal tendon. Impaired blinking and lagophthalmos may lead to exposure keratitis. If the condition causes symptoms, reconstruction may include lateral canthal repositioning along with suspension of the suborbicularis oculi fat to the lateral orbital rim to support the lower eyelid. If excess horizontal length is present, a lateral tarsal strip or eyelid margin resection may be required. Skin grafts may occasionally be necessary.

Ankyloblepharon

Ankyloblepharon is a partial *(ankyloblepharon filiforme adnatum)* or complete fusion of the eyelid margins (Fig 10-6). These webs of skin can usually be opened with scissors

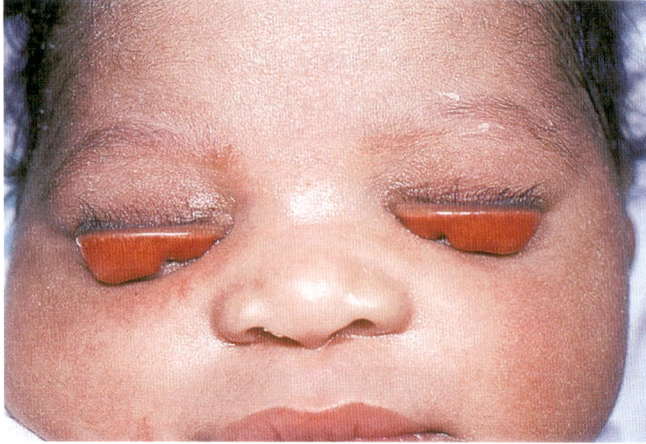

Figure 10-3   Congenital eyelid eversion. *(Courtesy of Thaddeus S. Nowinski, MD.)*

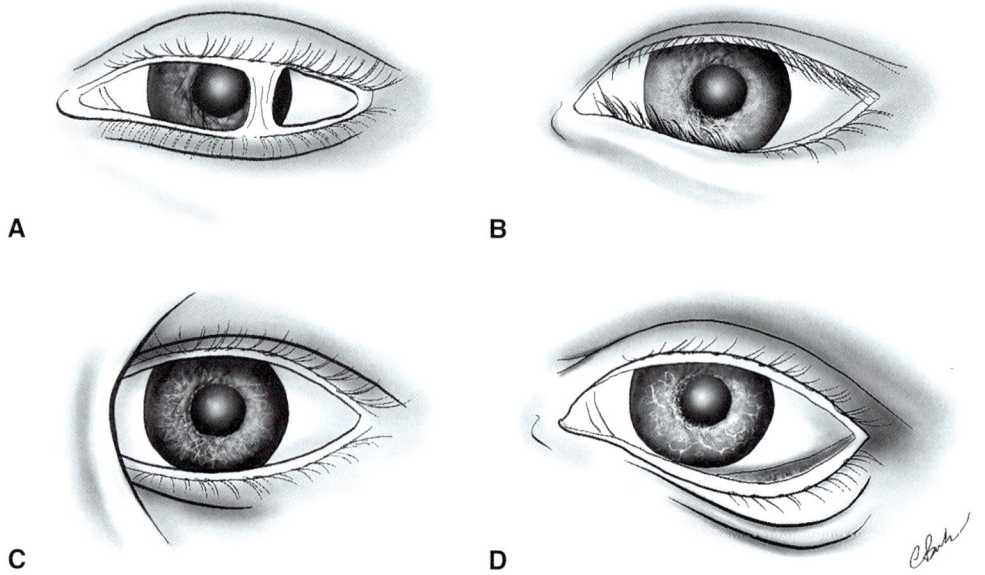

A

B

C

D

Figure 10-4   Congenital eyelid deformities. **A,** Ankyloblepharon. **B,** Epiblepharon. **C,** Epicanthus palpebralis. **D,** Euryblepharon. *(Illustration by Cat N. Burkat, MD.)*

after being clamped for a few seconds with a hemostat. In severe cases, underlying ocular abnormalities may exist.

Epicanthus

Epicanthus is a medial canthal fold that may result from immature midfacial bones or a fold of skin and subcutaneous tissue (see Fig 10-4C). The condition is usually bilateral, and an

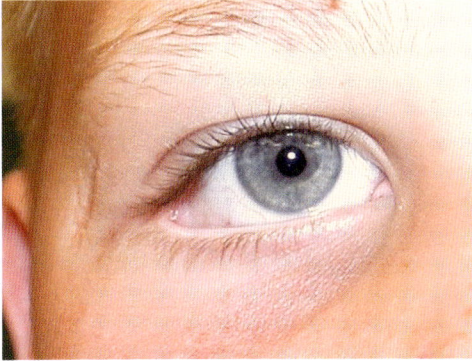

Figure 10-5 Patient with euryblepharon. *(Courtesy of Jill Foster, MD.)*

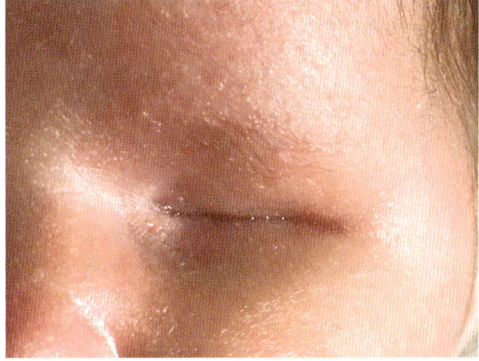

Figure 10-6 Newborn child with left ankyloblepharon. *(Courtesy of Cat N. Burkat, MD.)*

affected child may appear esotropic owing to decreased scleral exposure nasally *(pseudostrabismus)*. Traditionally, 4 types of epicanthus have been described:

- *epicanthus tarsalis,* in which the fold is most prominent in the upper eyelid
- *epicanthus inversus,* in which the fold is most prominent in the lower eyelid
- *epicanthus palpebralis,* in which the fold involves the upper and lower eyelids equally
- *epicanthus supraciliaris,* in which the fold extends from the eyebrow region to the lacrimal sac

Epicanthus tarsalis can be a normal variation of the Asian eyelid (Fig 10-7), whereas epicanthus inversus is often associated with BPES.

Most forms of epicanthus become less apparent with normal growth of the facial bones. If no associated eyelid anomalies are present, observation is recommended until the face achieves maturity. Epicanthus inversus, however, rarely resolves with facial growth. Most cases of isolated epicanthus requiring treatment are corrected by soft-tissue revisions such as Z-plasty or Y–V-plasty (Fig 10-8). Epicanthus tarsalis in an Asian patient may be eliminated by a Y–V-plasty with or without formation of an upper eyelid crease.

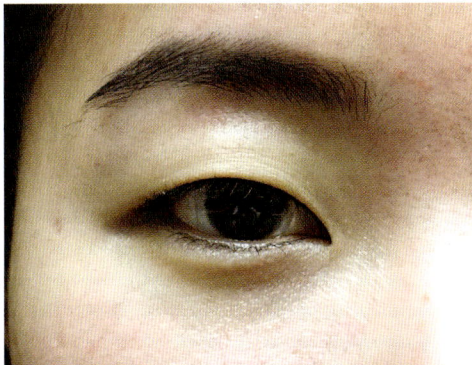

Figure 10-7 Epicanthus tarsalis. *(Courtesy of Cat N. Burkat, MD.)*

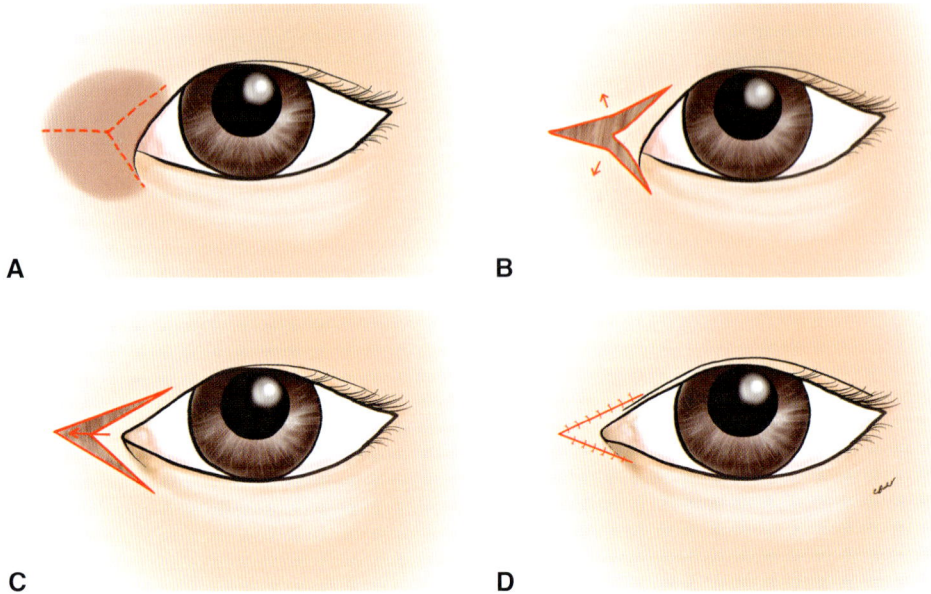

Figure 10-8 Epicanthus tarsalis Y-to-V repair. **A,** The letter "Y" is marked on the skin, with the stem placed horizontally inline with the medial canthal angle. The arms of the Y are marked along the edge of the epicanthal fold. **B,** The markings are incised and the shaded area undermined, which allows the tissue on both sides of the stem to recess into a "V" configuration. **C,** The skin at the center of the Y is advanced medially to meet the bottom of the stem. **D,** Final closure as a V shortens the epicanthal skin fold and exposes medial sclera. *(Illustration by Cat N. Burkat, MD.)*

Epiblepharon

Epiblepharon is most common in Asian children. In this condition, the lower eyelid pretarsal muscle and skin ride above the lower eyelid margin to form a horizontal fold of tissue, causing the cilia to assume a vertical position (Fig 10-9). Pathophysiologically, this condition results from a deficiency in the attachment of the lower eyelid retractors (capsulopalpebral fascia) to the skin.

The cilia often do not touch the cornea except in downgaze, and this rarely causes corneal staining. Epiblepharon may not require surgical treatment, as it tends to diminish with maturation of the facial bones. However, it occasionally results in acute or chronic corneal epithelial irritation; in that case, repair is performed by excision of

Figure 10-9 Bilateral lower eyelid epiblepharon with persistent corneal irritation. *(Courtesy of Cat N. Burkat, MD.)*

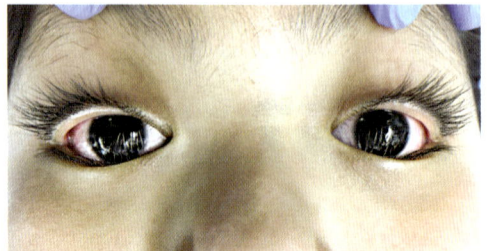

the excess skin and pretarsal orbicularis muscle combined with placement of marginal rotation sutures.

Woo KI, Kim YD. Management of epiblepharon: state of the art. *Curr Opin Ophthalmol.* 2016;27(5):433–438.

Congenital Entropion

In contrast to epiblepharon, eyelid margin inversion is present in congenital entropion. Developmental factors that lead to this rare condition include lower eyelid retractor dysgenesis, structural defects in the tarsal plate, and relative shortening of the posterior lamella. Unlike epiblepharon, congenital entropion is unlikely to improve spontaneously and may require surgical correction. Congenital entropion may be repaired by removing a small amount of the skin and orbicularis muscle along the subciliary portion of the eyelid, advancing the lower eyelid retractors to the tarsus, and lengthening the posterior lamella.

Tarsal kink (Fig 10-10) is an unusual form of congenital entropion in which the upper eyelid tarsal plate is folded, resulting in entropion. It may be repaired by removal of the kink in combination with a margin rotation. In some cases, skin grafting for the anterior lamella may be necessary.

Congenital Distichiasis

Distichiasis is a rare, sometimes hereditary condition in which an extra row of eyelashes is present in place of the meibomian gland orifices. Congenital distichiasis occurs when embryonic pilosebaceous units improperly differentiate into hair follicles (Fig 10-11). Treatment is indicated if the patient is symptomatic or if keratopathy develops. Lubricants and soft contact lenses may be sufficient; if not, electrolysis, radiofrequency ablation, and eyelid splitting with removal of the follicles are alternatives. Cryoepilation is used less often because of the risk of eyelid margin thinning or notching, eyelash loss, and skin hypopigmentation.

Congenital Coloboma

A *coloboma* is an embryologic cleft that is usually an isolated anomaly when it occurs in the medial upper eyelid. A true coloboma includes a defect in the eyelid margin (Fig 10-12).

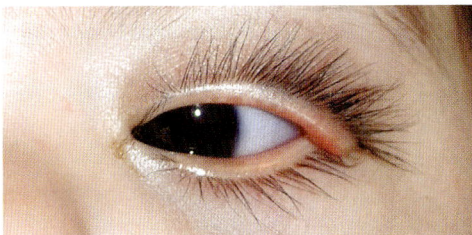

Figure 10-10 Congenital tarsal kink. *(Courtesy of Don O. Kikkawa, MD.)*

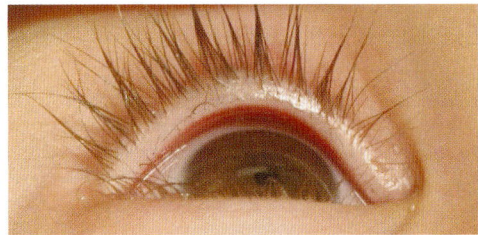

Figure 10-11 Congenital distichiasis. *(Courtesy of Jill Foster, MD.)*

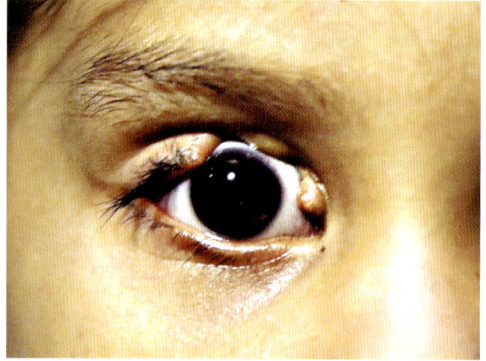

Figure 10-12 True coloboma of the upper eyelid. *(Courtesy of Cat N. Burkat, MD.)*

When located in the lower eyelid, however, a coloboma is frequently associated with other congenital conditions such as facial clefts (eg, Goldenhar syndrome) and lacrimal deformities.

Full-thickness defects affecting up to one-third of the eyelid can usually be repaired by creating raw vertical margins and sliding flaps along the eyelid crease. A lateral cantholysis may provide additional horizontal relaxation. Almost all large defects can be repaired with use of a variation of the lateral canthal semicircular flap technique (see Chapter 11 in this volume). Because of the risk of amblyopia, eyelid-sharing procedures that occlude the visual axis are avoided unless no other reconstructive options are possible.

Cryptophthalmos

Cryptophthalmos is a rare condition that presents with partial (Fig 10-13A) or complete (Fig 10-13B) absence of the eyebrow, palpebral fissure, eyelashes, and conjunctiva. The partially developed adnexa are fused to the anterior segment of the globe. Cryptophthalmos may be unilateral or bilateral. Histologically, the orbicularis oculi, levator muscle, tarsus, conjunctiva, and meibomian glands are attenuated or absent; thus, attempts at reconstruction are difficult. Severe ocular defects are present in the underlying eye, which can be microphthalmic or associated with an orbital cyst.

Congenital Eyelid Lesions: Infantile (Capillary) Hemangioma

Although infantile (capillary) hemangiomas sometimes occur as congenital eyelid lesions, most are not apparent at birth. In the typical natural course, the lesion usually develops within a few weeks or months after birth, increases in size over the first year, and gradually involutes over the next 3–7 years. Hemangiomas may also involve the orbit (see the section Vascular Tumors, Malformations, and Fistulas in Chapter 5 of this volume).

Management

Hemangiomas are associated with a high incidence of amblyopia; therefore, treatment is recommended for patients who present with occlusion of the visual axis, anisometropia, or strabismus, as well as for lesions causing significant disfigurement. Lesions limited to

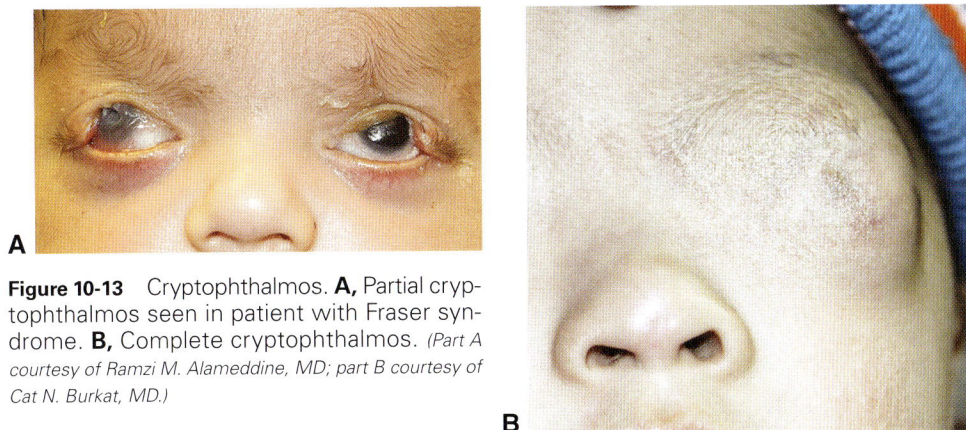

Figure 10-13 Cryptophthalmos. **A,** Partial cryptophthalmos seen in patient with Fraser syndrome. **B,** Complete cryptophthalmos. *(Part A courtesy of Ramzi M. Alameddine, MD; part B courtesy of Cat N. Burkat, MD.)*

the eyelid may be treated with topical timolol gel or intralesional steroids. Topical timolol gel appears to have minimal adverse effects. If vision is threatened or if there is more widespread or deeper orbital involvement, systemic propranolol or oral corticosteroids are typically required.

For patients who cannot take β-blockers or do not respond to timolol, intralesional steroids are considered. Intralesional steroids, which may act by rendering the tumor's vascular bed more sensitive to the body's circulating catecholamines, are relatively safe and effective. However, rare cases of eyelid necrosis, fat atrophy, embolic retinal vascular occlusion, and systemic adrenal suppression may occur after even a single injection. Although treatment with systemic steroids eliminates the risks of eyelid necrosis and vascular emboli, the dosage and risk of systemic adverse effects are increased.

Other treatment options may be considered for vision-compromising lesions that persist despite intervention. Topical treatment with clobetasol propionate has been reported to successfully shrink eyelid hemangiomas. Compared with oral or intralesional steroids, the topical route reduces, although does not eliminate, the risk of systemic exposure. Interferon-alfa is reserved for life-threatening or sight-threatening lesions unresponsive to other forms of treatment because of the risk of serious adverse effects. Surgical excision may be used for rare well-circumscribed lesions, but it requires meticulous control of hemostasis. Use of the carbon dioxide laser as an incisional device is helpful for controlling bleeding during removal of a lesion. Topical cutaneous lasers may be used on the superficial (1–2 mm) layers of the skin to diminish the redness of a lesion, but they do not penetrate deeply enough to shrink a visually disabling lesion.

Acquired Eyelid Disorders

Chalazion

A chalazion *(internal posterior hordeolum)* is a focal inflammation of the eyelids that results from an obstruction of the meibomian glands (Fig 10-14). This common disorder is

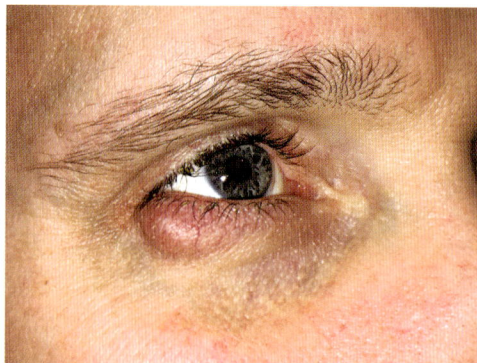

Figure 10-14 Chalazion on the right lower eyelid. *(Courtesy of Cat N. Burkat, MD.)*

often associated with rosacea and chronic blepharitis and may occasionally be confused with a malignant neoplasm.

The *meibomian glands* are oil-producing sebaceous glands located in the tarsal plate. The oil is an essential component of the tear film. If the gland orifices on the eyelid margin become plugged, the contents of the glands *(sebum)* are released into the tarsus and the surrounding eyelid soft tissue, eliciting an acute inflammatory response accompanied by pain and erythema. The exact role of bacterial agents (most commonly *Staphylococcus aureus*) in the production of chalazia is not clear. Histologically, these lesions are characterized by chronic lipogranulomatous inflammation.

Management

In the acute inflammatory phase, treatment consists of warm compresses and appropriate eyelid hygiene. Topical antibiotic or anti-inflammatory ocular medications may also be helpful. Acute secondary infection may be treated with an antibiotic directed at skin flora. Oral doxycycline, tetracycline, and azithromycin are commonly used, but there is insufficient supporting evidence from clinical studies. Tetracyclines and azithromycin have been shown in both in vitro and in vivo studies to modulate the expression of inflammatory mediators (matrix metalloproteinases, collagen production, interleukin-1, nitric oxide, and activated B cells), inhibiting bacterial lipase production and thereby improving the tear film balance. However, these medications are contraindicated in children and during pregnancy, and they require prolonged use that can be associated with allergy, gastrointestinal distress, photosensitivity, poor compliance, and multidrug resistance.

Occasionally, chronic, persistent chalazia require surgical management. In most cases, the greatest inflammatory response is on the posterior eyelid, and an incision through tarsus and conjunctiva is appropriate for drainage. Sharp dissection, curettage, and excision of all necrotic material, including the cyst wall, are indicated (Fig 10-15). This procedure results in a posterior marsupialization of the chalazion. Caution is required when removing inflammatory tissue at the eyelid margin or adjacent to the punctum. In rare cases, the inflammatory response is more severe on the anterior eyelid;

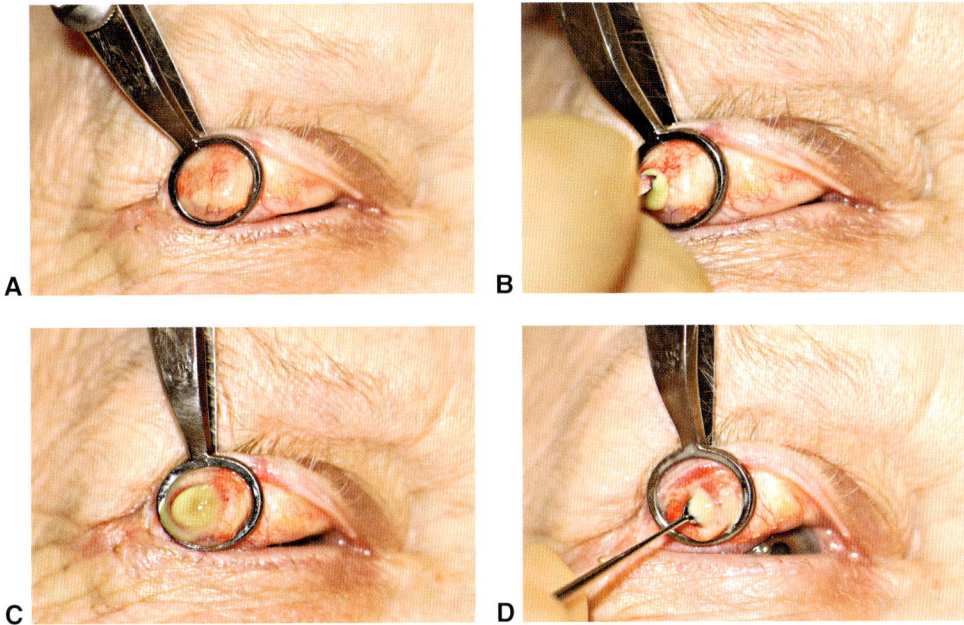

Figure 10-15 Incision and curettage of chalazion. **A,** The chalazion clamp is centered over the lesion and the eyelid everted. **B,** A number 11 blade scalpel is used to incise the tarsus vertically, stopping several millimeters from the eyelid margin. **C,** Lipogranulomatous material is drained. **D,** A curette can further remove the contents and excess fibrotic tissue or capsule can be excised. *(Courtesy of Cat N. Burkat, MD.)*

in such cases, a skin incision is used. Given the risk of masquerade conditions, including sebaceous cell carcinoma, pathologic examination is appropriate for atypical or recurrent chalazia.

Local intralesional injection of corticosteroids is sometimes employed as a less invasive option, but it can cause skin depigmentation and is less effective than surgical treatment. The combination of excision and steroid injection yields a 95% resolution rate.

Wladis EJ, Bradley EA, Bilyk JR, Yen MT, Mawn LA. Oral antibiotics for meibomian gland-related ocular surface disease: a report by the American Academy of Ophthalmology. *Ophthalmology.* 2016;123(3):492–496.

Hordeolum

An acute infection (usually staphylococcal) can involve the sebaceous secretions in the glands of Zeis *(external hordeolum,* or *stye)* or the meibomian glands *(internal hordeolum).* In the case of external hordeola, the infection may appear to center around an eyelash follicle, and the eyelash can be epilated to promote drainage (Fig 10-16). Most hordeola resolve spontaneously, but diligent application of hot compresses and topical antibiotic ointment may be helpful. In rare cases, hordeola may progress to superficial cellulitis, or

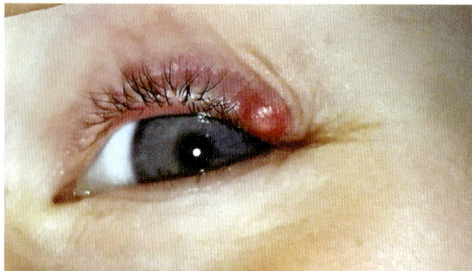

Figure 10-16 Hordeolum of the left upper eyelid. *(Courtesy of Cat N. Burkat, MD.)*

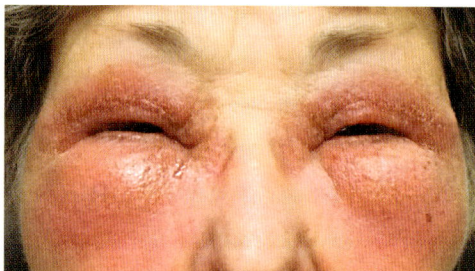

Figure 10-17 Eyelid swelling caused by allergy to ophthalmic ointment. *(Courtesy of Cat N. Burkat, MD.)*

even abscesses, of the eyelid. In such cases, systemic antibiotic therapy and possible surgical incision and drainage may be required.

Eyelid Edema

Eyelid swelling can be caused by local conditions, such as insect bites or allergy (Fig 10-17), or systemic conditions, such as cardiovascular disease, renal disease, thyroid eye disease, and collagen vascular disease. Cerebrospinal fluid leakage into the orbit and eyelids after trauma may mimic eyelid edema. Lymphedema may occur if the lymphatic drainage system from the eyelid is disrupted, such as after extensive lymph node dissection of the neck (Fig 10-18).

Floppy Eyelid Syndrome

Floppy eyelid syndrome is characterized by ocular irritation, redness, eyelash ptosis, loss of eyelash parallelism, and mild mucus discharge that is frequently worse on

Figure 10-18 Right periocular lymphedema after neck lymph node dissection. *(Courtesy of Cat N. Burkat, MD.)*

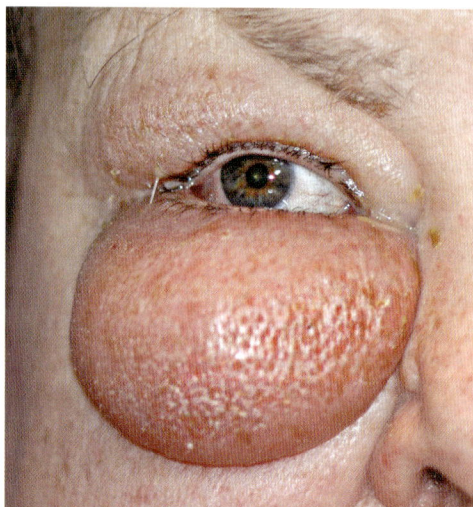

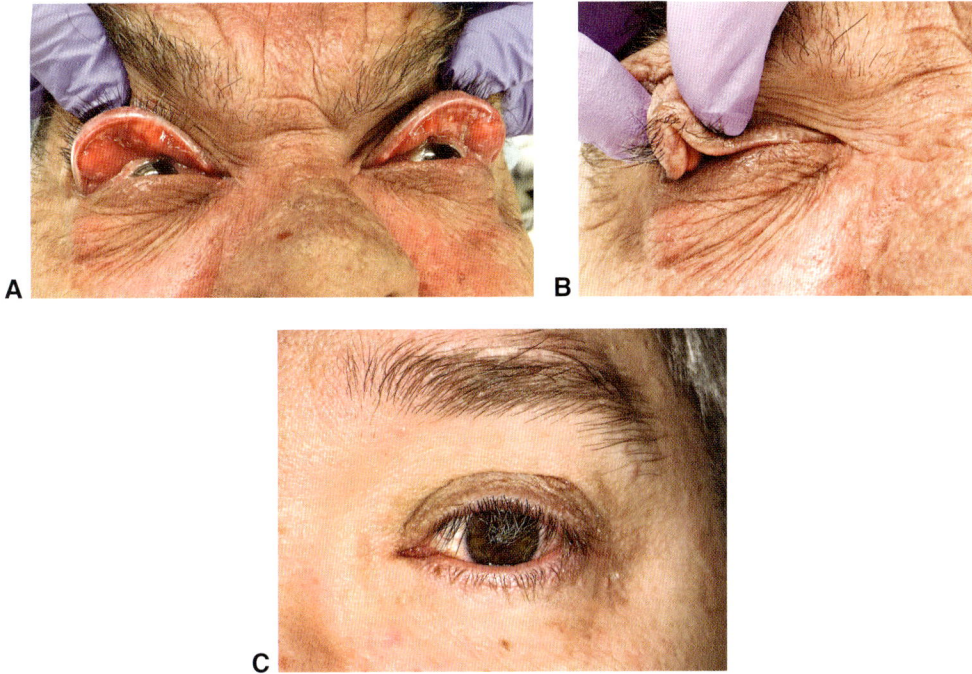

Figure 10-19 Floppy eyelid syndrome. **A,** Easily everted upper eyelids. **B,** Flaccid upper eyelid tone. **C,** Eyelash ptosis. *(Courtesy of Cat N. Burkat, MD.)*

awakening (Fig 10-19). Patients have chronic papillary conjunctivitis and a superior tarsal plate that is rubbery, flaccid, and easily everted. Histologic examination has demonstrated a marked decrease in the number of elastin fibers within the tarsus. During examination, the lax upper eyelid everts spontaneously, especially laterally, when pulled up toward the forehead. Patients often report sleeping in a prone position, which can cause mechanical upper eyelid eversion, with the superior palpebral conjunctiva rubbing against the pillow or bedding. Associations have been reported with obesity, sleep apnea, keratoconus, eyelid rubbing, and hyperglycemia. Sleep studies are recommended to rule out sleep apnea.

Initial conservative treatment consists of viscous lubrication and a patch or shield at night. Surgical correction, if warranted, consists of wedge resection and horizontal eyelid tightening. If the patient has been diagnosed with sleep apnea, use of a continuous positive airway pressure device may reduce prone position sleeping and minimize recurrence after surgical correction.

Ezra DG, Beaconsfield M, Sira M, et al. Long-term outcomes of surgical approaches to the treatment of floppy eyelid syndrome. *Ophthalmology.* 2010;117(4):839–846.

Eyelid Imbrication Syndrome

Eyelid imbrication syndrome occurs when a lax upper eyelid with a normal tarsal plate overrides the lower eyelid margin during closure; this results in chronic mechanical

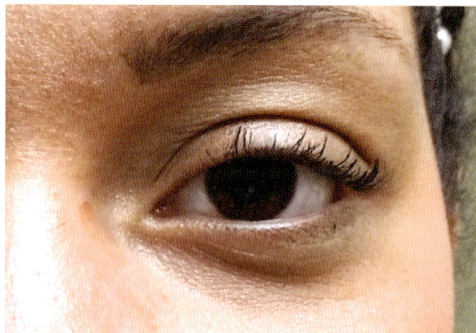

Figure 10-20 Trichotillomania, with character-istic finding of eyelashes of multiple different lengths. *(Courtesy of Cat N. Burkat, MD.)*

conjunctivitis. Management consists of topical lubrication in mild cases. In more severe cases, horizontal tightening of the upper eyelid is indicated.

Trichotillomania

Trichotillomania is an impulse-control disorder most commonly seen in preteen or teen-aged girls. It is characterized by the repeated desire to pull out hairs, frequently eyebrows or eyelashes. Diagnosis may be elusive, as affected patients usually deny the behavior; therefore, parental counseling or psychiatric consultation may be indicated. Characteristically, mul-tiple hairs are broken off and regrow at different lengths, a finding that guides the diagnosis (Fig 10-20).

Eyelid Neoplasms

Numerous benign and malignant cutaneous neoplasms can develop in the periocular skin, arising from the epidermis, dermis, or eyelid adnexal structures. Most lesions, whether be-nign or malignant, develop from the epidermis, the rapidly growing superficial layer of the skin. Although many of these lesions also occur elsewhere on the body, their appearance and behavior in the eyelids may be unique owing to the particular characteristics of eyelid skin and the specialized adnexal elements. The malignant lesions that most frequently affect the eyelids are basal cell carcinoma, squamous cell carcinoma, sebaceous cell carcinoma, and melanoma. Histologic examination of suspected cutaneous malignancies is recommended.

Clinical Evaluation of Eyelid Tumors

The history and physical examination of eyelid lesions offer important clues regarding the likelihood of malignancy. Predisposing factors in the development of skin cancer include

- a history of prior skin cancer
- excessive sun exposure, especially blistering sunburn
- previous radiation therapy
- a history of smoking
- Celtic or Scandinavian ancestry, with fair skin, red hair, and blue eyes
- immunosuppression

Signs suggesting malignancy are

- ulceration or chronic, nonhealing lesion
- bleeding, crusting, drainage
- destruction of normal eyelid margin architecture (especially meibomian orifices)
- loss of cilia *(madarosis)*
- heaped-up, pearly, translucent margins with central ulceration
- fine telangiectasias
- pigmentary changes
- loss of fine cutaneous wrinkles or vellus hair

Lesions near the puncta should be evaluated for punctal or canalicular involvement. Probing and irrigation may be required to exclude lacrimal system involvement or to prepare for surgical reconstruction.

Palpable induration extending beyond visibly apparent margins suggests tumor infiltration into the dermis and subcutaneous tissue. Large lesions should be assessed for evidence of fixation to deeper tissues or bone. In addition, regional lymph nodes should be palpated for evidence of metastases in cases of suspected squamous cell carcinoma, sebaceous cell carcinoma, melanoma, or Merkel cell carcinoma. Lymphatic tumor spread may produce rubbery swelling along the jawline or in front of the ear. Restriction of ocular motility and proptosis suggest orbital extension. Assessment of the function of cranial nerves V and VII can reveal deficiencies that may indicate perineural tumor spread. Perineural invasion is a characteristic of squamous cell carcinoma. Systemic evidence of liver, pulmonary, bone, or neurologic involvement should be sought in cases of sebaceous adenocarcinoma or melanoma of the eyelid. It is important to obtain photographs and measurements prior to treatment of the lesion.

For more extensive coverage, including additional clinical and pathology photographs, see BCSC Section 4, *Ophthalmic Pathology and Intraocular Tumors.*

> de la Garza AG, Kersten RC, Carter KD. Evaluation and treatment of benign eyelid lesions. *Focal Points: Clinical Modules for Ophthalmologists.* San Francisco: American Academy of Ophthalmology; 2010, module 5.

Benign Eyelid Lesions

Epithelial hyperplasias

The terminology used to describe benign epithelial proliferations, the most common type of benign eyelid lesions, continues to evolve. It is helpful to group these various benign epithelial proliferations under the clinical heading of *papillomas.* (This designation does not necessarily imply any association with the papillomavirus.) Clinical and histologic characterizations of these lesions overlap considerably. Included within this group are seborrheic keratosis, pseudoepitheliomatous hyperplasia, verruca vulgaris (wart), acrochordon (also called skin tag, fibroepithelial polyp, or squamous papilloma) (Fig 10-21), basosquamous acanthoma, squamous acanthoma, and many others. All of these benign proliferations can be managed with shave excision at the dermal–epidermal junction.

Seborrheic keratosis (Fig 10-22) is an example of an acquired benign eyelid papilloma that tends to affect middle-aged and elderly persons. Its clinical appearance varies; it may

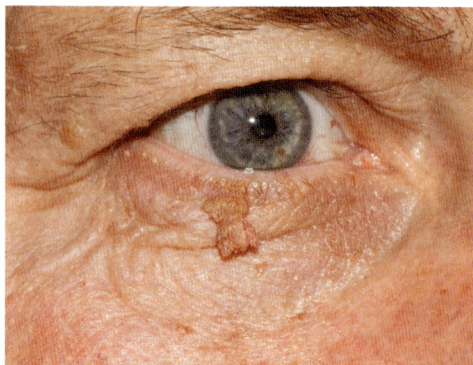

Figure 10-21 Acrochordon (also known as skin tag, fibroepithelial polyp, or squamous papilloma) of the right lower eyelid. *(Courtesy of Bobby S. Korn, MD, PhD.)*

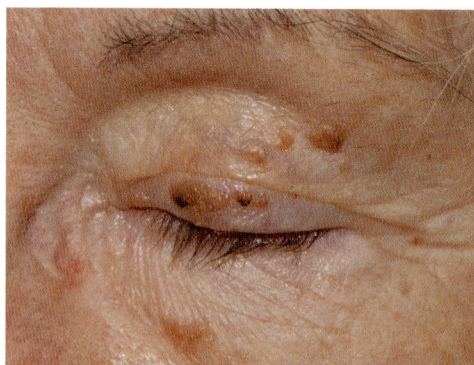

Figure 10-22 Seborrheic keratosis of the left upper eyelid. *(Courtesy of Bobby S. Korn, MD, PhD.)*

be sessile or pedunculated and have varying degrees of pigmentation and hyperkeratosis. On facial skin, seborrheic keratosis typically appears as a smooth, greasy, stuck-on lesion. On the thinner eyelid skin, however, it can be more lobulated, papillary, or pedunculated, with visible excrescences on its surface. These lesions can be managed by shave excision. A seborrheic keratosis involving a hair follicle, called an *irritated follicular keratosis,* may be more elevated and nodular (Fig 10-23) and can be confused with a keratoacanthoma or squamous cell carcinoma.

Pseudoepitheliomatous hyperplasia is not a discrete lesion but rather a pattern of reactive changes in the epidermis that may develop over areas of inflammation or neoplasia.

Verruca vulgaris (wart), caused by epidermal infection with the human papillomavirus (type 6 or 11), rarely occurs in thin eyelid skin (Fig 10-24). Cryotherapy or excision may eradicate the lesion and minimize the risk of viral spread.

Cutaneous horn is a descriptive, nondiagnostic term referring to *exuberant hyperkeratosis.* This lesion may be associated with various benign or malignant histologic processes,

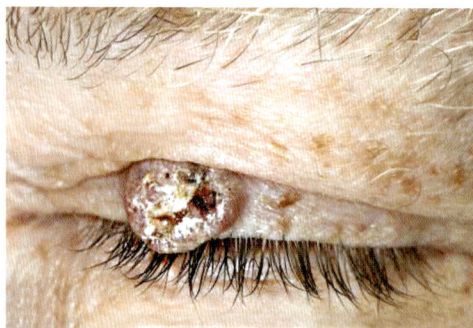

Figure 10-23 Follicular keratosis of the left upper eyelid. *(Courtesy of Cat N. Burkat, MD.)*

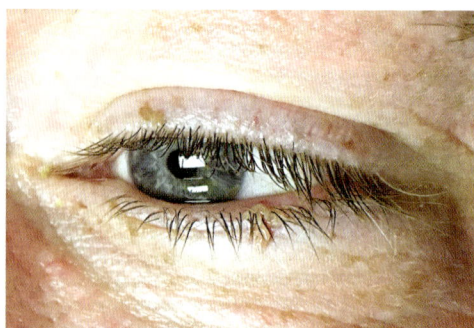

Figure 10-24 Verruca vulgaris (wart) of the left lower eyelid. *(Courtesy of Cat N. Burkat, MD.)*

including seborrheic keratosis, verruca vulgaris, and squamous or basal cell carcinoma. Biopsy of the base of the cutaneous horn is recommended.

Benign epithelial lesions

After papillomas, cysts of the epidermis are the second most common type of benign periocular cutaneous lesions, accounting for approximately 18% of excised benign lesions. Most of these are *epidermal inclusion cysts,* which arise from the infundibulum of the hair follicle, either spontaneously or following traumatic implantation of epidermal tissue into the dermis (Fig 10-25). The lesions are slow growing, elevated, round, and smooth. They often have a central pore, indicating the remaining pilar duct. Although these cysts are often called *sebaceous cysts,* they are actually filled with keratin. Rupture of the cyst wall may cause an inflammatory foreign-body reaction. The cysts may also become secondarily infected.

Recommended treatment for small cysts is excision or marsupialization, which involves excising around the periphery of the cyst but leaving the base of the cyst wall to serve as the new surface epithelium. Larger or deeper cysts may require complete excision, in which case the cyst wall should be removed intact to reduce the possibility of recurrence.

Multiple tiny epidermal inclusion cysts are called *milia* (Fig 10-26). They are particularly common in newborn infants. Generally, milia resolve spontaneously, but they may be marsupialized with a sharp blade or needle. Multiple confluent milia may be treated with topical retinoic acid cream.

A less common epidermal cyst is the *pilar,* or *trichilemmal, cyst.* Such cysts are clinically indistinguishable from epidermal inclusion cysts, but they tend to occur in areas containing large and numerous hair follicles. Approximately 90% of pilar cysts occur on the scalp; in the periocular region, they are generally found in the eyebrows. The cysts are filled with desquamated epithelium, and calcification occurs in approximately 25% of cases.

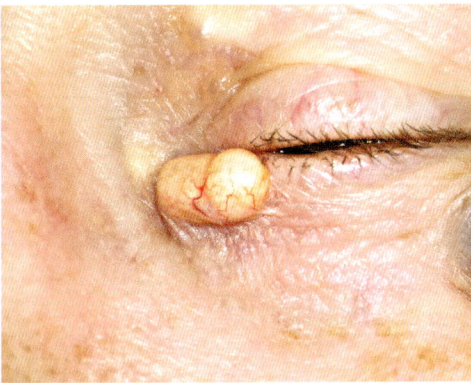

Figure 10-25 Epidermal inclusion cyst of the left lower eyelid. *(Courtesy of Cat N. Burkat, MD.)*

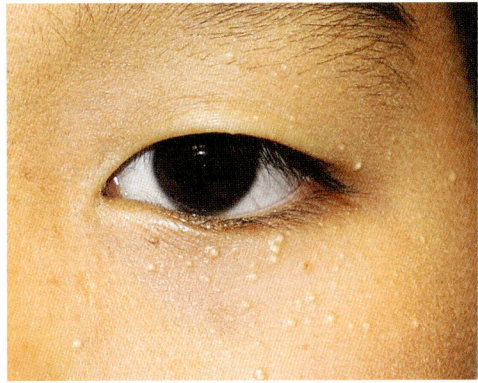

Figure 10-26 Milia of the left upper and lower eyelid. *(Courtesy of Bobby S. Korn, MD, PhD.)*

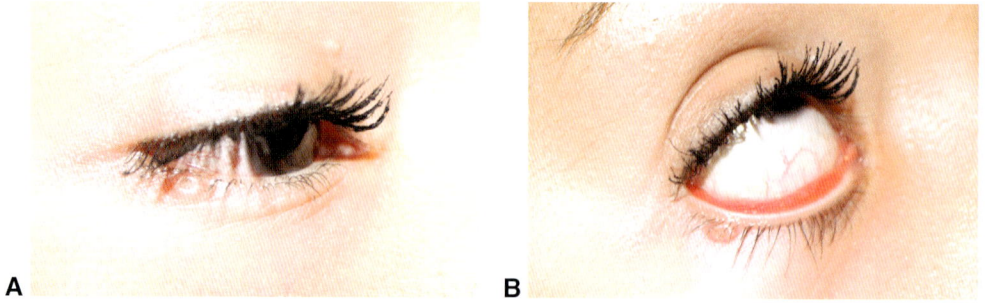

Figure 10-27 Molluscum contagiosum. **A,** Umbilicated eyelid lesion. **B,** Molluscum lesions can cause conjunctivitis, which typically resolves after removal of the lesion. *(Courtesy of Vikram Durairaj, MD.)*

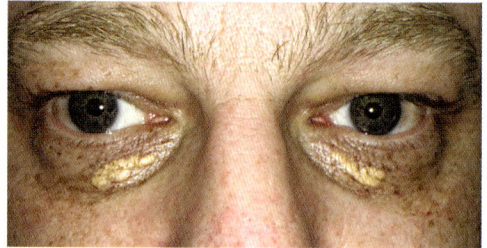

Figure 10-28 Xanthelasmas of the lower eyelids. *(Courtesy of Cat N. Burkat, MD.)*

Molluscum contagiosum is a viral infection of the epidermis that often involves the eyelid in children with an associated follicular conjunctivitis (Fig 10-27). Occasionally, multiple exuberant lesions appear in adult patients with AIDS. The lesions are characteristically waxy and nodular, with a central umbilication. They may produce an associated follicular conjunctivitis. Treatment is observation, oral cimetadine, excision, controlled cryotherapy, or curettage.

Xanthelasmas are yellowish plaques that occur commonly in the medial canthal areas of the upper and lower eyelids (Fig 10-28). They represent lipid-laden macrophages in the superficial dermis and subdermal tissues. Deep extension into the orbicularis oculi muscle can occur. In rare instances, xanthelasmas are associated with hyperlipidemia or congenital disorders of lipid metabolism, so patients whose lipid levels are unknown may benefit from having them checked by their primary care physician. When excising these lesions, the surgeon must be careful to avoid causing cicatricial ectropion or eyelid retraction. Other treatment options include serial excision, laser ablation, and topical trichloroacetic acid. Xanthelasmas may commonly recur after excision.

Benign Adnexal Lesions

In this context, the term *adnexa* refers to skin appendages that are located within the dermis but communicate through the epidermis to the surface. They include oil glands, sweat glands, and hair follicles. The eyelids contain both the specialized eyelashes and the normal vellus hairs found on skin throughout the body. Periocular adnexal oil glands include

- the *meibomian glands* within the tarsal plate
- the *glands of Zeis,* associated with eyelash follicles
- normal *sebaceous glands* that are present as part of the pilosebaceous units in the skin hair

Sweat glands in the periocular region include the *eccrine sweat glands,* which have a general distribution throughout the body and are responsible for thermal regulation, and the ciliary glands with apocrine secretion (the *glands of Moll*), which are located in the eyelid margin.

Lesions of oil gland origin

Chalazion and hordeolum These common eyelid lesions are discussed earlier in this chapter in the section Acquired Eyelid Disorders.

Sebaceous hyperplasia Sebaceous gland hyperplasia presents as multiple small yellow papules that may have central umbilication (Fig 10-29). They tend to occur on the forehead and cheeks and are common in patients older than 40 years. These lesions are sometimes mistaken for basal cell carcinoma because they may have central umbilication and fine telangiectasias. Patients with multiple acquired sebaceous gland adenomas, adenomatoid sebaceous hyperplasia, or basal cell carcinomas with sebaceous differentiation have an increased incidence of visceral malignancy *(Muir-Torre syndrome [MTS])* and should be evaluated accordingly.

Sebaceous adenoma This rare tumor appears as a yellowish papule on the face, scalp, or trunk and may mimic a basal cell carcinoma or seborrheic keratosis. As noted above, sebaceous adenoma may be associated with MTS.

Tumors of eccrine sweat gland origin

Eccrine hidrocystoma Eccrine hidrocystomas are common cystic lesions 1–3 mm in diameter that occur in groups and tend to cluster around the lower eyelids and canthi and on the face. They are considered to be ductal retention cysts, and they often enlarge in conditions such as heat and increased humidity, which stimulate perspiration. Treatment consists of surgical excision.

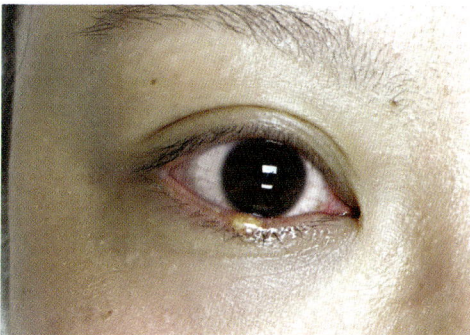

Figure 10-29 Sebaceous hyperplasia of the right lower eyelid. *(Courtesy of Cat N. Burkat, MD.)*

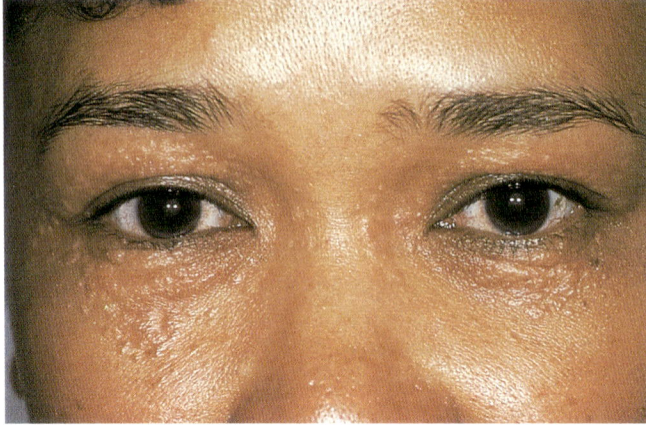

Figure 10-30 Syringomas. *(Courtesy of Robert C. Kersten, MD.)*

Syringoma Benign eccrine sweat gland tumors found commonly in young females, syringomas present as multiple small, waxy, elevated nodules 1–2 mm in diameter on the lower eyelids (Fig 10-30). Syringomas can also be found in the axilla and sternal region. They become more apparent during puberty. Because the eccrine glands are located within the dermis, these lesions are too deep to allow shave excision. Removal requires complete surgical excision.

A less common variant, *chondroid syringoma,* occurs most commonly in middle-aged men and can enlarge to 3 cm. It is composed of sweat gland components within a mixed cartilaginous stroma.

Pleomorphic adenoma This rare benign tumor occurs most commonly in the head and neck region and may involve the eyelids (Fig 10-31). Histologically, the tumor is identical to pleomorphic adenoma of the salivary and lacrimal glands (discussed in Chapter 5). Treatment is complete surgical excision.

Figure 10-31 Pleomorphic adenoma (benign mixed tumor) of the left eyebrow. *(Courtesy of Bobby S. Korn, MD, PhD.)*

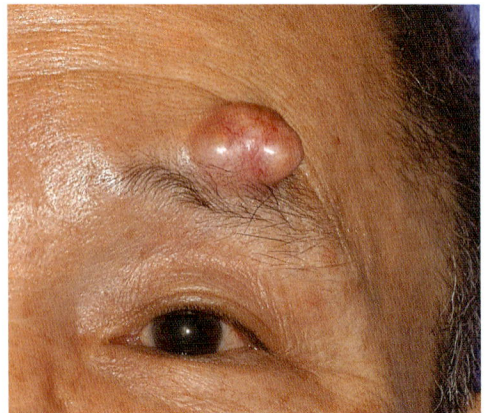

Tumors of apocrine sweat gland origin

Apocrine hidrocystoma A very common, smooth cyst arising from the glands of Moll along the eyelid margin, apocrine hidrocystoma is considered to be an adenoma of the secretory cells of Moll rather than a retention cyst (Fig 10-32). These lesions are typically translucent or bluish, and they transilluminate. They may be multiple and often extend deep beneath the surface, especially in the canthal regions. Treatment for superficial cysts is marsupialization. Deep cysts require complete excision of the cyst wall.

Cylindroma Cylindromas *(eccrine spiradenomas)* are rare tumors that can be solitary or multiple and may be dominantly inherited. Lesions are dome-shaped, smooth, flesh-colored nodules of varying size that tend to affect the scalp and face (Fig 10-33). They may occur so profusely in the scalp that it is entirely covered with lesions, in which case they are called *turban tumors.* Treatment is surgical excision, which may be difficult if multiple lesions involve a large surface area.

Tumors of hair follicle origin

Several rare benign lesions may arise from the eyelashes, eyebrows, or vellus hairs in the periocular region.

Trichoepithelioma These lesions are small, flesh-colored papules with occasional telan-giectasias that occur on the eyelids (Fig 10-34) or forehead. Histologically, trichoepithe-liomas appear as basaloid islands and keratin cysts with immature hair follicle structures. If keratin is abundant, these lesions may clinically resemble an epidermal inclusion cyst. The individual histologic picture may be difficult to differentiate from that of basal cell carcinoma. Simple excision is curative.

Trichofolliculoma A trichofolliculoma is a single, sometimes umbilicated lesion found mainly in adults. Histologically, it represents a squamous cystic structure containing kera-tin and hair shaft components (Fig 10-35).

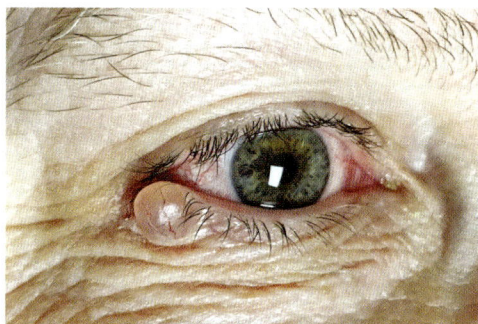

Figure 10-32 Apocrine hidrocystoma of the right lower eyelid. *(Courtesy of Cat N. Burkat, MD.)*

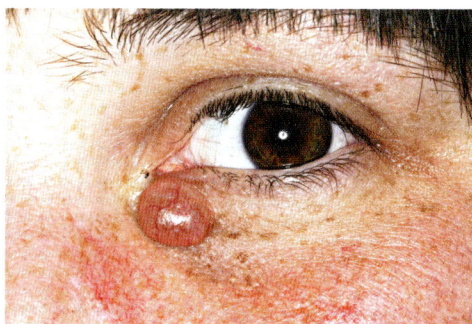

Figure 10-33 Cylindroma (eccrine spiradenoma) of the left lower eyelid. *(Courtesy of Stephen R. Klapper, MD.)*

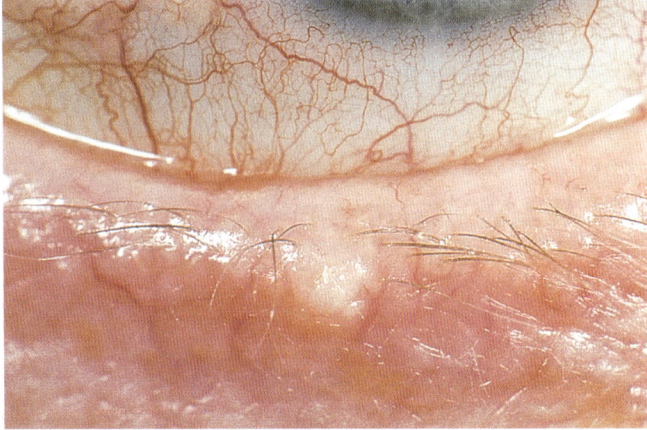

Figure 10-34 Trichoepithelioma. *(Courtesy of Jeffrey A. Nerad, MD.)*

Figure 10-35 Trichofolliculoma of the right upper eyelid. *(Courtesy of Cat N. Burkat, MD.)*

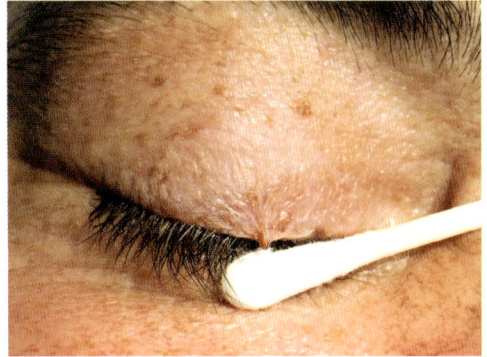

Trichilemmoma Another type of solitary lesion that occurs predominantly in adults, trichilemmomas resemble verrucae. Histologically, they show glycogen-rich cells oriented around hair follicles.

Pilomatricoma Also known as *pilomatrixoma,* this lesion most often affects children and young adults. It usually occurs in the eyebrow and central upper eyelid as a nontender, reddish purple subcutaneous mass attached to the overlying skin (Fig 10-36). Pilomatricomas may become quite large, measuring up to 5 cm or more. The tumor is composed of islands of epithelial cells surrounded by basophilic cells with shadow cells. Multiple lesions or familial cases may be associated with Gardner syndrome, familial adenomatous polyposis, Turner syndrome, myotonic dystrophy, and Rubinstein-Taybi syndrome. Excision is usually curative, and recurrence is rare.

Benign Melanocytic Lesions

Melanocytic lesions of the skin arise from 3 sources: nevus cells, dermal melanocytes, and epidermal melanocytes. Virtually any benign or malignant lesion may be pigmented, and

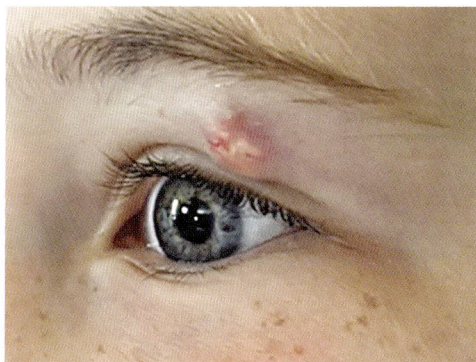

Figure 10-36 Pilomatricoma of the left upper eyelid. *(Courtesy of Cat N. Burkat, MD.)*

lesions of melanocytic origin do not necessarily have visible pigmentation. For example, seborrheic keratoses are frequently pigmented, and basal cell carcinomas are occasionally pigmented, especially if they arise in persons with darker skin. In contrast, dermal nevi typically have no pigmentation in white individuals. Melanocytes are normally found distributed at the dermal–epidermal junction throughout the skin. Nevus cells are similar to melanocytes in that both produce melanin, but nevus cells are arranged in clusters and nests, and they lack dendritic processes (except for blue nevus cells). Both nevus cells and melanocytes give rise to several types of benign lesions (Table 10-1). In addition to the individual lesions described in the following paragraphs, diffuse eyelid skin hyperpigmentation called *melasma,* or *chloasma,* can occur in women who are pregnant or using oral contraceptives; in families with an autosomal dominant trait; and in patients with chronic atopic eczema, rosacea, and other inflammatory dermatoses.

Nevi

Nevi are the third most common benign lesions encountered in the periocular region (after papillomas and epidermal inclusion cysts). They arise from *nevus cells,* which are grouped as clusters in the basal epidermis and dermis and in the junction zone between these 2 layers. Nevi are not apparent clinically at birth but begin to appear during childhood and often develop increased pigmentation during puberty.

Table 10-1 Melanocytic Skin Lesions of the Face

Benign Melanocytic Lesions	Premalignant Melanocytic Lesions	Malignant Melanocytic Lesions
Nevi	Lentigo maligna	Cutaneous melanoma:
Freckle (ephelis)		• Lentigo maligna melanoma
Lentigo simplex		• Nodular melanoma
Solar lentigo		• Superficial spreading melanoma
Blue nevi		• Acrolentiginous melanoma
Dermal melanocytosis (nevus of Ota)		
Melasma		

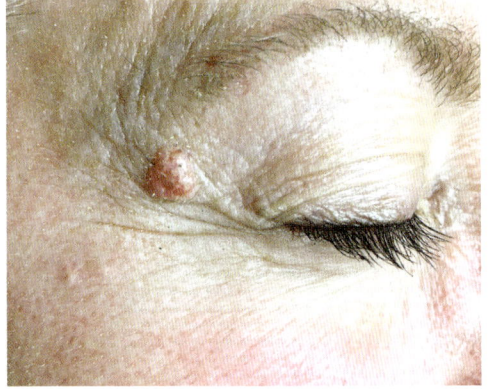

Figure 10-37 Compound nevus of the right lateral canthus. *(Courtesy of Cat N. Burkat, MD.)*

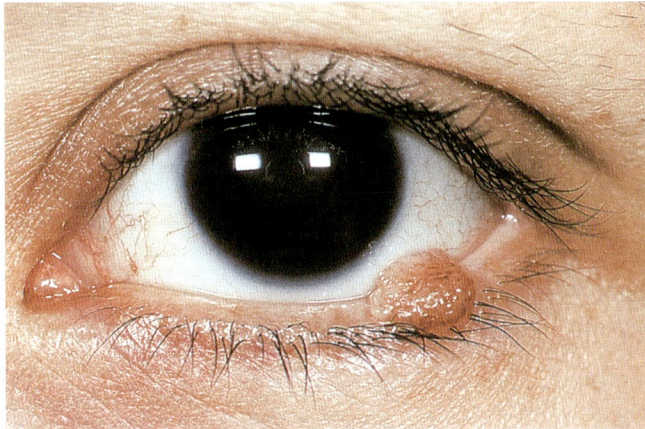

Figure 10-38 Eyelid margin nevus.

Over the course of a lifetime, nevi evolve through 3 stages: (1) *junctional* (located in the basal layer of the epidermis at the dermal–epidermal junction), (2) *compound* (extending from the junctional zone up into the epidermis and down into the dermis), and (3) *dermal* (caused by involution of the epidermal component and persistence of the dermal component). In children, nevi arise initially as junctional nevi, which are typically flat, pigmented macules. Beyond the second decade, most nevi become compound, at which stage they appear as elevated, pigmented papules. Later in life, the pigmentation is lost, and the compound nevus remains as a minimally pigmented or amelanotic lesion (Fig 10-37). By age 70 years, virtually all nevi have become dermal nevi and have lost pigmentation.

Nevi are frequently found on the eyelid margin, characteristically molded to the ocular surface (Fig 10-38). Asymptomatic benign nevi require no treatment, but malignant transformation of a junctional or compound nevus can occur in rare cases. Nevi can also involve both the upper and lower eyelid margins (*kissing nevus,* Fig 10-39). Nevi may become symptomatic if they rub on the ocular surface or enlarge and obstruct vision or

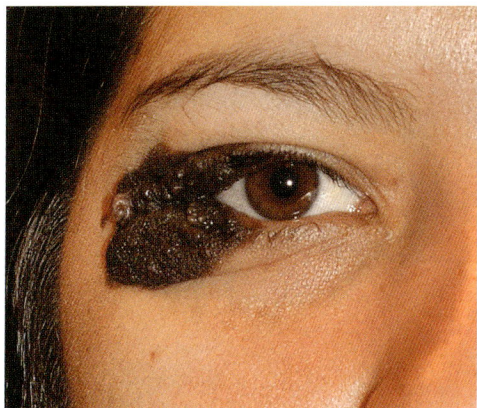

Figure 10-39 Kissing nevus of the right upper and lower eyelids. *(Courtesy of Bobby S. Korn, MD, PhD.)*

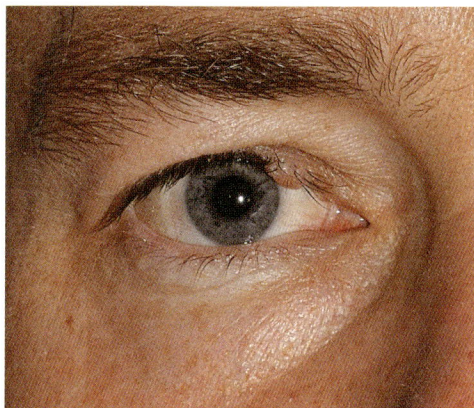

Figure 10-40 Amelanotic benign intradermal nevus of the right upper eyelid. *(Courtesy of Bobby S. Korn, MD, PhD.)*

lacrimal outflow. When amelanotic, they can be confused with basal cell tumors (Fig 10-40). They are managed with shave excision or wedge resection.

Ephelis (freckle)

An *ephelis*, or *freckle*, is a small, flat, brown spot that can occur on various areas of the body and facial skin, including malar areas, nose, and eyelids, or the conjunctiva. Ephelides arise from hyperpigmentation of the basal layer of the epidermis. Although the number of epidermal melanocytes is not increased, they extrude more than the usual amount of pigment into the epidermal basal cell layer. Ephelides are common in fair-skinned persons, and the hue of the ephelis darkens with sunlight exposure. No treatment is necessary other than sun protection.

Lentigo simplex

Simple lentigines are flat, pigmented spots that are larger in diameter than ephelides. Lentigo simplex can occur at any age and is not related to sun exposure. The condition also differs from ephelides in that the number of epidermal melanocytes is increased, and melanin is found in adjacent basal keratinocytes. Individual lesions are evenly pigmented and measure a few millimeters in diameter. Eyelid lentigines may be associated with *Peutz-Jeghers syndrome (autosomal dominant polyposis of the intestinal tract)*. No treatment is necessary; however, melanin-bleaching topical agents may improve cosmesis.

Solar lentigo

Multiple solar lentigines may occur in older persons, in which case they are called *senile lentigo* (Fig 10-41). Chronic sun exposure produces pigmented macules with an increased number of melanocytes. Solar lentigines are uniformly hyperpigmented and somewhat larger than simple lentigines. The dorsum of the hands and the forehead are the most frequently affected areas. No treatment is necessary, but sun protection is recommended. Melanin-bleaching

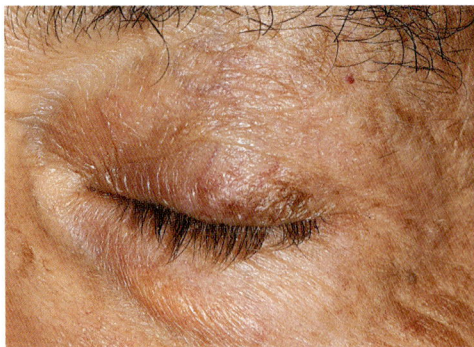

Figure 10-41 Solar lentigo of the left upper eyelid. *(Courtesy of Bobby S. Korn, MD, PhD.)*

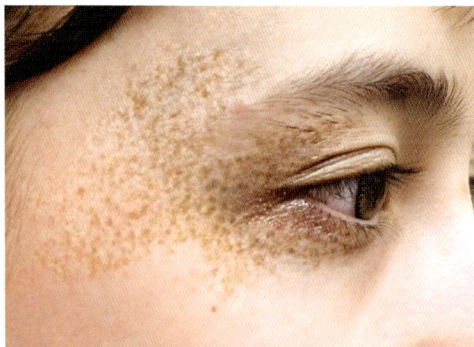

Figure 10-42 Right nevus of Ota. *(Courtesy of Cat N. Burkat, MD.)*

preparations, intense pulsed-light treatment, or cryotherapy may help fade the pigmentation of solar lentigines.

Blue nevi

Blue nevi are dark blue-gray to blue-black, slightly elevated lesions that may be congenital or may develop during childhood. They arise from a localized proliferation of dermal melanocytes. The dark, dome-shaped lesions beneath the epidermis are usually 10 mm or less in diameter. Although their malignant potential is extremely low, these lesions are generally excised.

Dermal melanocytosis

Also known as *nevus of Ota,* this diffuse, congenital blue nevus of the periocular skin most often affects persons of African, Hispanic, or Asian descent, especially females. Dermal melanocytes proliferate in the region of the first and second dermatomes of cranial nerve V. The eyelid skin is diffusely brown, gray, or blue, and pigmentation may extend to the adjacent forehead (Fig 10-42). Approximately 5% of cases are bilateral. When patchy slate-gray pigmentation also appears on the episclera and uvea, as occurs in two-thirds of affected patients, the condition is known as *oculodermal melanocytosis* (Fig 10-43). Although malignant transformation may occur, especially in white patients, no prophylactic treatment is recommended. Approximately 0.25% of patients with oculodermal melanocytosis develop a uveal melanoma. Patients should also be monitored for glaucoma, as 10% of patients with oculodermal melanocytosis also have glaucoma and pigmentation of the trabecular meshwork.

Premalignant Epidermal Lesions: Actinic Keratosis

Actinic keratosis is the most common precancerous skin lesion. It usually affects fair-skinned, elderly persons with a history of chronic sun exposure (Fig 10-44). These lesions are typically round, scaly, keratotic plaques that on palpation have the texture of sandpaper. They often develop on the face, head, neck, forearms, and dorsal hands. These lesions are in a state of continual flux, increasing in size and darkening in response to sunlight and remitting with reduced sun exposure. It has been reported that up to 25% of individual actinic keratoses

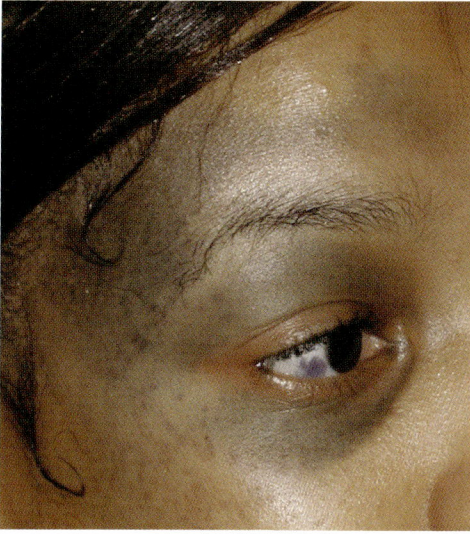

Figure 10-43 Oculodermal melanocytosis. *(Courtesy of Jill Foster, MD.)*

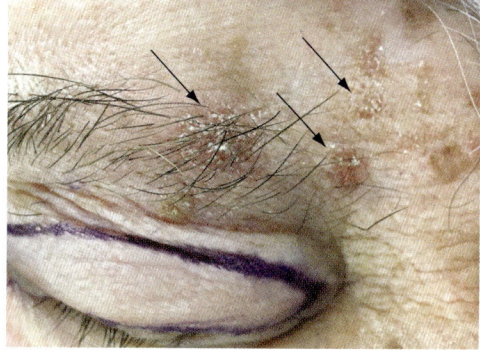

Figure 10-44 Multiple actinic keratoses *(arrows)* near the right eyebrow. *(Courtesy of Cat N. Burkat, MD.)*

spontaneously resolve over a 12-month period, although new lesions tend to develop continually. The risk of malignant transformation of an individual actinic keratosis is only 0.24% per year, but over extended follow-up, a person with multiple actinic keratoses has a 12%–20% risk of developing squamous cell carcinoma. Squamous cell carcinomas arising from actinic keratoses are thought to be less aggressive than those developing de novo. For lesions arising in the periocular region, incisional or excisional biopsy is recommended. Widespread lesions may be treated with topical 5-fluorouracil or imiquimod cream, cryotherapy, or photodynamic field therapy.

In Situ Epithelial Malignancies

Squamous cell carcinoma in situ

The term *Bowen disease* refers to squamous cell carcinoma in situ of the skin. These lesions typically appear as elevated, nonhealing, erythematous lesions. They may present with scaling, crusting, or pigmented keratotic plaques. Pathologically, the lesions demonstrate full-thickness epidermal atypia without dermal invasion, in contrast to the partial thickness atypia of actinic keratoses. In 5% of patients, Bowen disease may progress to vertically invasive squamous cell carcinoma; therefore, complete surgical excision is advised. Alternatively, electrodessication and curettage, cryotherapy, and 5-fluorouracil may be used, especially in larger areas of involvement.

Keratoacanthoma

Although keratoacanthoma was formerly considered to be a benign lesion, many authors now regard this entity as a low-grade squamous cell carcinoma. The lesion usually begins as a flesh-colored papule on the lower eyelid that develops rapidly into a dome-shaped nodule

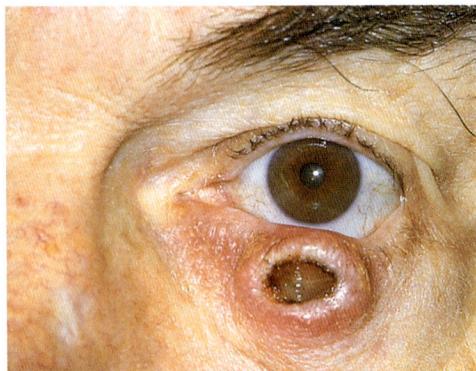

Figure 10-45   Keratoacanthoma.

with a central keratin-filled crater and elevated rolled margins (Fig 10-45). Keratoacanthomas typically occur in middle-aged and elderly individuals, and there is an increased incidence in immunosuppressed patients. Gradual involution over the course of 3–6 months has often been observed. The abundant keratin production in the center of the lesion may incite a surrounding inflammatory reaction, which may play a role in ultimate resolution. At present, incisional biopsy followed by complete surgical excision is recommended. Intralesional methotrexate or 5-fluorouracil may be options for patients who are not surgical candidates.

Premalignant Melanocytic Lesions: Lentigo Maligna

Also known as *Hutchinson melanotic freckle* or *precancerous melanosis* or *lentigo maligna melanoma in situ,* lentigo maligna is a flat, irregularly shaped, unevenly pigmented, slowly enlarging lesion that typically occurs on the malar regions in older white persons. Risk factors for development of lentigo maligna include advanced age, lighter skin types, tendency to develop solar lentigines, and a history of nonmelanoma skin malignancies. A history of intermittent severe sunburns, rather than cumulative sun exposure, is also considered a risk factor for lentigo maligna. Unlike senile or solar lentigo, lentigo maligna is characterized by significant pigmentary variation, irregular borders, and progressive enlargement. These characteristics reflect a radial, intraepidermal, uncontrolled growth phase of melanocytes, which can eventually progress to nodules of vertically invasive melanoma. The absolute risk of a lentigo maligna melanoma (at any location) after a histologically confirmed lentigo maligna is low, at 2.0%–2.6%.

The area of histologic abnormality frequently extends beyond the visible pigmented borders of the lesion; in the periocular region, cutaneous lentigo maligna of the eyelid may extend onto the conjunctival surface, where the lesion appears identical to primary acquired melanosis. Excision with adequate surgical margins is recommended, with permanent sections for final monitoring. Close observation for recurrence is warranted.

Malignant Eyelid Tumors

Basal cell carcinoma

Basal cell carcinoma, the most common eyelid malignancy, accounts for approximately 90%–95% of malignant eyelid tumors. A prospective series of 1295 patients found that basal

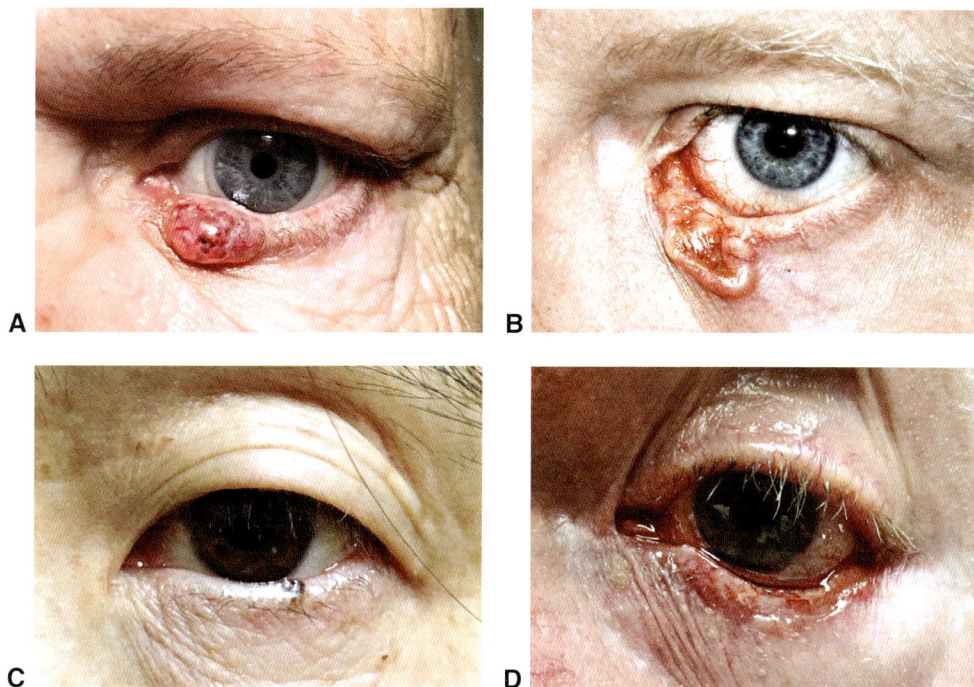

Figure 10-46 Basal cell carcinoma. **A,** Nodular. **B,** Ulcerative. **C,** Pigmented. **D,** Morpheaform. *(Courtesy of Cat N. Burkat, MD.)*

cell carcinomas are most often located on the medial canthus (48.3%), lower eyelid (47.5%), and upper eyelid (3.9%). Basal cell carcinomas can have many different clinical manifestations in the eyelid (Fig 10-46).

Patients at highest risk for basal cell carcinoma are fair-skinned, blue-eyed, red-haired or blond, and middle-aged and elderly persons with English, Irish, Scottish, or Scandinavian ancestry. A history of prolonged sun exposure during the first 2 decades of life and a history of cigarette smoking also increase the risk of basal cell carcinoma. Patients with prior basal cell carcinomas have a higher probability of developing additional skin cancers.

Basal cell carcinoma is being seen with increasing frequency in younger patients, and discovery of malignant eyelid lesions in these patients or those with a positive family history should prompt inquiry into possible systemic associations such as basal cell nevus syndrome or xeroderma pigmentosum:

- *Basal cell nevus syndrome (Gorlin syndrome)* is an uncommon autosomal dominant, multisystem disorder characterized by multiple nevoid basal cell carcinomas, which appear early in life and are associated with skeletal anomalies, especially of the mandible, maxilla, and vertebrae. Keratocystic odontogenic tumors (tooth-derived cysts arising from degeneration of the dental lamina) and palmar or plantar pits (punctiform reddish depressions in the skin caused by partial or complete absence of the stratum corneum) are typical findings (Fig 10-47).

A   B

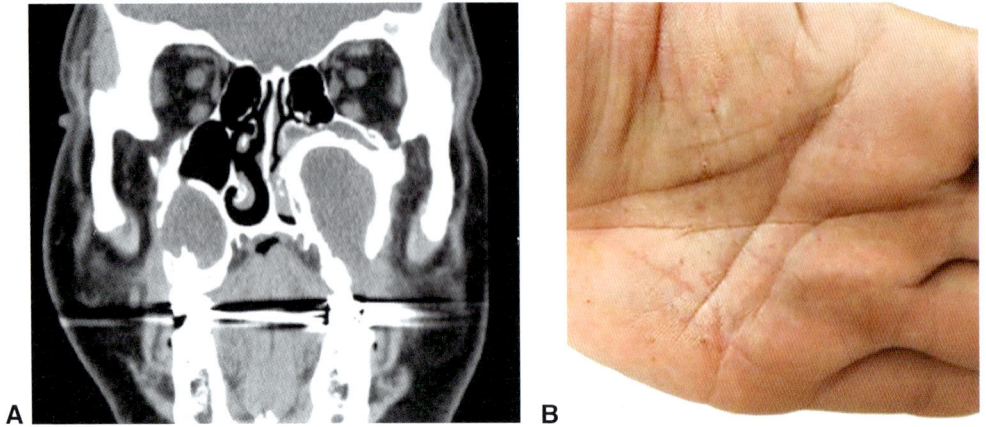

Figure 10-47   Odontogenic cysts and palmar pits seen in basal cell nevus syndrome (Gorlin syndrome). **A,** Bilateral keratocystic odontogenic tumors. **B,** Multiple punctate reddish palmar pits in the skin. *(Courtesy of Pete Setabutr, MD.)*

- *Xeroderma pigmentosum* is a rare autosomal recessive disorder characterized by extreme sun sensitivity and a defective repair mechanism for UV light–induced DNA damage in skin cells (Fig 10-48).

Nodular basal cell carcinoma, the most common type of basal cell carcinoma, is a firm, raised, pearly nodule that may be associated with telangiectasia and central ulceration (see Fig 10-46A, B). Histologically, this tumor type demonstrates nests of basal cells that originate from the basal cell layer of the epithelium and may show peripheral palisading. As the nests of atypical cells break through the epithelial surface, central necrosis and ulceration may occur.

The *morpheaform* tumor type is less common, and behaves more aggressively, than the nodular form of basal cell carcinoma. Morpheaform lesions may be firm and slightly elevated, with margins that may be indeterminate on clinical examination (Fig 10-49; see also Fig 10-46D). Histologically, these lesions show thin cords that radiate peripherally rather than peripheral palisading. The surrounding stroma may show fibrotic proliferation of connective tissue.

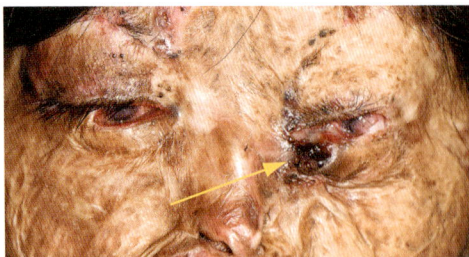

Figure 10-48   Xeroderma pigmentosum with an ulcerated basal cell carcinoma *(arrow)*. *(Courtesy of Bobby S. Korn, MD, PhD.)*

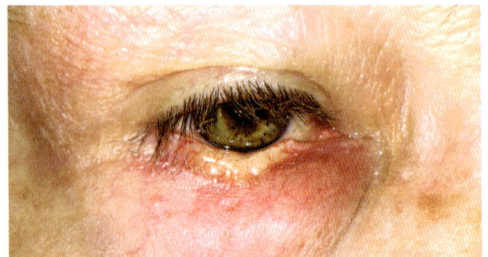

Figure 10-49   Madarosis of the right lower eyelid with morpheaform variant of basal cell carcinoma. *(Courtesy of Cat N. Burkat, MD.)*

Basal cell carcinoma may simulate chronic inflammation of the eyelid margin and is frequently associated with madarosis. *Multicentric* or *superficial* basal cell carcinoma may be mistaken for chronic blepharitis and can silently extend along the eyelid margin.

Malhotra R, Huilgol SC, Huynh NT, Selva D. The Australian Mohs database, part I: periocular basal cell carcinoma experience over 7 years. *Ophthalmology.* 2004;111(4): 624–630.

Management A biopsy is necessary to confirm any clinical suspicion of basal cell carcinoma (Fig 10-50). The most accurate diagnosis is facilitated by obtaining an incisional biopsy specimen that

- is representative of the clinically evident lesion
- is large enough for histologic processing
- is not excessively traumatized, cauterized, or crushed
- contains normal tissue at the margin to show the transitional area

The biopsy site should be first photographed, as the site often heals so well that the original location can be difficult to find for subsequent tumor removal.

An *incisional biopsy*, in which only a portion of the lesion is biopsied, can be used as a confirmatory office procedure if the suspected malignant tumor involves the eyelid margin or medial canthus or is especially large.

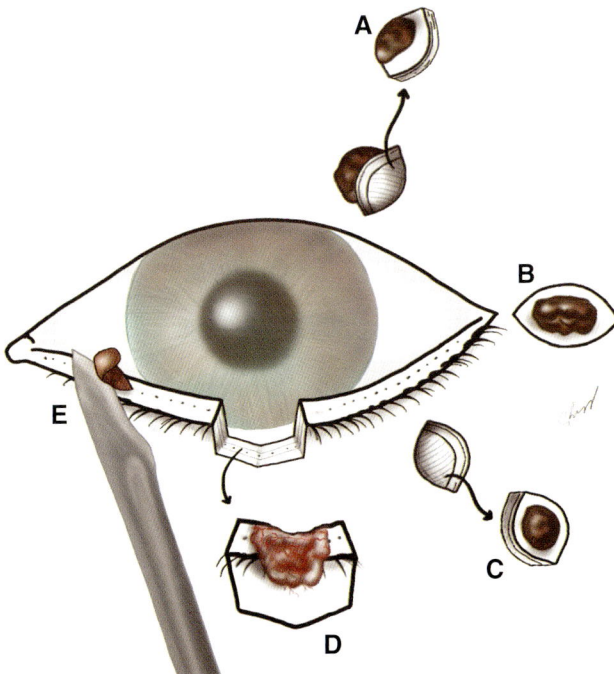

Figure 10-50 Techniques of eyelid biopsy. **A,** Incisional. **B,** Lateral canthal. **C,** Excisional. **D,** Full-thickness margin wedge resection. **E,** Shave. *(Illustration by Cat N. Burkat, MD.)*

An *excisional biopsy* is reasonable when lesions are small and do not involve the eyelid margin or when eyelid margin lesions are away from the lateral canthus or lacrimal punctum. However, histologic monitoring of tumor borders to ensure complete excision is critical. The borders of any excisional biopsy should be marked in case the excision is incomplete and further resection is necessary. Excisional biopsies should be oriented vertically so that closure avoids vertical traction on the eyelid that could lead to eyelid retraction or ectropion. If the margins of the excised portion are positive for residual tumor cells, the involved eyelid area should be excised again, with surgical monitoring of the margins by Mohs micrographic technique or frozen section technique.

Surgery is the treatment of choice for all basal cell carcinomas of the eyelid. Surgical excision affords the advantages of complete tumor removal with histologic control of the margins. The recurrence rate is lower with excision than with any other treatment modality. Surgical excision also offers superior cosmetic results in most cases.

When basal cell carcinomas involve the medial canthal area, the lacrimal drainage system may be excised in order to completely eradicate the tumor. If the lacrimal drainage system has been removed, reconstruction of the lacrimal outflow system is not undertaken until it is established that the patient is tumor free.

Incidence of orbital invasion of basal cell carcinoma is 2%–4% and occurs most commonly in cases that have been inadequately treated, in clinically neglected tumors, in morpheaform tumors, or in tumors with perineural spread. Orbital exenteration may be required in such cases. Retrospective studies show that the mortality rate from ocular adnexal basal cell carcinoma is 3%. The vast majority of patients who have died from basal cell carcinoma had disease that started in the canthal area, had undergone prior radiation therapy, or had clinically neglected tumors.

Histologic examination of the margins of an excised malignant tumor should confirm complete tumor removal. During surgery, frozen section techniques can be employed in which the clinically apparent tumor, along with 1–2 mm margins, is excised, oriented on a detailed drawing, and sent to pathology for immediate frozen section evaluation.

Reconstruction is undertaken when all margins are found to be free of tumor. Some tumors have subcutaneous extensions that are not recognized preoperatively. Consequently, the surgeon must always be prepared to do a much larger reconstruction than originally anticipated from the clinical appearance of the tumor.

To facilitate complete removal of recurrent, deeply infiltrated, or morpheaform tumors and tumors in the medial canthus, dermatologists with special training often use *Mohs micrographic surgery.* Tissue may be removed in thin layers that allow 3-dimensional mapping of the tumor excision. Mohs micrographic tumor resection is most commonly used for excision of squamous cell and morpheaform basal cell carcinoma.

Micrographic excision preserves the maximal amount of healthy tissue while providing the best assurance of complete cancer removal. Preoperative planning involving both the micrographic surgeon and the oculoplastic surgeon enables the most efficient patient care. In some cases, micrographic excision may allow the globe to be retained, whereas conventional surgical techniques might indicate the need for exenteration. However, a limitation of Mohs micrographic surgery is in identifying margins of the tumor if it has invaded orbital fat.

Following Mohs tumor resection, the eyelid should be reconstructed by the ophthalmologist. (Reconstruction techniques are reviewed in Chapter 11.) Although urgent reconstruction is not critical, the procedure should be performed expeditiously. Early surgery affords maximum globe protection and fresh eyelid tissue margins for optimal reconstruction. If immediate reconstruction is not possible, the cornea should be protected by patching or temporarily suturing the remaining eyelid closed over the globe. If defects are small, spontaneous granulation may be a treatment alternative.

The recurrence rate following *cryotherapy* is higher than that following surgical therapy for well-circumscribed nodular lesions. When cryotherapy is used to treat more diffuse sclerosing lesions, the recurrence rate is unacceptably high. In addition, histologic margins cannot be evaluated with cryotherapy. Consequently, this treatment modality is avoided for canthal lesions, recurrent lesions, lesions greater than 1 cm in diameter, and morpheaform lesions. Furthermore, cryotherapy may cause depigmentation and tissue atrophy, resulting in suboptimal final cosmesis. Therefore, cryotherapy for eyelid basal cell carcinoma is generally reserved for patients who are poor surgical candidates.

Radiation therapy should also be considered only as a palliative treatment that should generally be avoided for periorbital lesions. In particular, it should not be used for canthal lesions because of the risk of orbital recurrence. As with cryotherapy, histologic margins cannot be evaluated, and the recurrence rate is higher after radiation treatment than after surgical treatment. Moreover, recurrence after radiation is more difficult to detect, occurs at a longer interval after initial treatment, and is more challenging to manage surgically because of the altered healing of previously irradiated tissues.

Complications of radiation therapy include cicatricial changes in the eyelids, lacrimal drainage scarring with obstruction, keratitis sicca, and radiation-induced malignancy. Radiation may also cause injury to the globe if it is not shielded during treatment. See also BCSC Section 4, *Ophthalmic Pathology and Intraocular Tumors.*

Oral vismodegib or sonidegib may be useful treatments for advanced orbital infiltrative basal cell carcinoma that is not amenable to surgical resection or radiation. Initial studies show that these drugs are well tolerated and effective, although patients need to be carefully monitored for squamous cell carcinomas at uninvolved sites. Side effects include muscle spasm, alopecia, change in taste, and diarrhea.

Demirci H, Worden F, Nelson CC, Elner VM, Kahana A. Efficacy of vismodegib (Erivedge) for basal cell carcinoma involving the orbit and periocular area. *Ophthalmic Plast Reconstr Surg.* 2015;31(6):463–466.

Squamous cell carcinoma

Squamous cell carcinoma accounts for 20% of all cutaneous malignancies, but approximately 5%–10% of eyelid malignancies. Large longitudinal studies have shown that the age-adjusted incidence of squamous cell carcinoma has increased by 200% in the past 3 decades. Although less common than basal cell carcinoma of the eyelid, squamous cell carcinoma is clinically more aggressive (Fig 10-51). Tumors can arise spontaneously or from areas of solar

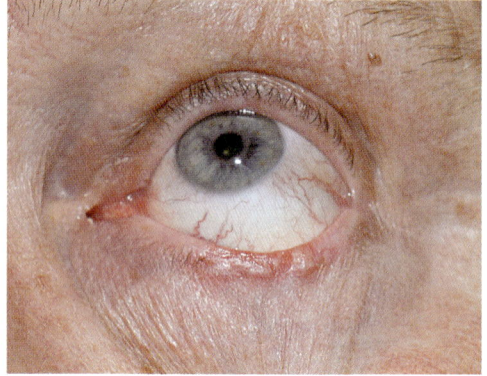

Figure 10-51 Squamous cell carcinoma of the left lower eyelid with diffuse madarosis. *(Courtesy of Bobby S. Korn, MD, PhD.)*

injury, and actinic keratosis and may be potentiated by immunodeficiency. Cutaneous squamous cell carcinoma is the most common malignancy to occur after solid organ transplant.

Treatment for squamous cell carcinoma is similar to that for basal cell carcinoma. Mohs micrographic resection or surgical excision with wide margins and frozen sections is preferred because of the potentially lethal nature of this tumor. Squamous cell carcinoma may metastasize through lymphatic transmission, blood-borne transmission, or direct extension, often along nerves. Recurrences should be treated with wide surgical resection, possibly including orbital exenteration or neck dissection, and may require collaboration with a head and neck cancer surgeon. Targeted therapy using immune-checkpoint inhibitors that disrupt programmed death 1 (PD-1) signaling (see later discussion of melanoma treatment) is a promising new option for patients who are not surgical candidates.

Ferris RL, Blumenschein G Jr, Fayette J, et al. Nivolumab for recurrent squamous cell carcinoma of the head and neck. *N Engl J Med.* 2016;375(19):1856–1867.

Sebaceous carcinoma

Sebaceous carcinoma (also called sebaceous gland carcinoma, sebaceous cell carcinoma, sebaceous adenocarcinoma, meibomian gland carcinoma) is a highly malignant and potentially lethal tumor that arises from the meibomian glands of the tarsal plate; from the glands of Zeis associated with the eyelashes; or from the sebaceous glands of the caruncle, eyebrow, or facial skin. Unlike basal cell or squamous cell carcinoma, sebaceous carcinoma occurs more frequently in women and originates twice as often in the upper eyelid as in the lower, reflecting the greater numbers of meibomian and Zeis glands in the upper eyelid. Multicentric origin is common, and separate upper and lower eyelid tumors occur in 6%–8% of patients. Patients are commonly older than 50 years, although tumors have been reported in younger patients. It represents approximately 1% of periorbital malignancies in the United States.

These tumors typically appear yellow due to lipid material within the neoplastic cells and often masquerade as benign eyelid diseases. Clinically, they may simulate chalazia, chronic blepharitis, basal cell or squamous cell carcinoma, mucous membrane (ocular cicatricial) pemphigoid, superior limbic keratoconjunctivitis, or pannus associated with adult inclusion conjunctivitis. Typically, effacement of the meibomian gland orifices with destruction of hair follicles occurs, leading to madarosis (Fig 10-52).

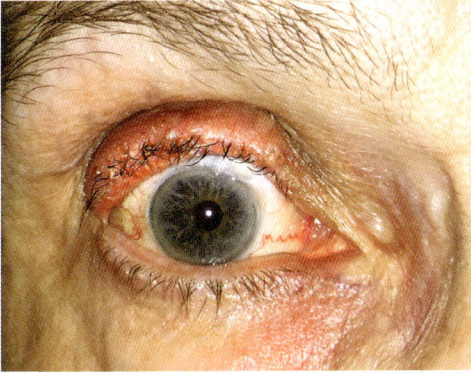

Figure 10-52 Sebaceous cell carcinoma of the right upper eyelid. *(Courtesy of Cat N. Burkat, MD.)*

In sebaceous carcinoma, the tumor within the tarsal plate tends to progress in an intraepidermal growth phase, which may extend over the palpebral and bulbar conjunctiva. A fine papillary elevation of the tarsal conjunctiva may indicate pagetoid spread of tumor cells; intraepithelial growth may replace corneal epithelium as well. Marked conjunctival inflammation and hyperemia may be present.

A nodule that initially simulates a chalazion but later causes eyelash loss and destruction of the meibomian gland orifices warrants biopsy, as this presentation is characteristic of sebaceous carcinoma. Solid material from a chalazion that has been excised more than once should be submitted for histologic examination. Because histologic misdiagnosis is not uncommon, the clinician should maintain suspicion based on clinical findings and request special stains (lipid) or additional histopathologic consultation if warranted. Any chronic unilateral blepharitis should raise suspicion of sebaceous carcinoma.

Muir-Torre syndrome (MTS) is an important consideration if a patient is diagnosed with sebaceous carcinoma. MTS is an autosomal dominant condition of sebaceous tumors (including sebaceous carcinoma, sebaceous adenoma, and basal cell epithelioma with sebaceous differentiation) involving the gastrointestinal, endometrial, or urologic systems.

Because eyelid margin sebaceous carcinomas originate in the tarsal plate or the eyelash margin, superficial shave biopsies may reveal chronic inflammation but miss the underlying tumor. Full-thickness eyelid biopsy with permanent sections or full-thickness punch biopsy of the tarsal plate may be required to obtain the correct diagnosis.

Management Wide surgical excision has historically been the standard treatment for sebaceous carcinoma, although Mohs micrographic surgery has been demonstrated to have lower local recurrence rates for periorbital sebaceous carcinoma. Overall, considerable caution is required due to the skip areas, pagetoid spread, and polycentric characteristic of these tumors. Map biopsies of the conjunctiva are helpful to assess for pagetoid spread. If pagetoid spread is present, adjunctive cryotherapy may be used. Orbital exenteration (see Chapter 8 in this volume) may be considered for recurrent or large tumors invading through the orbital septum. These tumors usually metastasize to regional lymph nodes but may in rare cases spread hematogenously or through direct extension. Radiation therapy is not appropriate as a primary treatment modality, as sebaceous carcinomas are relatively radioresistant.

Sentinel lymph node biopsy can be considered for patients with eyelid sebaceous cell carcinoma with high-risk features (recurrent lesions, or extensive involvement of the eyelid [>10 mm] or orbit), as well as for conjunctival or cutaneous melanoma with a Breslow thickness greater than 1 mm or Merkel cell carcinoma of the eyelid. With the exception of basal cell carcinoma, cancers of the eyelid and conjunctiva typically metastasize to the regional lymph nodes, and regional metastasis commonly occurs before metastasis to distant sites. Regional lymphadenectomy includes parotidectomy because of the lymphatic drainage routes of periorbital structures. Identification of regional nodal metastases may indicate that more extensive therapy is warranted, such as adjuvant radiation or chemotherapy, and can provide prognostic information to the physician and patient (Key Points 10-1).

KEY POINTS 10-1

Periorbital sebaceous carcinoma The following list highlights essential points for the ophthalmologist to remember about periorbital sebaceous carcinoma.

- Mohs micrographic surgery has been associated with lower local recurrence rates than wide local excision for periorbital lesions.
- Exenteration is considered for orbital invasion.
- Patients should be screened for Muir-Torre syndrome.
- Sentinel lymph node biopsy can be considered for sebaceous carcinomas >10 mm in diameter.
- Regional lymphadenectomy and parotidectomy with adjuvant radiation are indicated for regional metastasis.
- Radiation therapy and chemotherapy are considered for recurrent or metastatic disease, not as a primary treatment modality.

Ho VH, Ross MI, Prieto VG, Khaleeq A, Kim S, Esmaeli B. Sentinel lymph node biopsy for sebaceous cell carcinoma and melanoma of the ocular adnexa. *Arch Otolaryngol Head Neck Surg.* 2007;133(8):820–826.

Melanoma

Although melanoma accounts for approximately 1%–2% of cutaneous cancers, it causes about 75% of deaths due to skin cancer. Incidence of melanoma in the United States has been steadily increasing over the past 30 years. Risk factors include sunlight exposure, genetic predisposition, and environmental mutagens. Cutaneous melanomas may develop de novo or from preexisting melanocytic nevi or lentigo maligna. Primary cutaneous melanoma of the eyelid skin is rare (<0.1% of eyelid malignancies). Melanoma should be suspected in any patient over 20 years of age with an acquired pigmented lesion. Melanomas typically have variable pigmentation and irregular borders and may ulcerate and bleed.

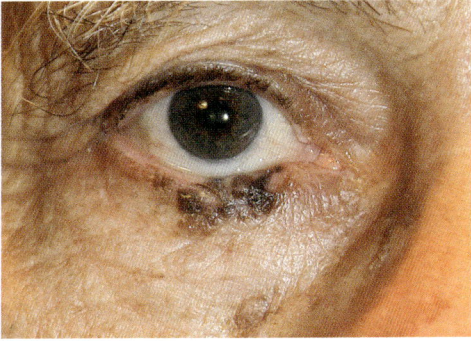

Figure 10-53 Lentigo maligna melanoma of the right lower eyelid. *(Courtesy of Bobby S. Korn, MD, PhD.)*

There are 4 clinicopathologic forms of cutaneous melanoma:

- lentigo maligna melanoma
- nodular melanoma
- superficial spreading melanoma
- acrolentiginous melanoma

The eyelid is most often involved by either lentigo maligna melanoma or nodular melanoma.

Lentigo maligna melanoma (Fig 10-53) represents the invasive vertical malignant growth phase that occurs in 2.0%–2.6% of patients with lentigo maligna. It accounts for 90% of head and neck melanomas. Clinically, the invasive areas are marked by nodule formation within the broader, flat, tan to brown irregular macule. The eyelid is usually involved by secondary extension from the malar region, and pigmentation may progress over the eyelid margin onto the conjunctival surface. Excision is recommended for a premalignant lentigo maligna and is mandatory in patients with lentigo maligna melanoma. Unlike the other types of melanoma, lentigo maligna melanoma has a higher incidence of *p53* mutations compared with BRAF mutations.

Nodular melanoma accounts for approximately 10% of cutaneous melanomas but is extremely rare on the eyelids (Fig 10-54). These tumors may be amelanotic. The vertical

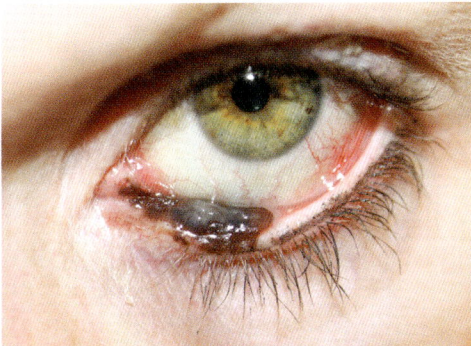

Figure 10-54 Lower eyelid melanoma spreading to the conjunctiva and caruncle. *(Courtesy of Jill Foster, MD.)*

invasive growth phase is the initial presentation of these lesions; thus, they are likely to have extended deeply by the time of diagnosis.

Management Treatment of cutaneous melanoma includes wide surgical excision with histo-logic confirmation (by means of permanent sections) of complete tumor removal. Random-ized trials have thus far provided insufficient information to determine optimal excision margins for primary cutaneous eyelid melanoma. In the periocular regions, margins less than 1 cm are often used to help preserve tissue needed for reconstruction and protection of the eye.

Regional lymph node dissection or sentinel lymph node biopsy may be performed for melanomas that have microscopic evidence of vascular or lymphatic involvement or Bre-slow thickness greater than 1 mm. Complete preoperative metastatic workup is indicated for tumors with thickness greater than 1.5 mm. Thin lesions (<0.75 mm) confer a 5-year survival rate of 98%, while thicker lesions (>4 mm) with ulceration have a survival rate of less than 50%. Because tumor thickness has strong prognostic implications, a punch biopsy that allows a core to be taken through the full tumor depth should be performed. Biopsy of these lesions does not increase the risk of metastatic spread.

Although cryotherapy may have a role in the treatment of acquired melanomas in the conjunctiva, it should not be considered for treatment of cutaneous melanoma. Topical im-iquimod cream can be considered in some cases of very early melanomas that are located in sensitive areas of the face where surgery may be disfiguring.

Immunotherapy can help stimulate the immune system or enhance the ability of im-mune cells to recognize and attack cancer cells. Because this modality can also affect healthy cells, side effects such as flulike symptoms, fatigue, skin rashes, and gastrointestinal prob-lems may occur. Immunotherapy drugs can be used as a first-line treatment for melanoma or in combination with chemotherapy or surgery.

Oncolytic virus therapy makes use of modified versions of viruses to trick the immune system into launching an attack. The US Food and Drug Administration (FDA) approved talimogene laherparepvec (T-VEC) in 2015 for local treatment of unresectable cutaneous, subcutaneous, and nodal lesions in patients with recurrent melanoma after initial surgery. T-VEC, a genetically modified herpes simplex virus type 1, is injected directly into mela-noma lesions or lymph nodes and is designed to replicate within tumors and cause tumor cell death.

Cytokines, such as interleukin-2 and peginterferon alfa-2b, are FDA-approved adju-vant therapies for metastatic melanoma that has been surgically resected but has a high risk of recurrence. These agents help stimulate the rapid growth and activity of immune cells. However, recent randomized trials of interferon used in an adjuvant setting show that it can lengthen the time to melanoma recurrence but does not appear to prolong survival. These drugs may also be given in conjunction with chemotherapy for metastatic melanoma.

Checkpoint inhibitors block signaling proteins that would otherwise prevent activated T cells from attacking the tumor, thus allowing the immune system to induce tumor regression in cases of advanced or metastatic melanoma. Ipilimumab, which stimulates T cells, was the first drug of this type to be approved. It was followed by pembrolizumab and nivolumab, which target PD-1, a protein on T cells that normally helps keep T cells from attacking other cells in the body. By blocking PD-1, these drugs boost the immune response against melanoma cells, causing tumor regression. Nivolumab has been approved as a single agent for first-line therapy in inoperable or metastatic melanoma, or as a second-line treatment following treatment with ipilimumab. Some trials showed nivolumab improved survival in treated patients when compared to chemotherapy. Combination therapy using nivolumab and ipilimumab have demonstrated improved responses; however, the risk of adverse effects, such as elevated liver enzymes, gastrointestinal toxicities, and severe pneumonitis, increases. Nivolumab has recently received accelerated approval as a single agent in the treatment of melanoma with a BRAF V600 mutation.

Sladden MJ, Balch C, Barzilai DA, et al. Surgical excision margins for primary cutaneous melanoma. *Cochrane Database Syst Rev.* 2009;4:CD004835.

Valentin-Nogueras SM, Brodland DG, Zitelli JA, González-Sepulveda L, Nazario CM. Mohs micrographic surgery using MART-1 immunostain in the treatment of invasive melanoma and melanoma in situ. *Dermatol Surg.* 2016;42(6):733–744.

Kaposi sarcoma

This tumor, which is associated with human herpesvirus 8, presents as a chronic reddish dermal mass (Fig 10-55) and is a frequent manifestation of AIDS, although it may also occur in elderly or immunocompromised patients, such as those who have received organ transplants. Conjunctival lesions can be mistaken for a foreign-body granuloma or cavernous hemangioma. The lesion is composed of spindle cells of probable endothelial origin. It may be treated with cryotherapy, excision, radiation, or intralesional chemotherapeutic agents. If Kaposi sarcoma is related to AIDS, it may regress with adequate antiviral treatment of the underlying HIV infection.

Shuler JD, Holland GN, Miles SA, Miller BJ, Grossman I. Kaposi sarcoma of the conjunctiva and eyelids associated with the acquired immunodeficiency syndrome. *Arch Ophthalmol.* 1989;107(6):858–862.

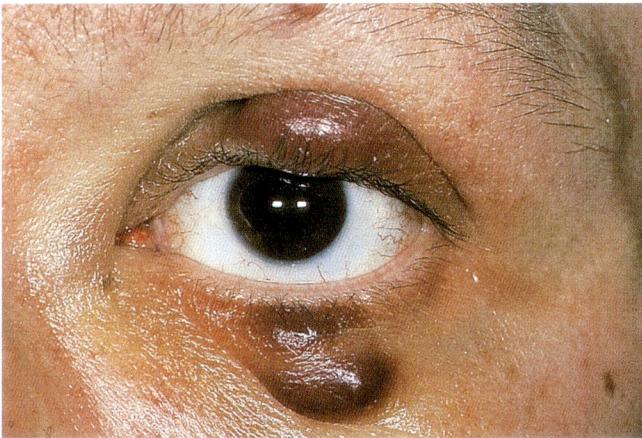

Figure 10-55 Kaposi sarcoma.

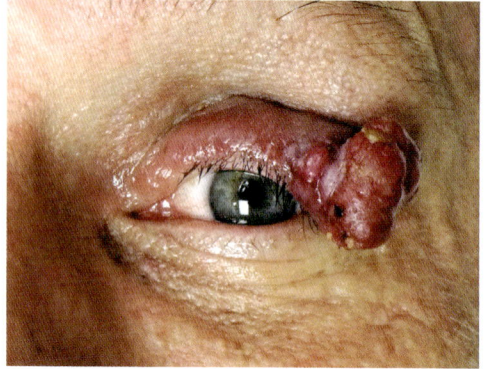

Figure 10-56 Merkel cell carcinoma of the left upper eyelid. *(Courtesy of Cat N. Burkat, MD.)*

Merkel cell carcinoma

The Merkel cell is part of the dendritic (neuroendocrine) cell population of the skin and plays a role in mediating the sense of touch. Merkel cells can give rise to malignant neoplasms, 10% of which occur in the eyelid and periocular area and manifest as painless, erythematous nodules with overlying telangiectasias (Fig 10-56). Merkel cell carcinoma can mimic other malignant lesions, making diagnosis difficult. One-third of the tumors recur after excision, and there is a high rate of metastasis. The estimated 5-year survival rate is 50%. Initial treatment should include aggressive wide surgical resection, with consideration of postoperative radiation and/or chemotherapy.

Herbert HM, Sun MT, Selva D, et al. Merkel cell carcinoma of the eyelid: management and prognosis. *JAMA Ophthalmol.* 2014;132(2):197–204.

CHAPTER 11

Reconstructive Eyelid Surgery

Highlights

- Precise anatomic tissue realignment can minimize the need for secondary repairs.
- Secondary repair of eyelid trauma often requires more complex tissue rearrangement to address the cicatricial changes.
- The location of a scar in relation to the relaxed skin tension lines determines the best combination of reconstructive techniques to utilize.
- Observation for several months may allow for spontaneous improvement prior to consideration of surgery for traumatic ptosis.
- Horizontal eyelid tension is preferred over vertical tightening during tissue closure in order to avoid postoperative eyelid retraction.

Eyelid Trauma

Injuries of the eyelid may be divided into 2 categories: blunt trauma and penetrating trauma. Cardinal rules in the management of eyelid trauma include the following:

- Take a careful history.
- Record the best visual acuity for each eye.
- Thoroughly evaluate the globe and orbit.
- Obtain appropriate radiologic studies.
- Have a detailed knowledge of eyelid and orbital anatomy.
- Ensure the best possible primary repair.

Blunt Trauma

Ecchymosis and edema are the most common presenting signs of blunt trauma. Patients should be evaluated for intraocular injury with a thorough biomicroscopic evaluation and dilated fundus examination. Computed tomography may be indicated to assess for an orbital fracture. See Chapter 6 in this volume for further discussion of orbital fractures.

Penetrating Trauma

The treatment of eyelid lacerations depends on the depth and location of the injury. Detailed knowledge of eyelid anatomy is required to optimize repair and reduce the need for secondary repairs.

Lacerations not involving the eyelid margin

Superficial eyelid lacerations involving just the skin and orbicularis oculi muscle usually require only skin sutures, with or without buried subcutaneous sutures. Unnecessary scarring can be avoided by following the basic principles of repair, including conservative wound debridement, use of small-caliber sutures, wound edge eversion, and early suture removal.

The presence of orbital fat in the wound indicates that the orbital septum has been violated (Fig 11-1). Prior to repair, any foreign bodies in the wound should be identified and removed, and the wound should be properly irrigated. Orbital fat prolapse in the wound is also an indication for exploration of the levator muscle and aponeurosis. If lacerated, the levator muscle or aponeurosis must be carefully repaired to enable the levator muscle to function normally. Upper eyelid retraction and tethering to the superior orbital rim are common if the orbital septum is inadvertently incorporated into the repair. Similarly, orbital septum lacerations should not be sutured to avoid eyelid retraction from vertical shortening of the sutured orbital septum.

Lacerations involving the eyelid margin

Repair of eyelid margin lacerations requires precise suture placement and suture tension to minimize notching of the eyelid margin. Tarsal approximation and anatomical alignment of the eyelid margin should be meticulous in order to precisely repair the eyelid margin (Figs 11-2, 11-3). The eyelid margin is typically aligned by placing interrupted silk sutures through the lash line, meibomian gland plane, and the gray line. Additional nonmarginal tarsal sutures are placed through the height of the lacerated tarsus to strengthen the margin closure, as well as to avoid imbrication of the tarsal edges. To prevent corneal abrasion, the sutures should be partial thickness through the tarsus without extension through the conjunctival surface, and the suture tails should be directed away from the ocular surface. Eyelid margin closure should result in a moderate eversion of the well-approximated wound edges. Resorbable, buried, vertical mattress sutures may be used in the margin as an alternative to externally tied sutures.

Trauma involving the canthal soft tissue

Trauma to the medial or lateral canthal areas is usually the result of horizontal traction on the eyelid, which causes avulsion at the eyelid's weakest points, the medial or lateral canthal

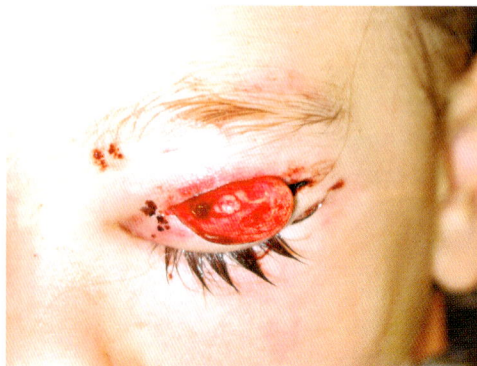

Figure 11-1 Left upper eyelid laceration not involving the margin shows orbital fat prolapse. *(Courtesy of Cat N. Burkat, MD.)*

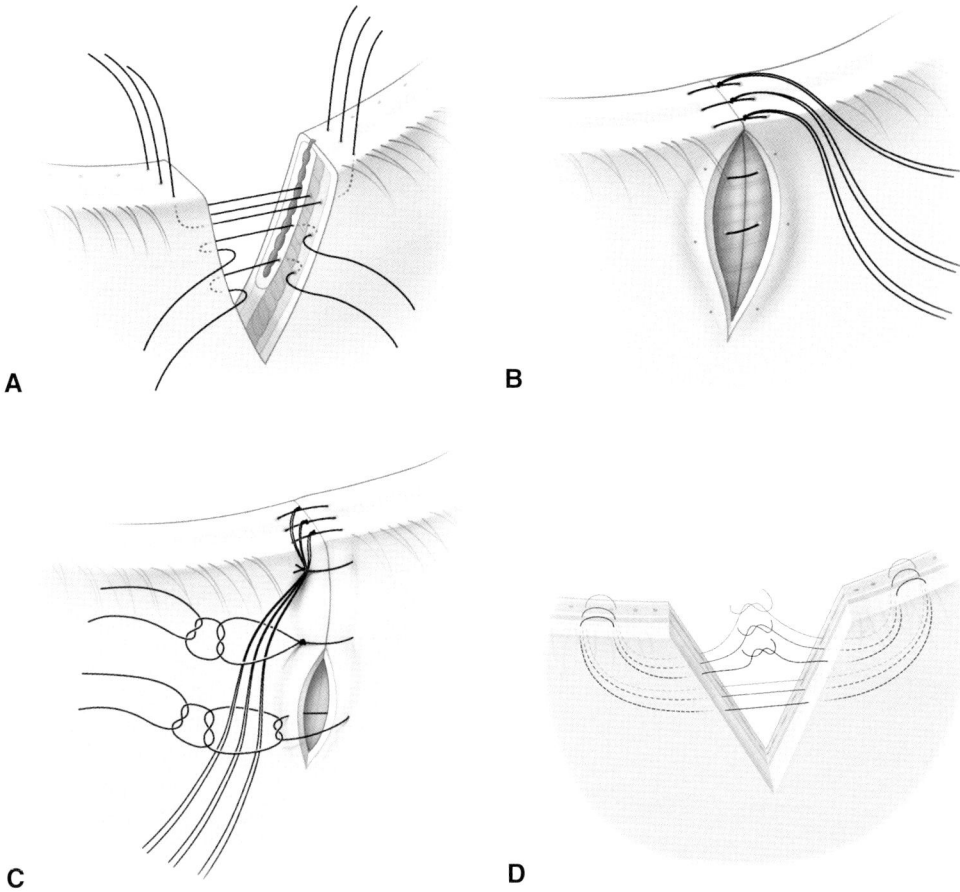

Figure 11-2 Eyelid margin repair. **A,** The eyelid margin is aligned with resorbable tarsus-to-tarsus sutures, and the lash line, gray line, and mucocutaneous junction are aligned with silk sutures. **B,** The tarsal sutures are tied and cut; the eyelid margin sutures are tied and left long. **C,** The skin surface of the eyelid is sewn closed, with the skin sutures used to tie down the tails of the margin sutures. **D,** An alternative approach is to place vertical mattress sutures in the lash line, gray line, and mucocutaneous junction, so that the knots are buried below the eyelid margin. This approach uses resorbable sutures that do not require removal. *(Parts A–C illustration by Christine Gralapp, part D illustration by Mark Miller.)*

tendon. Lacerations in the medial canthal area require evaluation of the lacrimal drainage apparatus, with canalicular involvement confirmed by inspection and gentle probing (Fig 11-4). These lacerations are discussed in more detail in Chapter 15 in this volume.

The integrity of the inferior and superior limbs of the medial or lateral canthal tendon can be assessed by grasping each eyelid with toothed forceps and tugging away from the injury while palpating the insertion of the tendon. Medial canthal tendon avulsion should be suspected when there is rounding of the medial canthal angle and acquired telecanthus. Treatment of medial canthal tendon avulsions depends on the extent of the avulsion. Attention to the posterior tendinous attachment to the posterior lacrimal crest is critical. If the upper or lower limb is avulsed but the posterior attachment of the tendon is intact,

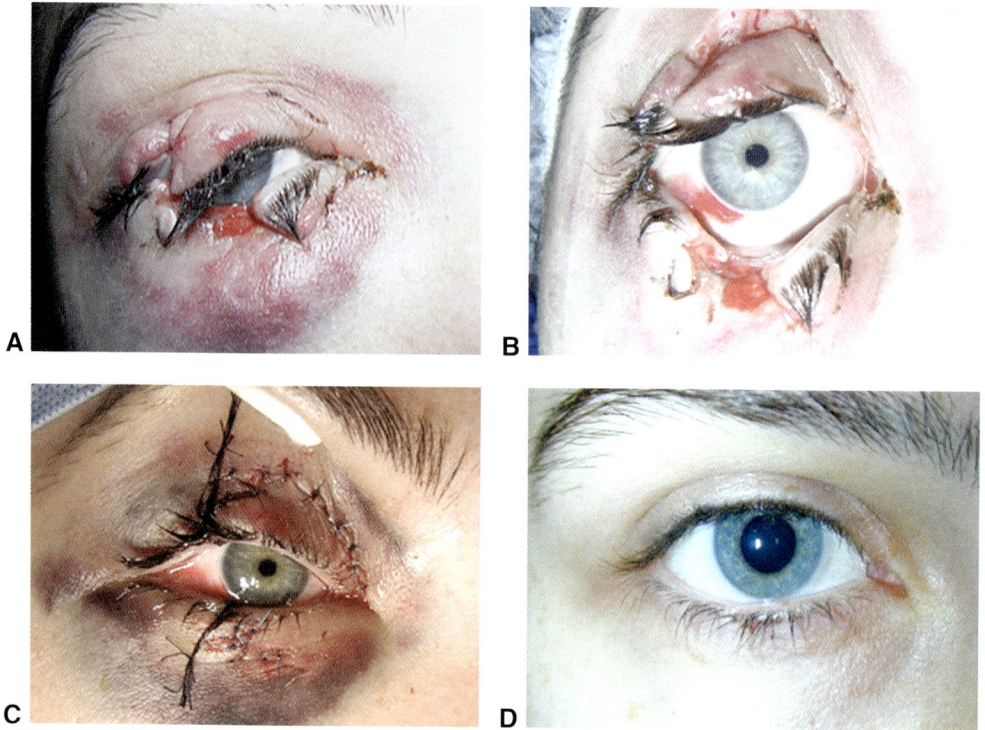

Figure 11-3 Complex full-thickness eyelid margin laceration repair. **A** and **B,** Full-thickness eyelid laceration involving the margin. **C,** Intraoperative repair with silk sutures at the eyelid margin to minimize corneal irritation. **D,** Postoperative result at 3 months. *(Courtesy of Bobby S. Korn, MD, PhD.)*

the avulsed limb may be sutured to its stump or to the periosteum overlying the anterior lacrimal crest. If the entire tendon, including the posterior portion, is avulsed but there is no naso-orbital fracture, the avulsed tendon may be wired through small drill holes in the ipsilateral posterior lacrimal crest. If the entire tendon is avulsed and there is a naso-orbital fracture, transnasal wiring or plating is necessary after fracture reduction. A Y-shaped miniplate may be fixed anteriorly on the nasal bone, extending posteriorly into the orbit. The suture is sewn through the transected tendon and passed through holes in the miniplate. This technique is particularly helpful when the bone of the posterior lacrimal crest is absent.

Secondary Repair

Secondary repair of eyelid trauma usually requires treatment of cicatricial changes that resulted from either the initial trauma or the surgical repair (Fig 11-5). Scar revision may require a simple excision with primary closure or a more complex tissue rearrangement. The location of a scar in relation to the relaxed skin tension lines determines the best technique or combination of techniques to use. An elliptical scar excision is most useful for revising scars that follow the relaxed skin tension lines. Single or multiple Z-plasty flap techniques can be used to revise scars that do not conform to relaxed skin tension lines.

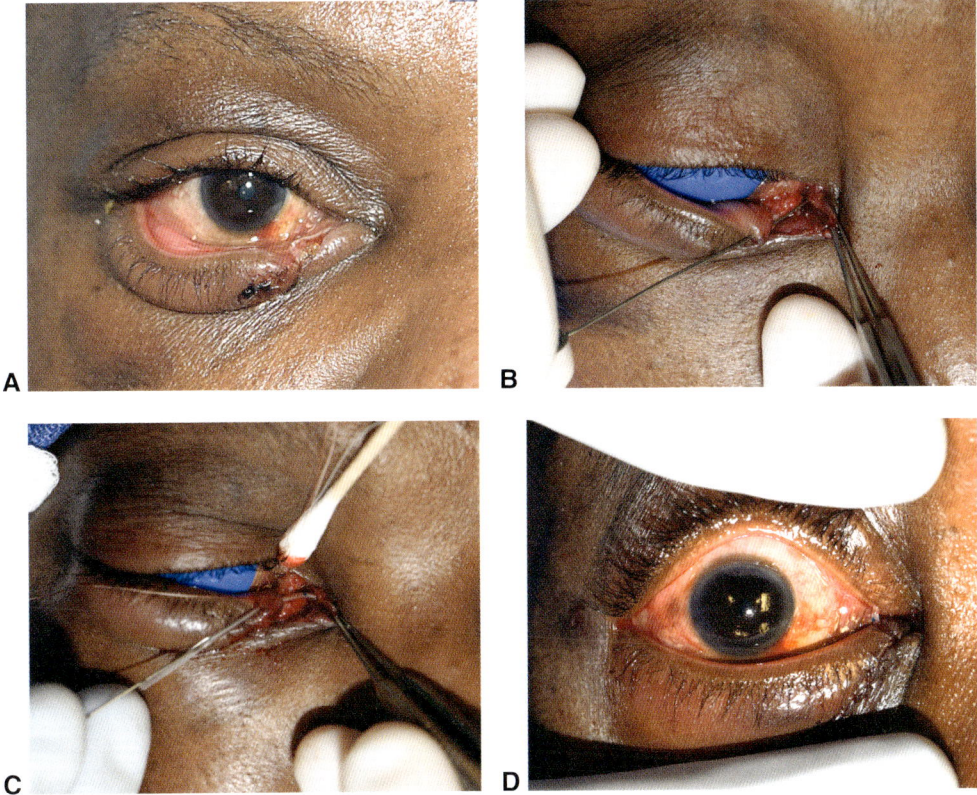

Figure 11-4 Repair of right lower eyelid laceration involving the canaliculus. **A,** Avulsion injury of the right lower eyelid. **B,** Lacrimal probe placed demonstrating the canalicular involvement. **C,** Lacrimal stent placement through the lacerated eyelid. **D,** Immediate postoperative result after reconstruction. *(Courtesy of Bobby S. Korn, MD, PhD.)*

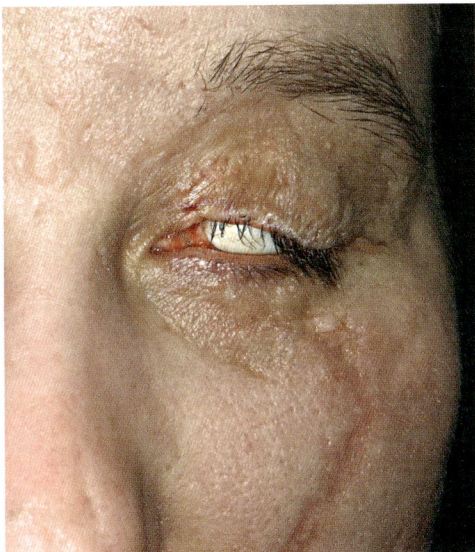

Figure 11-5 Anterior lamella cicatrix after trauma resulting in lagophthalmos. *(Courtesy of Cat N. Burkat, MD.)*

Free skin grafts, performed alone or in combination with various flaps, are used when tissue has been lost or when lengthening of the anterior lamella is required. Although any non–hair-bearing skin can be used, the ideal donor site for eyelid reconstruction is full-thickness upper eyelid skin. Harvested skin should be similar in color and thickness to the skin it is replacing, and it should also be hairless and supple, with minimal actinic damage.

Tarsoconjunctival flaps are good substitutes for posterior lamella eyelid defects when both the tarsal plate and conjunctiva are deficient. Buccal mucosa may be used when only the conjunctiva is missing. Hard palate composite grafts can be used for posterior lamella tarsal defects in the lower eyelid; however, these grafts should be avoided in the upper eyelid due to the presence of keratinized epithelium, which can irritate the cornea.

Before treatment is considered for traumatic ptosis, the patient can be observed for 3–6 months to allow for spontaneous improvement. An exception to this rule may be amblyogenic ptosis in a young child.

Dog and Human Bites

Tearing and crushing injuries occur secondary to dog or human bites. Partial-thickness and full-thickness eyelid lacerations, canthal avulsions, and canalicular lacerations are common. Tissue loss is uncommon but may occur. Irrigation and early wound repair are preferred, and tetanus and rabies protocols should be observed. Systemic antibiotics are recommended for mixed organism flora specific to dog bites, which most often include *Pasteurella canis*, as well as aerobes (streptococci, staphylococci, *Moraxella*, and *Neisseria*), and anaerobes *(Fusobacterium, Bacteroides, Porphyromonas)*. Ocular and canalicular injuries are seen most commonly in children, and more often in association with dog bites from mixed breeds, German shepherds, Labrador retrievers, pit bull terriers, and rottweilers.

Prendes MA, Jian-Amadi A, Chang SH, Shaftel SS. Ocular trauma from dog bites: characterization, associations, and treatment patterns at a regional level I trauma center over 11 years. *Ophthalmic Plast Reconstr Surg.* 2016;32(4):279–283.

Burns

Burns of the eyelid are rare and are generally seen in patients who have sustained significant burns over large areas of the body. Often, these patients are semiconscious or heavily sedated and require ocular surface protection to prevent corneal exposure, ulceration, and infection (Fig 11-6). Lubricating antibiotic ointments, moisture chambers, and frequent evaluation of

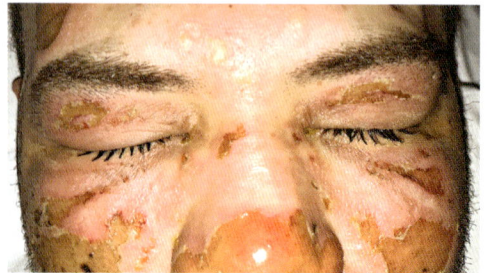

Figure 11-6 Facial burns with no corneal exposure. *(Courtesy of Cat N. Burkat, MD.)*

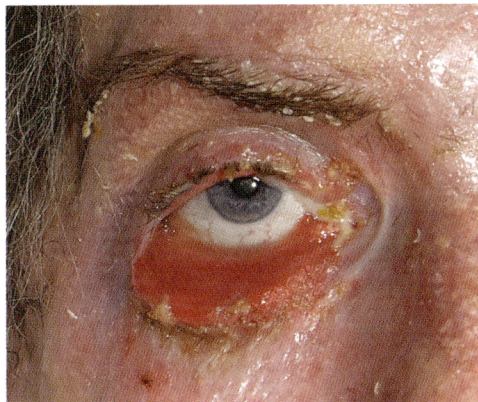

Figure 11-7 Cicatricial right lower eyelid ectropion after extensive facial burns. *(Courtesy of Bobby S. Korn, MD, PhD.)*

both the globes and the eyelids are part of the early treatment of these patients. Once cicatricial changes begin in the eyelids, relentless and rapid deterioration of the patient's ocular status often ensues secondary to cicatricial ectropion and eyelid retraction (Fig 11-7), lagophthalmos, and corneal exposure. If tarsorrhaphies are used, they should always be more extensive than seems to be immediately necessary. Unfortunately, with progression of the cicatricial traction, even the most aggressive eyelid adhesions may dehisce. In the past, skin grafting was usually delayed until the cicatricial changes stabilized, but the early use of full-thickness skin grafts, amniotic membrane, and various types of flaps can effectively reduce ocular morbidity in select patients. Cicatrization may also be reduced with the early use of ablative fractional laser and wound modulators (5-fluorouracil).

Lee BW, Levitt AE, Erickson BP, et al. Ablative fractional laser resurfacing with laser-assisted delivery of 5-fluorouracil for the treatment of cicatricial ectropion and periocular scarring. *Ophthalmic Plast Reconstr Surg.* 2018;34(3):274–279.

Eyelid and Canthal Reconstruction

The following discussion of eyelid reconstruction applies to defects resulting from tumor resection as well as congenital and traumatic defects. Several techniques may be appropriate for reconstruction of a particular eyelid defect. The choice of procedure depends on multiple factors, including the patient's age and comorbidities, the condition of the eyelids, the size and position of the defect, and the surgeon's personal preference. Priorities in eyelid reconstruction are

- preserving eyelid function
- developing a stable eyelid margin
- ensuring adequate eyelid closure for ocular protection
- maintaining adequate vertical eyelid height
- creating a smooth, epithelialized internal surface
- maximizing cosmesis and symmetry

The following general principles guide the practice of eyelid reconstruction:

- One may reconstruct either the anterior or the posterior eyelid lamella, but not both, with a graft; 1 of the layers must provide a blood supply *(pedicle flap)*.
- Direct the tension horizontally, while minimizing vertical tension.
- Maintain sufficient and anatomical canthal fixation.
- Match tissue similar in color and thickness to each other.
- Minimize the defect area as much as possible before sizing a graft.
- Request assistance from a subspecialist if necessary.

Eyelid Defects Not Involving the Eyelid Margin

Defects not involving the eyelid margins can be repaired by direct closure if the repair does not distort the eyelid margin. If undermining of the surrounding tissue does not allow direct closure, advancement or transposition of skin flaps may be used. The tension of closure should be directed horizontally, because vertical tension may cause eyelid retraction or ectropion. Vertical tension may be avoided by placement of vertically oriented incision lines.

If the defect is too large to be closed primarily, techniques utilizing advancement or transposition of local skin flaps may be employed. The flaps most commonly used are rectangular advancement, rotation, and transposition. Flaps usually provide the best tissue match and aesthetic result, but they require planning in order to minimize secondary deformities. Upper eyelid skin is often an acceptable option for lower eyelid anterior lamellar defect repair. The final texture, contour, and cosmesis are typically better with flaps as compared to skin grafts from sites other than eyelid skin.

Anterior lamella upper eyelid defects are best repaired with full-thickness skin grafts from the contralateral upper eyelid (Fig 11-8). Preauricular or postauricular skin grafts may be used, but their greater thickness may limit upper eyelid mobility. If flaps are not sufficient, lower eyelid defects are best filled with preauricular or postauricular skin grafts. If skin is not available from the upper eyelid or auricular areas, full-thickness grafts may be harvested from the supraclavicular fossa or the inner upper arm. Grafts should be slightly oversized, because contraction is likely to occur.

Use of split-thickness grafts should also be avoided in eyelid reconstruction. They are recommended only in the treatment of severe facial burns when adequate full-thickness skin is not available.

Eyelid Defects Involving the Eyelid Margin

Small upper eyelid defects

Small defects involving the upper eyelid margin can be repaired by primary closure if this technique does not place too much tension on the wound (Fig 11-9). Primary closure is usually employed when one-third or less of the eyelid margin is involved; if a larger area is involved, advancement of adjacent tissue or grafting of distant tissue may be required. The superior limb of the lateral canthal tendon can be released to allow 3–5 mm of medial mobilization of the remaining lateral eyelid margin. Care must be taken to avoid the lacrimal ductules in the lateral upper eyelid; removal or destruction of these ductules may lead to

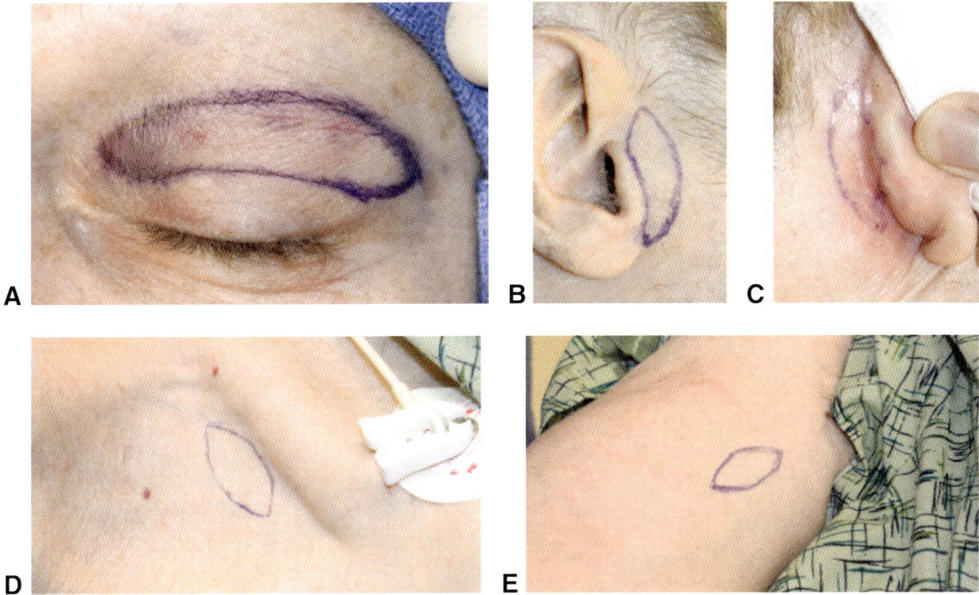

Figure 11-8 Possible donor sites for a full-thickness skin graft. **A,** Upper eyelid. **B,** Preauricular. **C,** Postauricular. **D,** Supraclavicular. **E,** Inner arm. *(Courtesy of Bobby S. Korn, MD, PhD.)*

chronic dry eye problems in the patient. Postoperatively, the eyelid may appear tight and ptotic due to traction, but it typically relaxes over several weeks.

Moderate upper eyelid defects

Moderate defects of the upper eyelid margin (33%–50% margin involvement) can be repaired by advancement of the lateral eyelid segment and temporal tissue. The lateral canthal tendon is released, and a semicircular skin flap is made below the lateral eyebrow extending from the canthus to allow for further eyelid mobilization. The temporal branch of the facial nerve should be avoided when incising the flap. Tarsal-sharing procedures involving the lower eyelid may be required in younger patients with less eyelid laxity.

Large upper eyelid defects

Upper eyelid defects involving more than half of the upper eyelid margin are likely to require eyelid-sharing techniques. After a horizontal subciliary incision in the lower eyelid tarsus, a full-thickness lower eyelid flap is advanced into the defect of the upper eyelid behind the remaining lower eyelid margin (*Cutler-Beard flap*; Fig 11-10). This procedure requires a second procedure to open the eyelids, and often results in a thick and relatively immobile upper eyelid. Alternatively, a tarsoconjunctival flap from the lower eyelid used in conjunction with an overlying skin graft may result in better cosmesis. Eyelid-sharing procedures are less optimal in monocular patients or in children in whom deprivation amblyopia may be a concern. A free tarsoconjunctival graft taken from the contralateral upper eyelid and covered with a skin–muscle flap may be an option if adequate redundant upper eyelid skin is present.

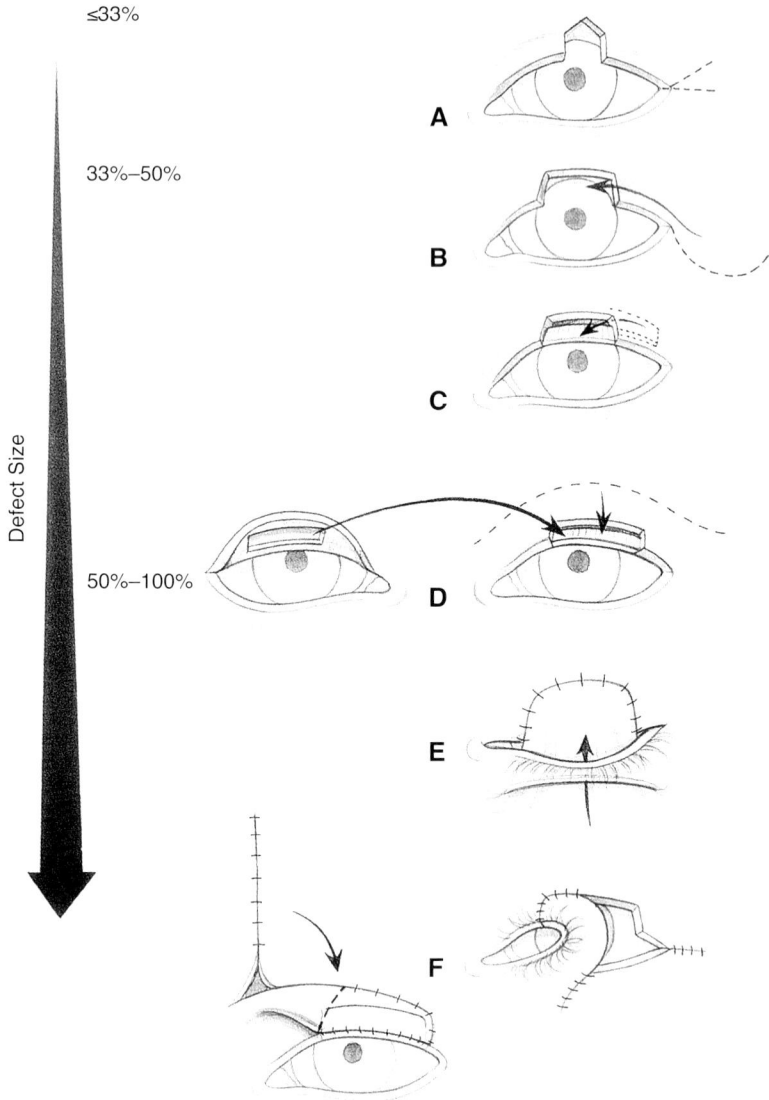

Figure 11-9 Reconstructive ladder for upper eyelid defect. **A,** Primary closure with or without lateral canthotomy or superior cantholysis. **B,** Semicircular flap. **C,** Adjacent tarsoconjunctival flap and full-thickness skin graft. **D,** Free tarsoconjunctival graft and skin flap. **E,** Full-thickness lower eyelid advancement flap (Cutler-Beard flap). **F,** Lower eyelid switch flap or median forehead flap. *(Illustration by Christine Gralapp.)*

Small lower eyelid defects

Small defects of the lower eyelid (margin involvement of less than one-third) can be repaired by primary closure (Fig 11-11). In addition, the inferior crus of the lateral canthal tendon can be internally or externally released so that there is an additional 3–5 mm of medial mobilization of the remaining lateral eyelid margin.

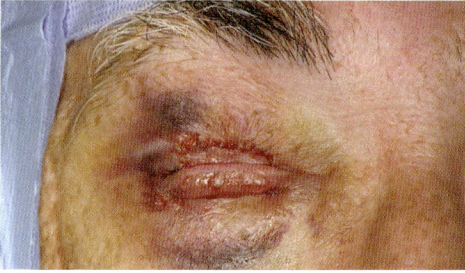

Figure 11-10 Upper eyelid reconstruction using a lower eyelid skin and orbicularis flap (Cutler-Beard flap). *(Courtesy of Bobby S. Korn, MD, PhD.)*

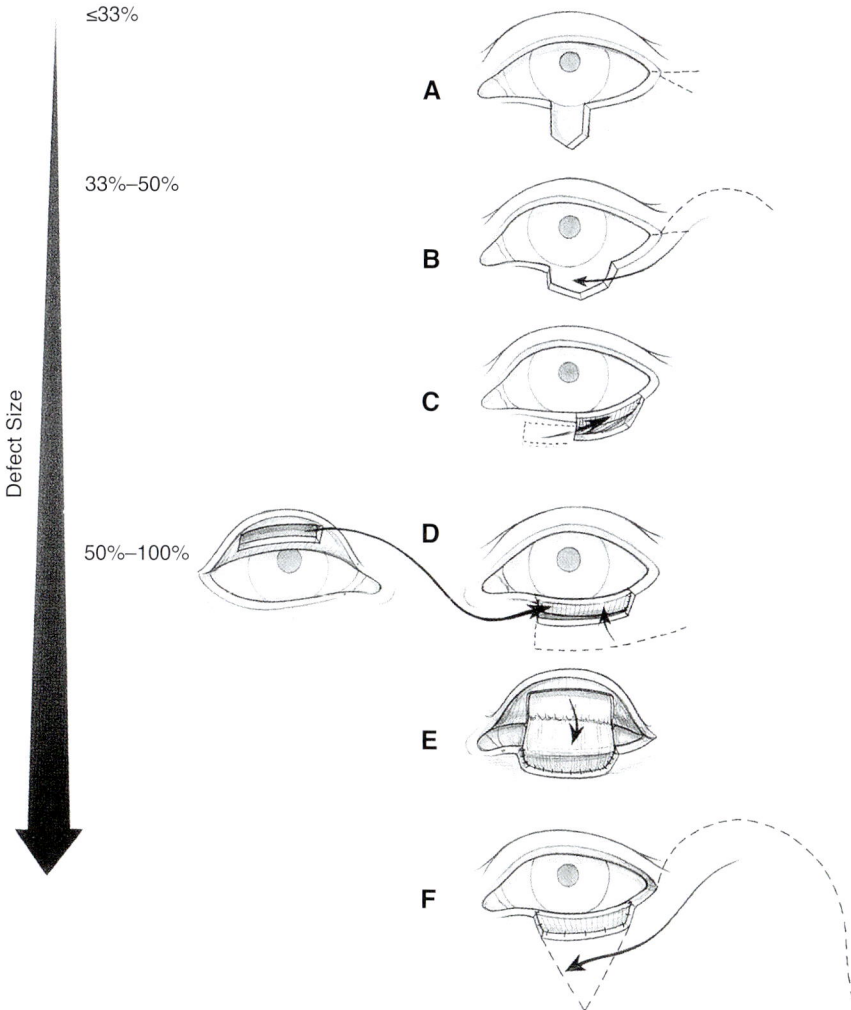

Figure 11-11 Reconstructive ladder for lower eyelid defect. **A,** Primary closure with or without lateral canthotomy or superior cantholysis. **B,** Semicircular flap. **C,** Adjacent tarsoconjunctival flap and full-thickness skin graft. **D,** Free tarsoconjunctival graft and skin flap. **E,** Tarsoconjunctival flap from upper eyelid and skin graft (modified Hughes flap). **F,** Composite graft with cheek advancement flap (Mustardé flap). *(Illustration by Christine Gralapp.)*

Moderate lower eyelid defects

Semicircular advancement or rotation flaps, which have been described for upper eyelid repair, can also be used for reconstruction of moderate defects in the lower eyelid. The most commonly used flap in such cases is a modification of the Tenzel semicircular rotation flap. Tarsoconjunctival autografts harvested from the underside of the upper eyelid may be transplanted into the lower eyelid defect for reconstruction of the posterior lamella of the eyelid. When tarsal grafts are harvested, the marginal 4–5 mm height of the tarsus is preserved to prevent distortion of the donor eyelid margin. Tarsoconjunctival autografts may be covered with skin flaps or skin–muscle flaps. Cheek elevation (suborbicularis oculi fat lift) may be required to avoid ectropion and vertical traction on the eyelid. Alternatively, a tarsoconjunctival flap developed from the upper eyelid and a full-thickness skin graft can be used (discussed in the next subsection).

Large lower eyelid defects

Defects involving more than half of the lower eyelid margin can be repaired by advancement of a tarsoconjunctival flap from the upper eyelid into the posterior lamellar defect of the lower eyelid. The anterior lamella of the reconstructed eyelid is then created with an advancement skin flap or, in most cases, a free skin graft taken from the preauricular area, the postauricular area, or the contralateral upper eyelid (modified Hughes flap). The modified Hughes flap therefore results in placement of a bridge of conjunctiva from the upper eyelid across the pupil for several weeks (Fig 11-12). The vascularized pedicle of conjunctiva is then released in a staged, second procedure once the lower eyelid flap is revascularized, typically 3–4 weeks later. Eyelid-sharing techniques should be used cautiously in children, because deprivation amblyopia may develop. Large rotating cheek flaps (Mustardé flap; Fig 11-13) can work well for repair of large anterior lamellar defects, but they may require a tarsal substitute such as a free tarsoconjunctival autograft, hard-palate mucosa, or a Hughes flap for posterior lamella replacement. Both the cheek rotation flap and the semicircular rotation flap frequently result in a rounded lateral canthus, which can be mitigated by creating a very high incision toward the lateral end of the eyebrow, in which the incision emanates from the lateral commissure. Free tarsoconjunctival autografts from the upper eyelid covered with

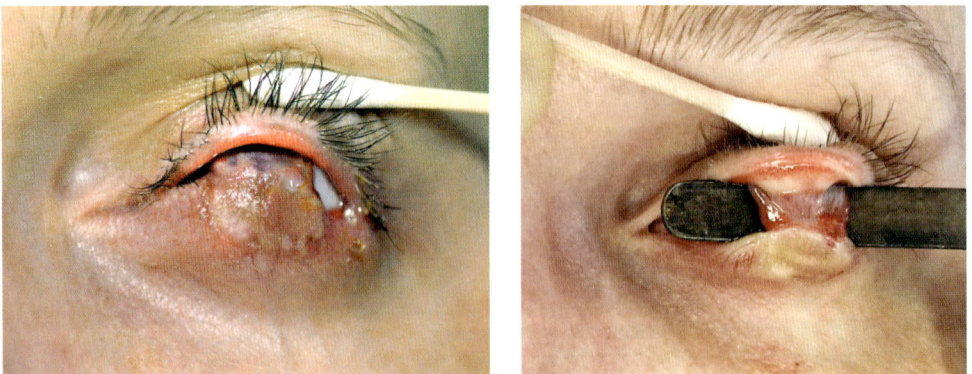

Figure 11-12 Lower eyelid reconstruction with tarsoconjunctival flap (modified Hughes flap) and full-thickness skin graft. *(Courtesy of Cat N. Burkat, MD.)*

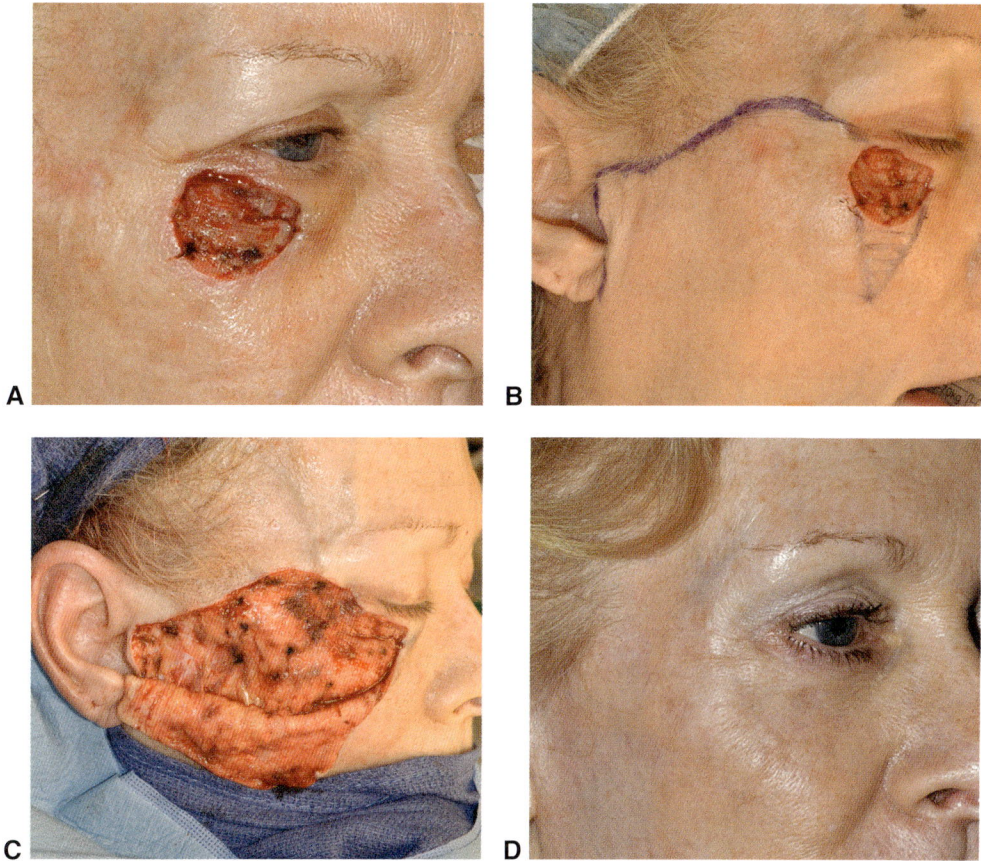

Figure 11-13 Reconstruction of large right anterior lamellar defect with rotational cheek flap (Mustardé flap). **A,** Defect after excision of basal cell carcinoma. **B,** Skin marking for rotational flap. **C,** Subcutaneous elevation of the flap showing the underlying superficial musculoaponeurotic system (SMAS). **D,** Postoperative result 6 months after surgery. *(Courtesy of Bobby S. Korn, MD, PhD.)*

a vascularized skin flap have also been used to repair large defects. This type of procedure has the advantage of requiring only 1 surgical stage and prevents temporary occlusion of the visual axis.

Lateral Canthal Defects

Laterally based transposition flaps of upper eyelid tarsus and conjunctiva can be used for large lower eyelid defects extending to the lateral canthus. These flaps can be covered with free skin grafts. Semicircular advancement or rhomboid flaps (Fig 11-14) can also be used to repair defects extending to the lateral canthal area. Horizontal strips of periosteum and/or deep temporal fascia left attached at the lateral orbital rim can be swung over and attached to the remaining eyelid margins for reconstruction of the entire lateral canthal posterior lamella (Fig 11-15). A Y-shaped pedicle flap of periosteum can be used for reconstruction of the entire lateral canthal posterior lamella of the upper and lower eyelids.

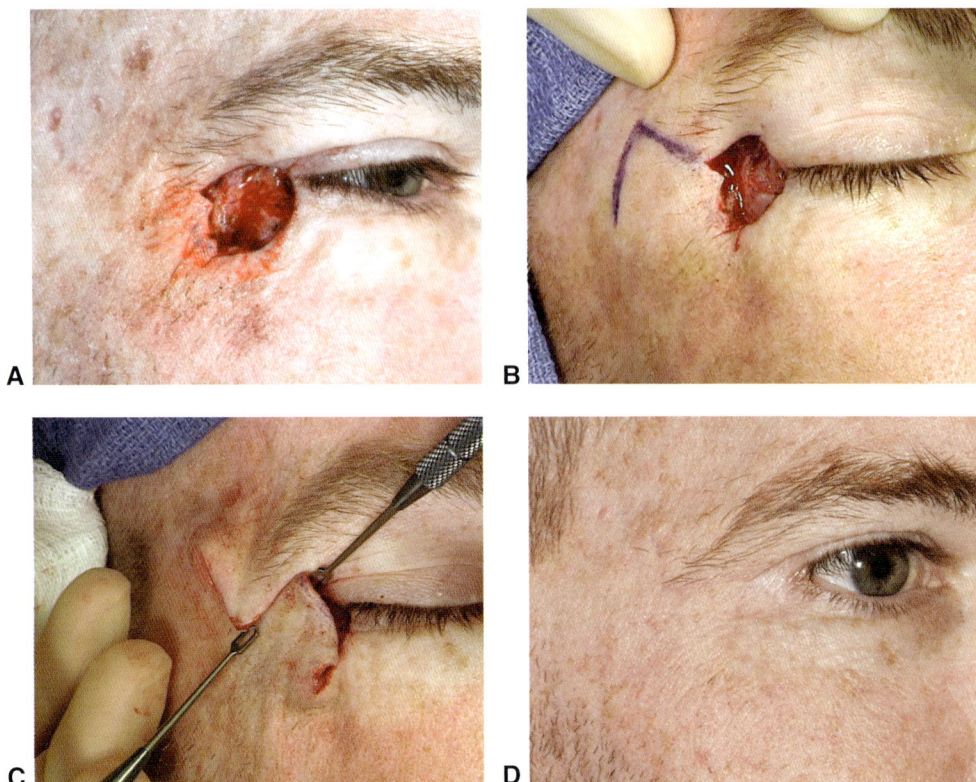

Figure 11-14 Reconstruction of lateral canthal defect with rhomboid flap. **A,** Lateral canthal defect after excision of squamous cell carcinoma. **B,** Rhomboid flap marking. **C,** Transposition of flaps after tissue undermining. **D,** Postoperative result 6 months after surgery. *(Courtesy of Bobby S. Korn, MD, PhD.)*

Medial Canthal Defects

The medial canthal area is typically repaired with full-thickness skin grafting (Fig 11-16) or via various flap techniques, although spontaneous granulation of anterior lamellar defects has demonstrated variable success. When full-thickness medial eyelid defects are present, the medial canthal attachments of the remaining eyelid margin must be fixed to firm periosteum or bone. This fixation may be accomplished with heavy permanent suture, wire, or titanium miniplates. Defects involving the lacrimal drainage apparatus are more complex, requiring simultaneous microsurgical reconstruction and possible lacrimal intubation or marsupialization. If extensive sacrifice of the canaliculi has occurred in the resection of a tumor, the patient may have to tolerate epiphora until tumor recurrence is deemed unlikely, after which a conjunctivodacryocystorhinostomy can be considered (see Chapter 15).

Full-thickness skin grafts offer an excellent way to reconstruct the medial canthus compared with the cicatrix resulting from spontaneous granulation, and they are thin enough to allow for early detection of tumor recurrence. Frozen sections and wide margins or Mohs micrographic resection techniques should be performed at the time of initial tumor resection to minimize the risk of recurrent medial canthal tumors and the risk of orbital or

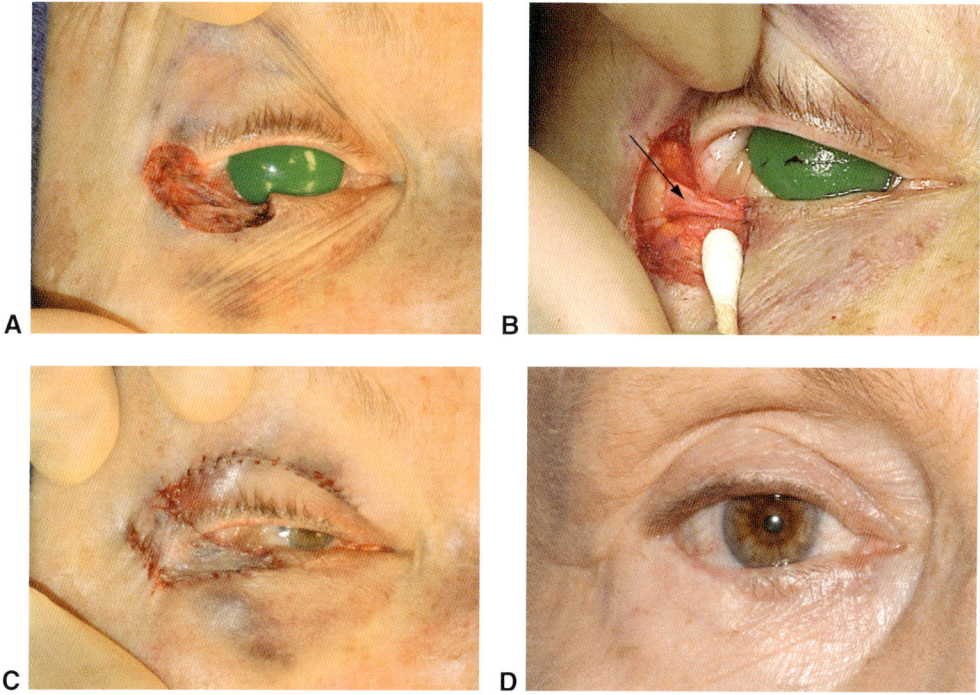

Figure 11-15 Reconstruction of lateral canthal defect and full-thickness lower eyelid defect with periosteal flap and rotational upper eyelid pedicle flap. **A,** Extensive eyelid defect after excision of basal cell carcinoma. **B,** Elevation of periosteal flap used to reconstruct lower eyelid posterior lamella *(arrow)*. **C,** Upper eyelid pedicle advancement flap to reconstruct anterior lamella of the lower eyelid. **D,** Postoperative result 6 months after surgery. *(Courtesy of Bobby S. Korn, MD, PhD.)*

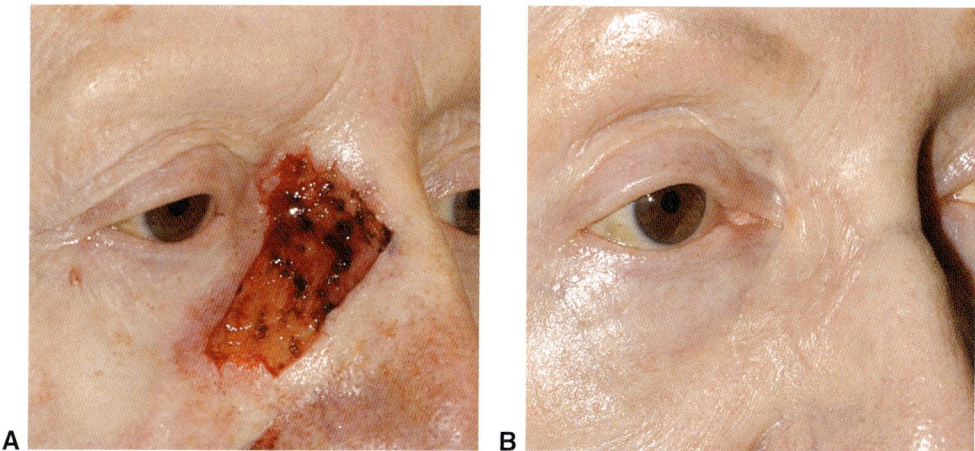

Figure 11-16 Reconstruction of medial canthal defect with full-thickness skin graft. **A,** Large medial canthal defect after excision of basal cell carcinoma. **B,** Postoperative result 6 months after full-thickness skin graft from the inner arm. *(Courtesy of Bobby S. Korn, MD, PhD.)*

lacrimal tumor extension. Large medial canthal defects of anterior lamellar structures may be properly reconstructed through the careful transposition of forehead or glabellar flaps. However, such flaps can have the disadvantage of being thick, thereby making early detection of recurrences difficult. In addition, they may require second-stage thinning or laser resurfacing to achieve the optimal cosmetic result. Mohs micrographic resection of tumors offers the highest cure rates for eradication of medial canthal epithelial malignancies.

CHAPTER **12**

Periocular Malpositions and Involutional Changes

▶ *This chapter includes related videos, which can be accessed by scanning the QR codes provided in the text or going to www.aao.org/bcscvideo_section07.*

Highlights

- Proper treatment of ectropion and entropion of the eyelids requires accurate identification of the underlying cause of the malposition.
- Successful blepharoptosis repair requires correct diagnosis, thorough understanding of eyelid anatomy, thoughtful planning, and good surgical technique.
- Important clinical measurements for evaluation of a patient with blepharoptosis include margin–reflex distance, vertical palpebral fissure height, upper eyelid crease position, levator function, and presence of lagophthalmos.
- Chemodenervation with botulinum toxin is the mainstay of treatment for benign essential blepharospasm, with surgical myectomy considered in refractory cases.
- Treatment options for brow ptosis include browpexy, direct eyebrow elevation, endoscopic forehead-lift, and pretrichial brow-lift.

History and Examination

Whether their concerns are functional or cosmetic, patients with eyelid malpositions require careful evaluation, including a history of the presenting condition and a general medical history. A detailed ocular exam including visual acuity, ocular motility, slit-lamp examination, and testing of tearing and protective mechanisms should be performed. The presenting morphology must be compared with normal, and photographs and visual field testing are obtained as appropriate. For a general discussion of the perioperative management of ocular surgery, see BCSC Section 1, *Update on General Medicine.*

Ectropion

Ectropion (Fig 12-1) is an outward turning of the eyelid margin and may be classified as

- congenital
- involutional

229

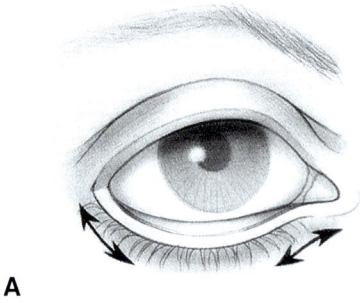

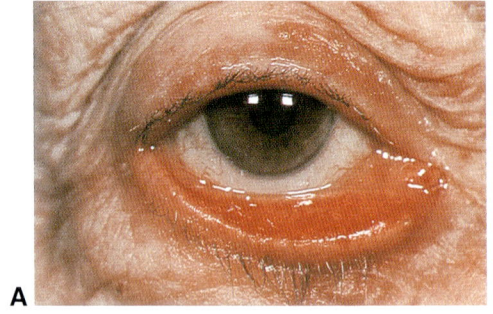

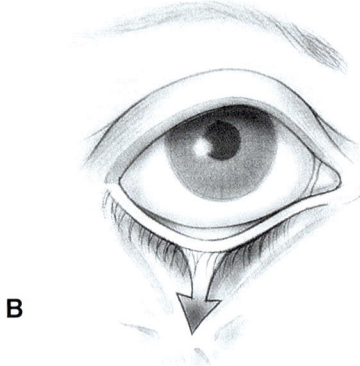

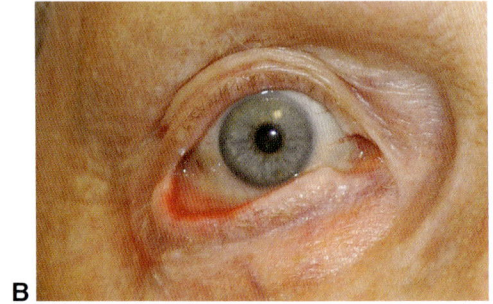

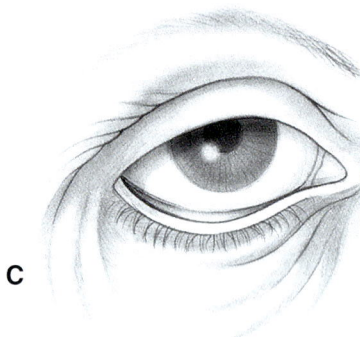

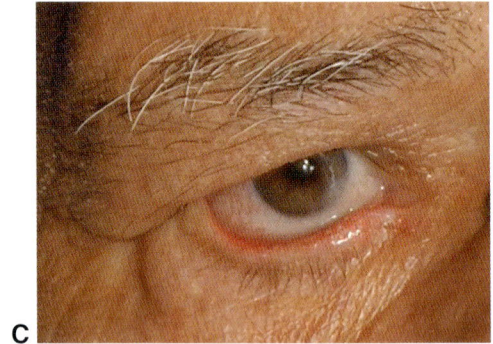

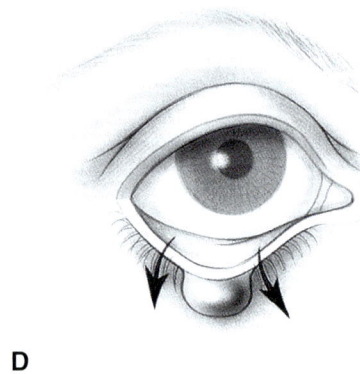

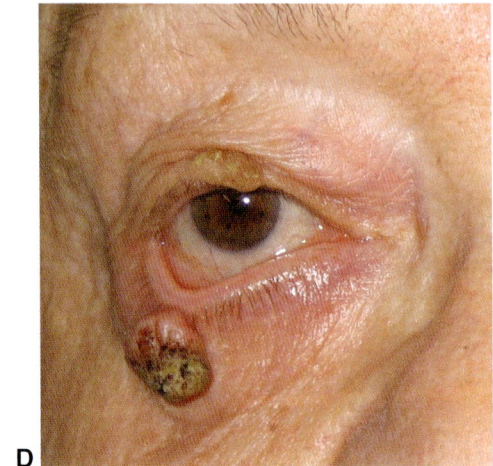

Figure 12-1 Types of ectropion. **A,** Involutional. **B,** Cicatricial. **C,** Paralytic. **D,** Mechanical. *(Illustrations by Christine Gralapp. Photographs courtesy of James R. Patrinely, MD [part A]; Bobby S. Korn, MD, PhD [parts B, C]; Morris E. Hartstein, MD [part D].)*

- cicatricial
- paralytic
- mechanical

Most cases seen in a general ophthalmology practice are involutional, with horizontal eyelid laxity being the primary cause. Horizontal lower eyelid tightening is the common component in surgical repair of the various types of ectropion (see the section "Horizontal eyelid tightening"). Congenital ectropion of the eyelid is rare and is discussed in Chapter 10 of this volume and in BCSC Section 6, *Pediatric Ophthalmology and Strabismus*.

Involutional Ectropion

Involutional ectropion results from horizontal eyelid laxity in the medial or lateral canthal tendons or both. Untreated, this condition leads to loss of eyelid apposition to the globe and eversion of the eyelid margin. Chronic conjunctival inflammation with hypertrophy and keratinization results from mechanical irritation and drying of the conjunctival surface. Involutional ectropion usually occurs in the lower eyelid because of the effects of gravity on a horizontally lax lower eyelid.

Horizontal eyelid tightening

The lower eyelid can be tightened by a variety of surgeries. Horizontal laxity can be detected by the *snapback test* or the *distraction test.* Lateral stretching of the eyelid at the time of the preoperative evaluation helps the surgeon assess whether lateral canthal resuspension would return the eyelid to its normal anatomic position (Fig 12-2A). In the *lateral tarsal strip procedure,* the tarsus is sutured directly to the lateral orbital rim periosteum (Fig 12-2B). The goal of this procedure is to correct the position of the eyelid while maintaining the horizontal dimension of the palpebral fissure and a sharp, correctly positioned lateral canthal angle (Video 12-1).

VIDEO 12-1 Lateral tarsal strip procedure.
Courtesy of Bobby S. Korn, MD, PhD.
Access all Section 7 videos at www.aao.org/bcscvideo_section07.

Laxity of the lower limb of the medial canthal tendon can be diagnosed by demonstration of excessive lateral movement of the lower punctum with lateral eyelid traction. Repair of medial canthal laxity is more challenging than repair of horizontal lower eyelid laxity, as the anterior and posterior limbs of the medial canthal tendon surround the lacrimal sac. The repair may be complicated by a kinking of the canaliculus or distraction of the punctum away from the globe, with resultant epiphora.

Medial spindle procedure

In cases of mild medial ectropion with punctal eversion, a *medial spindle procedure* can be performed. The procedure involves a horizontal fusiform excision of conjunctiva and eyelid retractors 4 mm inferior to the puncta, followed by inverting sutures for closure (Fig 12-2C). In cases with associated horizontal eyelid laxity, lateral canthal tightening (see Fig 12-2B) may be used in conjunction with this procedure.

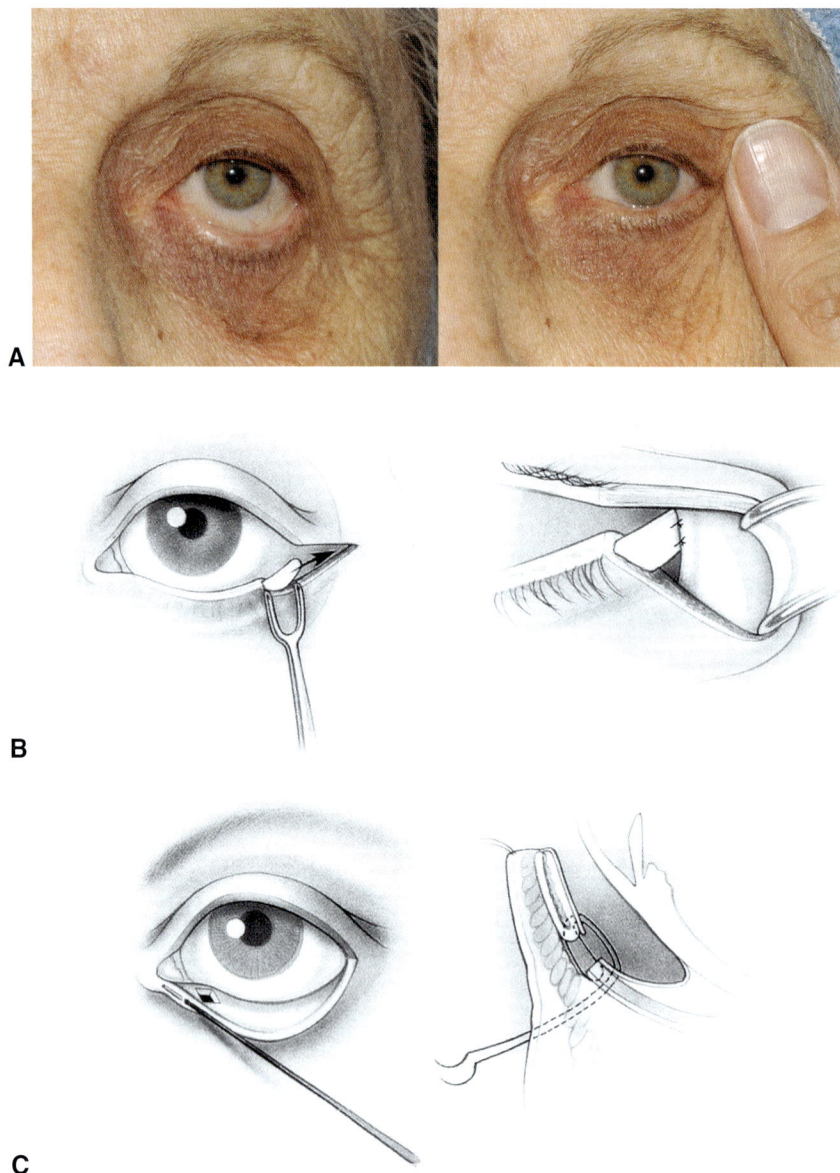

Figure 12-2 Lower eyelid tightening. **A,** Lateral stretching of the eyelid demonstrates the potential of lower eyelid tightening. **B,** Lateral tarsal strip procedure: anchoring the tarsal strip to periosteum inside the lateral orbital rim. **C,** Medial spindle procedure: outline of excision of conjunctiva and retractors. *(Part A courtesy of Bobby S. Korn, MD, PhD; illustrations by Christine Gralapp.)*

Repair of lower eyelid retractors

Retractor laxity, disinsertion, or dehiscence may be associated with ectropion, especially when the eyelid is completely everted, a condition known as *tarsal ectropion.* Attenuation or disinsertion of the inferior retractors may occur as an isolated defect or may accompany horizontal laxity in involutional ectropion. When both defects are present, repair of the retractors is combined with horizontal tightening of the eyelid.

Korn BS. Ectropion and entropion. *Focal Points: Clinical Modules for Ophthalmologists.* San Francisco: American Academy of Ophthalmology; 2014, module 2.

Paralytic Ectropion

See the section Facial Paralysis in this chapter.

Cicatricial Ectropion

Cicatricial ectropion of the upper or lower eyelid occurs when there is a deficiency of skin secondary to thermal or chemical burns, mechanical trauma, surgical trauma, or chronic actinic skin damage. Cicatricial ectropion can also be caused by chronic inflammation of the eyelid from dermatologic conditions such as rosacea, atopic dermatitis, or eczematoid dermatitis or by scarring from herpes zoster infections. Management consists of addressing the underlying cause, along with conservative medical protection of the cornea. Cicatricial ectropion of the lower eyelid is usually treated in a 3-step procedure (Fig 12-3):

1. Vertical cicatricial traction is surgically released through an anterior approach.
2. The eyelid is horizontally tightened.

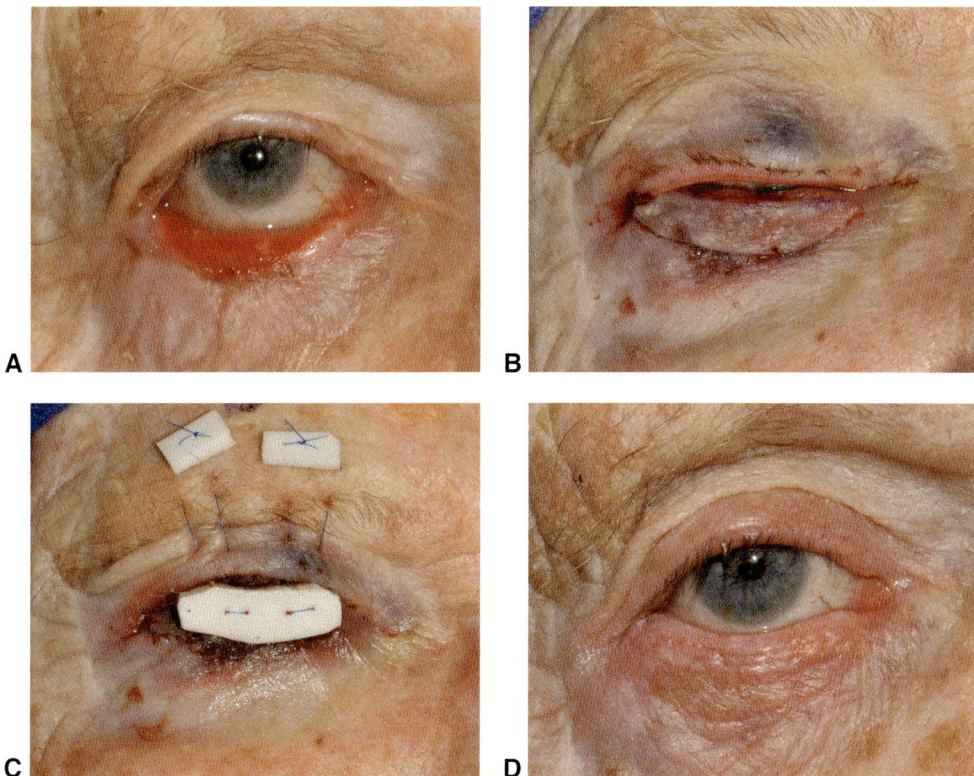

Figure 12-3 Repair of cicatricial ectropion. **A,** Preoperative appearance. **B,** Release of vertical cicatricial traction and placement of full-thickness skin graft in association with lateral canthal tightening. **C,** Immobilization of skin graft with Frost suture. **D,** Final appearance after skin graft placement and lateral tarsal strip. *(Courtesy of Bobby S. Korn, MD, PhD.)*

3. The anterior lamella is vertically augmented by means of a midface-lift, full-thickness skin graft, or adjacent tissue transfer, and the eyelid is placed on superior traction with a suture.

Treatment of cicatricial ectropion or retraction of the upper eyelid usually requires only release of traction and augmentation of the vertically shortened anterior lamella with a full-thickness skin graft.

Although upper eyelid skin from the fellow eye would be ideal for grafting, there is rarely enough tissue available from this source. The postauricular, preauricular, supraclavicular, and medial upper arm areas are other potential donor sites (see Chapter 11, Fig 11-8).

Mechanical Ectropion

Mechanical ectropion is usually caused by the gravitational effect of a bulky eyelid mass. Other causes include fluid accumulation, herniated orbital fat, or poorly fitted spectacles. Treatment is focused on addressing the underlying etiology.

Entropion

Entropion is an inversion of the eyelid margin. Lower eyelid entropion (usually involutional) is much more common than upper eyelid entropion (usually cicatricial). Entropion may be unilateral or bilateral and is often classified as follows:

- congenital
- involutional
- acute spastic
- cicatricial

Congenital Entropion

Congenital entropion is discussed in Chapter 10.

Involutional Entropion

Involutional entropion occurs in the lower eyelids (Fig 12-4). Causative factors include horizontal laxity of the eyelid, attenuation or disinsertion of eyelid retractors, and overriding by the preseptal orbicularis oculi muscle. Horizontal laxity can be assessed with snapback and distraction testing. Such laxity is a result of senescence, with stretching of the eyelid and canthal tendons. Typically, the lower eyelid retractors maintain the eyelid margin in proper orientation. However, attenuation of the eyelid retractors (capsulopalpebral fascia and inferior tarsal muscle), in conjunction with preseptal orbicularis override, allows the inferior border of the tarsus to roll forward and superiorly, resulting in inward rotation of the margin. Several clinical clues may suggest disinsertion of the retractors:

- a white subconjunctival line several millimeters below the inferior tarsal border caused by the leading edge of the detached retractors
- a deeper-than-normal inferior fornix

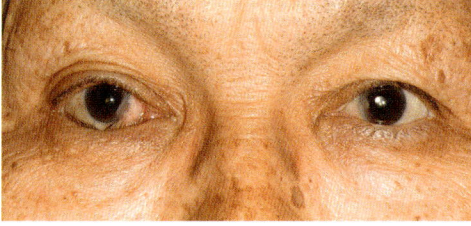

Figure 12-4 Involutional entropion of the right lower eyelid. *(Courtesy of Bobby S. Korn, MD, PhD.)*

- elevation of the lower eyelid
- minimal movement of the lower eyelid on downgaze

After the entropic eyelid has been placed in its normal position, the clinician can detect superior override of the preseptal orbicularis by instructing the patient to forcefully close the eyelids. This maneuver accentuates the inward rotation of the lower eyelid margin. Procedures to repair involutional entropion of the lower eyelid fall into 3 groups: temporizing measures, horizontal tightening procedures, and retractor repair. Often, a combination of procedures is necessary. If trichiasis is present, it may require specific treatment, either in conjunction with the entropion repair or subsequently, if the eyelashes remain misdirected after proper positioning of the eyelid margin (see the Trichiasis section).

Temporizing measures

Lubrication and a bandage contact lens may be used to protect the cornea from mechanical abrasion by the misdirected eyelashes. Rotational suture techniques (Fig 12-5) are

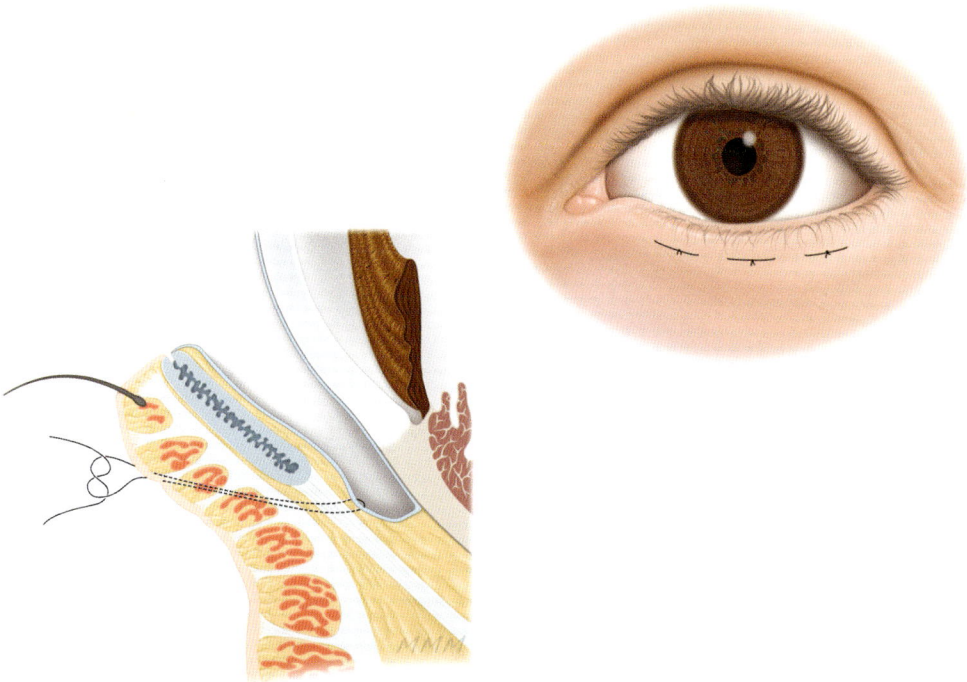

Figure 12-5 Rotational suture repair of spastic entropion. *(Illustration by Mark Miller.)*

occasionally helpful as temporizing measures in involutional entropion; however, when these techniques are used in isolation, recurrence is anticipated.

Surgical repair

Direct repair of lower eyelid retractor defects through a skin incision (Fig 12-6A) or a transconjunctival approach (Fig 12-6B) can be performed to stabilize the inferior border of the tarsus. In addition, a small amount of preseptal orbicularis oculi muscle can be removed in selected patients who have preseptal orbicularis overriding the pretarsal orbicularis. Reinsertion of the eyelid retractors and limited myectomy of the orbicularis in conjunction with a lower eyelid shortening procedure such as a lateral tarsal strip operation or wedge resection (see Fig 12-2B) correct all 3 etiologic factors in involutional entropion (Video 12-2).

VIDEO 12-2 Transconjunctival lower eyelid entropion repair.
Courtesy of Bobby S. Korn, MD, PhD.

Erb MH, Uzcategui N, Dresner SC. Efficacy and complications of the transconjunctival entropion repair for lower eyelid involutional entropion. *Ophthalmology.* 2006;113(12):2351–2356.

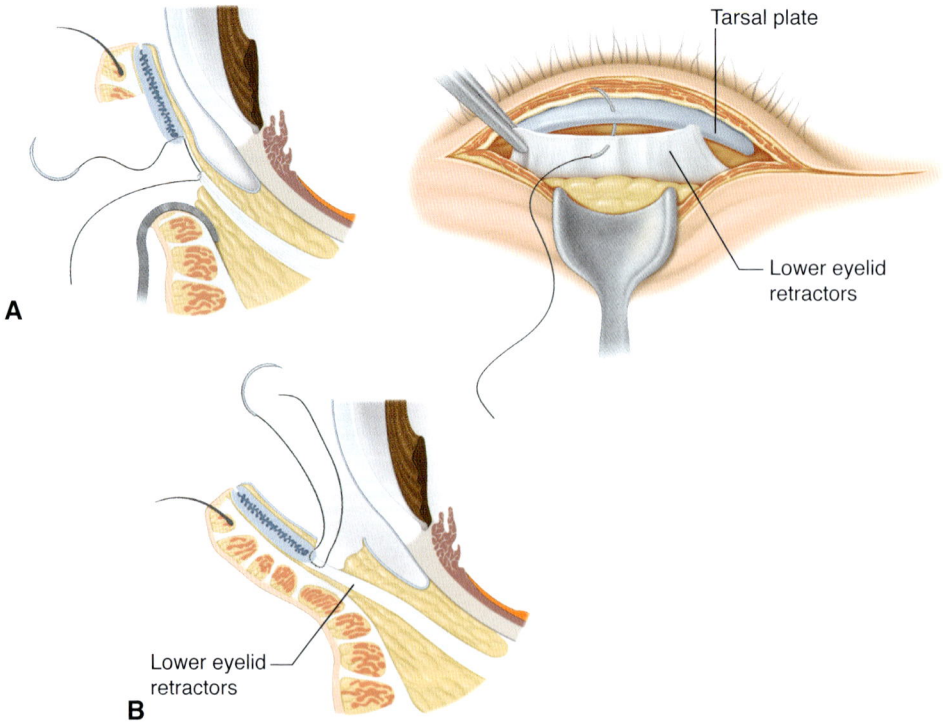

Figure 12-6 Retractor repair of lower eyelid involutional entropion. **A,** Transcutaneous approach. **B,** Transconjunctival approach. *(Illustration by Mark Miller.)*

Acute Spastic Entropion

Acute spastic entropion arises from ocular irritation or inflammation. Sustained contraction of the orbicularis oculi muscle leads to inward rotation of the eyelid margin. A cycle of increasing frequency of orbicularis muscle spasm caused by corneal irritation perpetuates the problem. The acute entropion usually resolves when the cycle is broken by treatment of the underlying cause.

Taping of the entropic eyelid to evert the margin, cautery, or various rotational suture techniques (see Fig 12-5) afford temporary relief for most patients. In selected cases, botulinum toxin injection can be used to temporarily paralyze the overriding preseptal orbicularis muscle. However, involutional changes are often present in the eyelid; therefore, definitive surgical repair may be required.

Cicatricial Entropion

Cicatricial entropion is caused by vertical tarsoconjunctival contracture and internal rotation of the eyelid margin, with resulting irritation of the globe from inturned cilia or the keratinized eyelid margin (Fig 12-7). Various conditions may lead to cicatricial entropion, including *autoimmune* (mucous membrane [ocular cicatricial] pemphigoid), *inflammatory* (Stevens-Johnson syndrome, Fig 12-8), *infectious* (trachoma, herpes zoster), *surgical* (enucleation, posterior approach ptosis correction, transconjunctival surgery), and *traumatic* (thermal or chemical burns, scarring) conditions. The long-term use of topical glaucoma medications, especially miotics and prostaglandins, may cause chronic conjunctivitis with vertical conjunctival shortening and secondary cicatricial entropion.

The patient's history, along with a simple diagnostic test *(digital eversion),* usually distinguishes cicatricial entropion from involutional entropion. Attempting to return the eyelid to a normal anatomic position using digital traction will correct the abnormal margin position in involutional entropion but not in cicatricial entropion. In addition, inspection of the posterior lamella may reveal scarring of the tarsal conjunctiva in cases of cicatricial entropion.

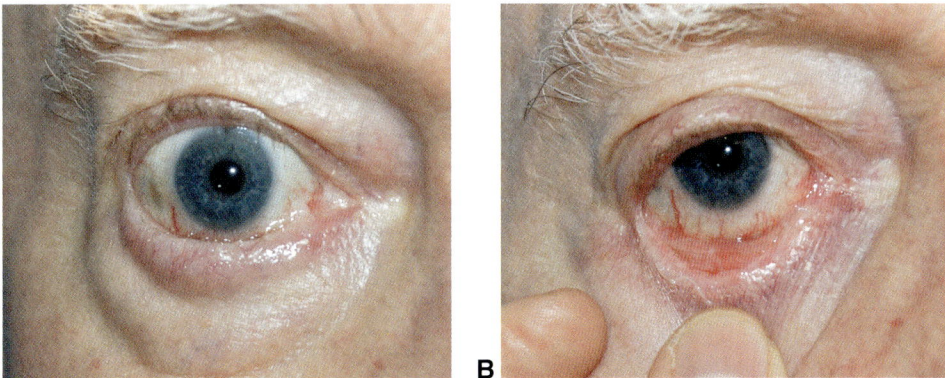

Figure 12-7 Cicatricial entropion. **A,** Entropion of the right lower eyelid. **B,** Eyelid everted, showing conjunctival scarring and shortening of the fornix. *(Courtesy of Don O. Kikkawa, MD.)*

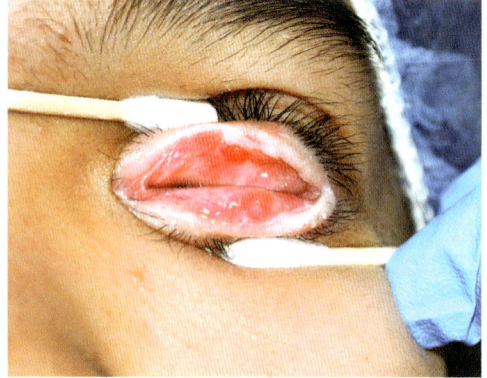

Figure 12-8 Stevens-Johnson syndrome with conjunctival scarring and eyelid margin keratinization. *(Courtesy of Bobby S. Korn, MD, PhD.)*

Management

Successful management of cicatricial entropion depends on careful preoperative evaluation to determine the cause, severity, and prominent features in each patient. When the etiology is autoimmune or inflammatory disease, the prognosis is guarded because of frequent disease progression.

Cicatricial entropion usually requires surgery, but lubricating drops and ointments, barriers to symblepharon formation, and eyelash ablation with lash cautery are sometimes useful. Indeed, surgery is contraindicated during the acute phase of autoimmune diseases, and medical management of the inflammatory condition with topical and systemic medications is more appropriate until the disease stabilizes. When surgery is indicated, maximal inflammatory suppression is achieved with pulsed systemic anti-inflammatory medications (corticosteroids and immunosuppressive agents).

The *tarsal fracture operation* is useful in cases of mild to moderate cicatricial entropion *(marginal entropion)* of the upper or lower eyelid (Fig 12-9). In this situation, lashes abrade the cornea, and careful examination shows that the eyelid margin has lost its square edges and is rotated posteriorly. A posterior horizontal tarsal incision is made 2 mm distal to the eyelid margin. This incision through the full thickness of the tarsus allows the

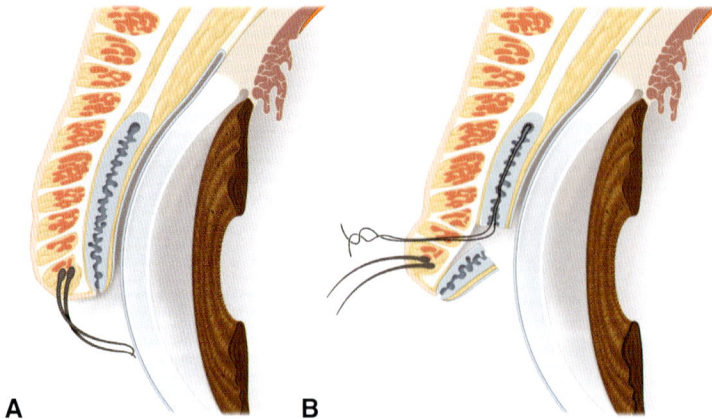

A   B

Figure 12-9 Tarsal fracture operation. **A,** Tarsotomy. **B,** Margin rotation for cicatricial entropion. *(Illustration by Mark Miller.)*

eyelid margin to be rotated away from the globe. The eyelid position is stabilized with everting sutures.

For margin rotation to be effective, the tarsus should be intact and of reasonably good quality. In patients with severe cicatricial entropion, the involved tarsus is usually scarred and distorted and generally needs to be replaced. In the upper eyelid, tarsoconjunctival and other mucosal grafts are useful tarsal substitutes; in the lower eyelid, autogenous ear cartilage, preserved scleral grafts, and hard-palate mucosa have been used.

> Bleyen I, Dolman PJ. The Wies procedure for management of trichiasis or cicatricial entropion of either upper or lower eyelids. *Br J Ophthalmol.* 2009;93(12):1612–1615.

Symblepharon

Symblepharon is an adhesion between conjunctival surfaces. It can occur as a result of inflammation, infection, trauma, or previous surgery. Conjunctival Z-plasties are sometimes effective for localized contracted linear adhesions when vertical lengthening of the involved tissue is the primary objective. More extensive symblepharon formation requires a full-thickness conjunctival graft or flap, a partial-thickness buccal mucous membrane graft, or an amniotic membrane graft.

Trichiasis

Trichiasis is an acquired misdirection of eyelashes (Fig 12-10). The treatment method is usually determined by the pattern (segmental or diffuse) of the misdirected lashes and the quality of the posterior lamella of the involved eyelid. Inturned lashes not associated with involutional entropion are usually seen in cases of chronic eyelid inflammation and posterior lamellar scarring *(marginal cicatricial entropion)*. If the eyelid margin is misdirected, treatment should focus on correcting the entropion.

Management

Trichiasis may be initially treated with *mechanical epilation*. Because of eyelash regrowth, recurrence can be expected 3–8 weeks after epilation. Broken cilia are often more irritating to the cornea than mature longer lashes.

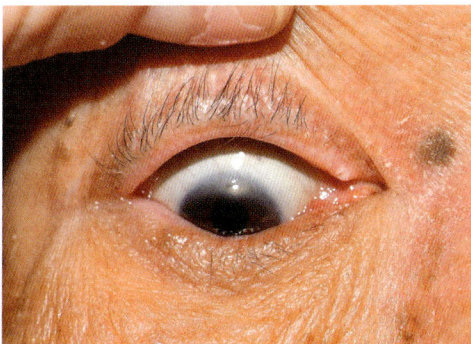

Figure 12-10 Trichiasis of the right upper eyelid. *(Courtesy of Bobby S. Korn, MD, PhD.)*

Standard *electrolysis* or *radiofrequency ablation* is used for definitive treatment of trichiasis. The energy is delivered through an insulated needle to destroy the hair follicle. When the needle tip is removed, the lash is easily extracted. However, the recurrence rate is high, adjacent normal lashes may be damaged, and scarring of the adjacent eyelid margin tissue can worsen the problem.

Segmental trichiasis can be treated with *cryotherapy* in an office procedure that requires only local infiltrative anesthesia. The involved area is frozen for approximately 25 seconds, allowed to thaw, and then refrozen for 20 seconds *(double freeze–thaw technique).* The lashes are mechanically removed with forceps after treatment. Edema lasting several days, loss of skin pigmentation, notching of the eyelid margin, and possible interference with goblet cell function are disadvantages of cryotherapy.

Argon laser treatment of trichiasis can be useful when only a few scattered eyelashes require ablation or when the stimulation of larger areas of inflammation is undesirable. Some pigment is required in the base of the lash to absorb the laser energy and ablate the lash, making this technique sensitive to hair color.

In all of these procedures, success rates vary, and additional treatment sessions are commonly necessary. An ophthalmic microtrephine can also be used to extract misdirected eyelash units. *Full-thickness pentagonal resection* with primary closure may be considered when trichiasis is confined to a segment of the eyelid.

Dutton JJ, Tawfik HA, DeBacker CM, Lipham WJ. Direct internal eyelash bulb extirpation for trichiasis. *Ophthalmic Plast Reconstr Surg.* 2000;16(2):142–145.

McCracken MS, Kikkawa DO, Vasani SN. Treatment of trichiasis and distichiasis by eyelash trephination. *Ophthalmic Plast Reconstr Surg.* 2006;22(5):349–351.

Rosner M, Bourla N, Rosen N. Eyelid splitting and extirpation of hair follicles using a radiosurgical technique for treatment of trichiasis. *Ophthalmic Surg Lasers Imaging.* 2004;35(2):116–122.

Blepharoptosis

Blepharoptosis, also referred to as *ptosis,* is the inferior displacement of the upper eyelid. It is a common cause of reversible peripheral vision loss. Although the superior visual field is most often involved, central vision can also be affected. Many patients with ptosis report difficulty with reading because the ptosis worsens in downgaze. Ptosis has also been shown to decrease the overall amount of light reaching the macula and, therefore, can reduce visual acuity, especially at night.

Upper eyelid ptosis can be classified by onset as *congenital* or *acquired.* It can be further categorized by the cause: *myogenic, aponeurotic, neurogenic, mechanical,* or *traumatic.* The most common type of congenital ptosis is myogenic, resulting from a poorly developed levator palpebrae superioris muscle; the most common type of acquired ptosis is aponeurotic and is caused by stretching or disinsertion of the levator aponeurosis.

Cahill KV, Bradley EA, Meyer DR, et al. Functional indications for upper eyelid ptosis and blepharoplasty surgery: a report by the American Academy of Ophthalmology. *Ophthalmology.* 2011;118(12):2510–2517.

Evaluation

Many elements are involved in the evaluation of blepharoptosis. The history can provide pertinent clues, such as variability in the degree of ptosis, which suggests myasthenia gravis. Affected family members may highlight potential heritable conditions such as oculopharyngeal or myotonic dystrophy. The physical examination further elucidates etiology through eyelid measurements, assessment of surrounding orbital and facial structures, and observation of head positioning and possible synkinetic movements. The pupils and tear film are also assessed. Further ancillary testing may be guided by additional history and clinical exam findings.

Eyelid measurements

Physical examination of the ptosis patient begins with 5 clinical measurements (Video 12-3, Fig 12-11):

- margin–reflex distances 1 and 2
- vertical palpebral fissure height
- upper eyelid crease position
- levator function (upper eyelid excursion)
- presence of lagophthalmos

VIDEO 12-3 Eyelid measurements.
Courtesy of Richard C. Allen, MD, PhD.

The *margin–reflex distance 1 (MRD$_1$)*, which is the distance from the upper eyelid margin to the corneal light reflex in primary position, is the single most important measurement in describing the amount of ptosis. In severe ptosis, the light reflex may be obstructed by the eyelid, and the MRD$_1$ has a zero or negative value. The more ptotic eyelid should be

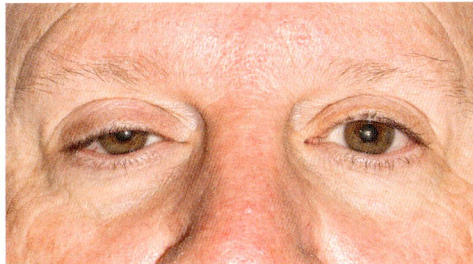

Margin–reflex distance 1	+0.5	+3.5
Margin–reflex distance 2	+5.5	+5.5
Palpebral fissure height	6.0	9.0
Upper eyelid crease	12	8
Levator function	15	15
Lagophthalmos	0	0

Figure 12-11 Evaluation of ptosis. Patient appearance and example of a ptosis data collection sheet. *(Courtesy of Bobby S. Korn, MD, PhD.)*

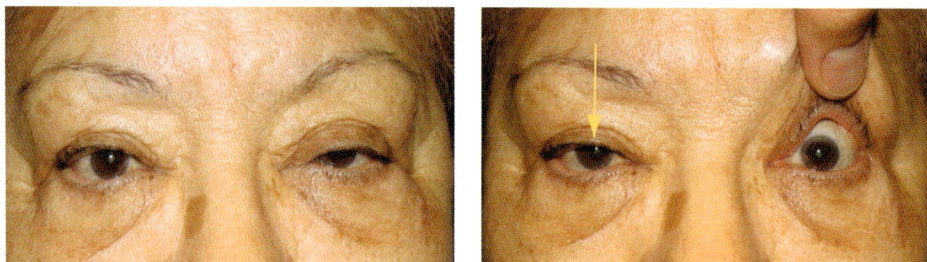

Figure 12-12 Unmasking of right upper eyelid ptosis *(arrow)* with elevation of ptotic left upper eyelid, demonstrating the effect of Hering's law of equal innervation. *(Courtesy of Don O. Kikkawa, MD.)*

elevated to unmask occult contralateral ptosis according to Hering's law of equal innervation (Fig 12-12). If the patient reports visual obstruction while reading, the eyelid position in downgaze is checked. Lower eyelid retraction (or scleral show) should be noted separately as the *margin–reflex distance 2 (MRD$_2$)*. The MRD$_2$ is the distance from the corneal light reflex to the lower eyelid margin. The sum of the MRD$_1$ and the MRD$_2$ should equal the vertical palpebral fissure height.

The *vertical palpebral fissure* is measured at the widest point between the lower eyelid and the upper eyelid. This measurement is taken with the patient fixating on a distant object in primary gaze.

The distance from the *upper eyelid crease* to the eyelid margin is measured. Because the insertion of fibers from the levator muscle into the skin contributes to formation of the upper eyelid crease, high, duplicated, or asymmetric creases may indicate an abnormal position of the levator aponeurosis. In the typical non-Asian eyelid, the upper eyelid crease is 8–9 mm in males and 9–11 mm in females. The crease is often elevated in patients with involutional ptosis and is often shallow or absent in patients with congenital ptosis. As a normal anatomic finding, the upper eyelid crease is typically lower or obscured in the Asian eyelid, with or without ptosis.

Levator function is estimated by measuring the *upper eyelid excursion* from downgaze to upgaze with frontalis muscle function negated. Fixating the brow with digital pressure minimizes contributions from accessory elevators of the eyelids such as the frontalis muscle. Failure to negate the influence of the frontalis muscle results in overestimation of levator function, which may affect the diagnosis and treatment plan.

Finally, the patient should be assessed for *lagophthalmos;* if it is present, the gap between the eyelids should be measured and the amount noted (in millimeters). Lagophthalmos and poor tear film quantity or quality may predispose the patient to complications of ptosis repair such as dryness and exposure keratopathy.

Allen RC. Surgical management of ptosis and brow ptosis. *Focal Points: Clinical Practice Perspectives.* San Francisco: American Academy of Ophthalmology; 2017, module 5.

Additional assessments

Physical examination also includes checking *head position, chin elevation, brow position,* and *brow action* in attempted upgaze. These features help to show the patient how ptosis affects function. Quantity and quality of the tear film is documented in the initial examination.

The examiner should also note the presence or absence of supraduction of the globe with eyelid closure *(Bell phenomenon)* and assess corneal sensation; these factors may affect the treatment plan.

Variation in the amount of ptosis with extraocular muscle or jaw muscle movements *(synkinesis)* occurs in several conditions, including Marcus Gunn jaw-winking ptosis, aberrant regeneration of the oculomotor nerve or the facial nerve, and some types of Duane retraction syndrome. The examiner should attempt to elicit synkinesis as part of the evaluation of patients with congenital blepharoptosis or those with possible aberrant regeneration.

The *position of the ptotic eyelid in downgaze* (palpebral fissure in downgaze) can help differentiate between congenital and acquired causes. The congenitally ptotic eyelid is typically higher in downgaze than the contralateral normal eyelid. The congenitally ptotic eyelid may also manifest lagophthalmos. By contrast, in acquired involutional ptosis the affected eyelid remains ptotic in all positions of gaze and may even worsen in downgaze with relaxation of the frontalis muscle.

The ophthalmologist must assess *visual function* and *refractive error* in all cases of congenital or childhood ptosis in order to identify and treat the child with concomitant amblyopia resulting from anisometropia, high astigmatism, strabismus, or occlusion of the pupil. Amblyopia occurs in approximately 20% of patients with congenital ptosis. *Extraocular muscle function* should also be assessed because extraocular muscle dysfunction associated with ptosis occurs in various congenital conditions (combined superior rectus/levator muscle maldevelopment, congenital oculomotor palsy) and acquired conditions (ocular or systemic myasthenia gravis, chronic progressive external ophthalmoplegia, oculopharyngeal dystrophy, and oculomotor palsy with or without aberrant regeneration).

In addition, *pupillary examination* is important in the evaluation of ptosis. Pupil abnormalities are present in some acquired and congenital conditions associated with ptosis (eg, Horner syndrome, cranial nerve III palsy). Miosis that is most apparent in dim illumination is a finding in Horner syndrome; mydriasis is seen in some cases of oculomotor nerve palsy.

External examination may reveal other abnormalities as well. For example, severe bilateral congenital ptosis may be associated with telecanthus, epicanthus inversus, hypoplasia of the superior orbital rims, horizontal shortening of the eyelids, ear deformities, hypertelorism, and hypoplasia of the nasal bridge. These findings are classically seen in *blepharophimosis–ptosis–epicanthus inversus syndrome* (BPES; discussed in Chapter 10).

Ancillary testing

Visual field testing may be used to quantitate the patient's level of functional visual impairment. Comparison of visual fields with eyelids elevated with tape to those with eyelids in their natural ptotic state gives an estimate of the superior visual field improvement that can be anticipated following surgery. Visual field testing and external full-face photography may be required by third-party payers for insurance coverage.

Pharmacologic testing, pupillary evaluation in light and dark, and *lower eyelid elevation (smaller MRD_2)* may be helpful in confirming the clinical diagnosis of *Horner syndrome* and in localizing the causative lesion (see BCSC Section 5, *Neuro-Ophthalmology*). Third-order neuron dysfunction resulting in Horner syndrome is typically benign. However, neuron dysfunction of the first or second order is sometimes associated with malignant neoplasms such as an apical lung (Pancoast) tumor, aneurysm, or dissection of the carotid artery.

Pharmacologic testing may also be used in the diagnosis of myasthenia gravis (MG), a disease in which ptosis is the most common presenting sign. Fluctuating ptosis that seems to worsen with fatigue or prolonged upgaze—especially when accompanied by diplopia or other clinical signs of systemic MG such as dysphonia, dyspnea, dysphagia, or proximal muscle weakness—is an indication for further diagnostic evaluation with the edrophonium chloride, ice-pack, or acetylcholine receptor antibody tests. (Also see the section "Myasthenia gravis.")

Classification

Myogenic ptosis

The patient's history usually distinguishes congenital from acquired ptosis. *Congenital myogenic ptosis* results from dysgenesis of the levator muscle. Instead of normal muscle fibers, fibrous or adipose tissue is present in the muscle belly, diminishing the ability of the levator to contract and relax. Therefore, most congenital ptosis caused by maldevelopment of the levator muscle is characterized by decreased levator function, lid lag, and, sometimes, lagophthalmos (Fig 12-13). The upper eyelid crease is often absent or poorly formed, especially in patients with more severe ptosis. Congenital myogenic ptosis associated with a poor Bell phenomenon or with vertical strabismus may indicate concomitant

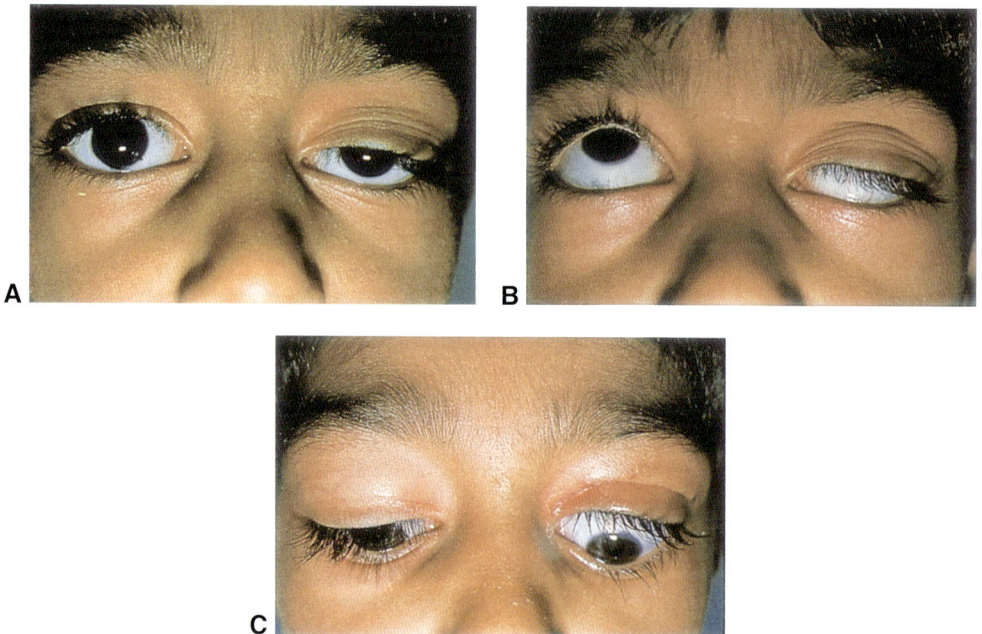

Figure 12-13 Left congenital ptosis. **A,** Patient's margin–reflex distance 1 is 6.0 mm OD and 0.5 mm OS (normal is 4–5 mm). **B,** Upgaze accentuates ptosis. **C,** Downgaze reveals lid lag. *(Courtesy of Robert C. Kersten, MD.)*

maldevelopment of the superior rectus and levator muscles (*monocular elevation deficiency,* formerly called *double-elevator palsy*).

Acquired myogenic ptosis results from localized or diffuse muscular disease such as muscular dystrophy, chronic progressive external ophthalmoplegia, MG, or oculopharyngeal dystrophy. Because of the underlying muscle dysfunction, surgical correction may be difficult and require a frontalis sling procedure.

> Allen RC, Zimmerman MB, Watterberg EA, Morrison LA, Carter KD. Primary bilateral silicone frontalis suspension for good levator function ptosis in oculopharyngeal muscular dystrophy. *Br J Ophthalmol.* 2012;96(6):841–845.

Aponeurotic ptosis

The levator aponeurosis transmits levator palpebrae superioris muscle force to the eyelid. Thus, any disruption in its anatomy or function can lead to ptosis.

Acquired aponeurotic ptosis is the most common form of ptosis. It results from stretching or dehiscence of the levator aponeurosis or disinsertion from its normal position. Common causes are involutional attenuation or repetitive traction on the eyelid, which may occur with frequent eye rubbing or prolonged use of rigid contact lenses. Aponeurotic ptosis may also be caused or exacerbated by intraocular surgery or eyelid surgery (Fig 12-14).

Eyelids with aponeurotic defects characteristically have a high or an absent upper eyelid crease secondary to upward displacement or loss of the insertion of levator fibers into the skin. Thinning of the eyelid superior to the upper tarsal plate is often an associated finding. Because the levator muscle itself is healthy, levator function in aponeurotic ptosis is usually normal (15 mm). Acquired aponeurotic ptosis may worsen in downgaze, thus interfering with the patient's ability to read, as well as limiting the superior visual field. Table 12-1 compares acquired aponeurotic ptosis with congenital myogenic ptosis.

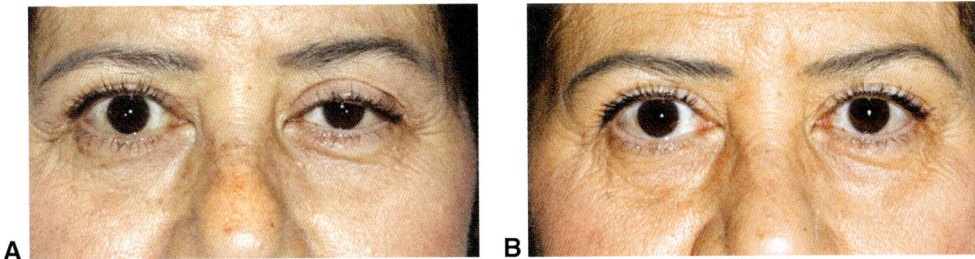

Figure 12-14 Aponeurotic ptosis. **A,** Aponeurotic ptosis of the left upper eyelid after cataract surgery. Similar aponeurotic ptosis can occur following various other intraocular and eyelid surgical procedures. **B,** After repair, the symmetry of the eyelid creases and folds is improved, as well as the position of the left eyelid margin. *(Courtesy of Bobby S. Korn, MD, PhD.)*

Table 12-1 Blepharoptosis Comparison

	Congenital Myogenic Ptosis	Acquired Aponeurotic Ptosis
Upper eyelid crease	Poorly formed	Higher than normal or absent
Levator function	Reduced	Near normal
Downgaze	Lid lag	Eyelid drop

Neurogenic ptosis

Congenital conditions *Congenital neurogenic ptosis* is caused by innervational defects that occur during embryonic development. This condition is relatively rare and is most commonly associated with congenital cranial nerve III (CN III) palsy, congenital Horner syndrome, or Marcus Gunn jaw-winking syndrome.

Congenital oculomotor nerve (CN III) palsy is manifested as ptosis together with inability to elevate, depress, or adduct the globe. The pupils may also be dilated. This palsy may be partial or complete, but ptosis is very rarely an isolated finding. It is uncommon to find aberrant innervation in congenital CN III palsies. Management of strabismus and amblyopia is difficult in many cases of congenital CN III palsy. Treatment of the associated ptosis is also complicated, usually requiring a frontalis suspension procedure, which often leads to some degree of lagophthalmos. As a result of lagophthalmos, poor ocular motility, and poor postoperative eyelid excursion, postoperative management may be complicated by diplopia, exposure keratopathy, and corneal ulceration.

Congenital Horner syndrome is a manifestation of an interruption in the sympathetic nerve chain. It can cause mild ptosis associated with miosis, anhidrosis, and decreased pigmentation of the iris on the involved side. The mild ptosis of Horner syndrome results from an innervational deficit to the Müller muscle. Decreased sympathetic tone to the inferior tarsal muscle in the lower eyelid results in elevation of the lower eyelid, sometimes referred to as *reverse ptosis.* The combination of upper ptosis and lower eyelid elevation decreases the vertical palpebral fissure and may falsely suggest enophthalmos. The pupillary miosis is most apparent in dim illumination, when the contralateral pupil dilates more.

Congenital neurogenic ptosis may also be synkinetic. *Marcus Gunn jaw-winking syndrome* is the most common form of congenital synkinetic neurogenic ptosis (Video 12-4, Fig 12-15). In this synkinetic syndrome, the unilaterally ptotic eyelid elevates with jaw movements. The movement that most commonly causes elevation of the ptotic eyelid is lateral mandibular movement to the contralateral side. This phenomenon is usually first noticed by the mother when she is feeding or nursing the baby. This synkinesis is thought to be caused by aberrant connections between the motor division of CN V and the levator muscle. Infrequently, this syndrome is associated with abnormal connections between CN III and other cranial nerves. Some forms of Duane retraction syndrome also cause elevation of a ptotic eyelid with movement of the globe. This congenital syndrome is also thought to result from aberrant nerve connections.

VIDEO 12-4 Marcus Gunn jaw-winking.
Courtesy of Pete Setabutr, MD.

Demirci H, Frueh BR, Nelson CC. Marcus Gunn jaw-winking synkinesis: clinical features and management. *Ophthalmology.* 2010;117(7):1447–1452.

Acquired conditions *Acquired neurogenic ptosis* results from interruption of normally developed innervation and is most often secondary to an acquired CN III palsy, Horner syndrome, or MG.

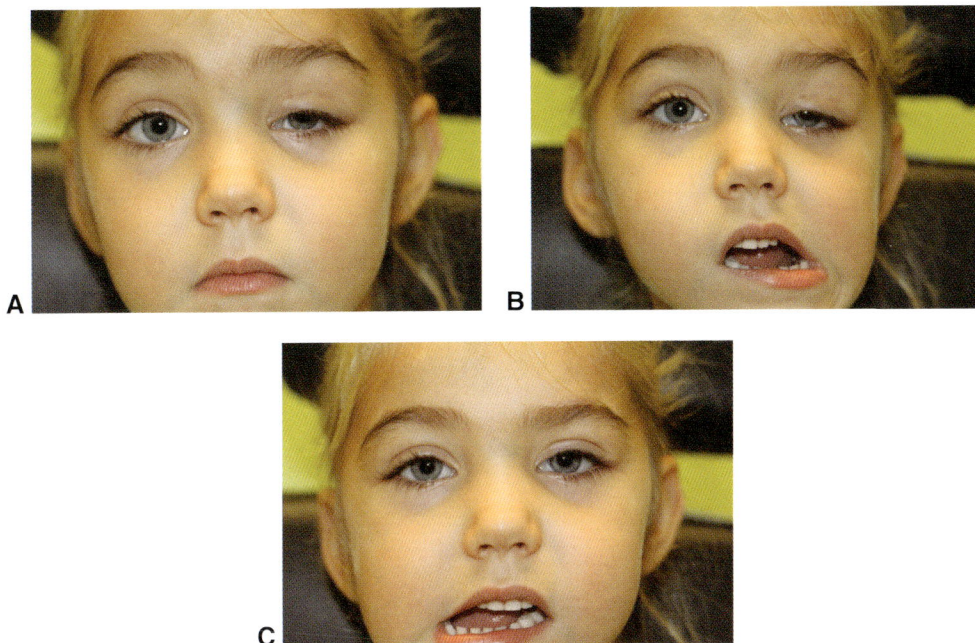

Figure 12-15 Marcus Gunn jaw-winking ptosis (synkinesis linking cranial nerve V to cranial nerve III). **A,** Relaxed position with ptosis of the left upper eyelid. **B,** When the mandible is moved to the left, the eyelid position remains low. **C,** Moving the mandible to the right elevates the left upper eyelid. *(Courtesy of Jill Foster, MD.)*

Delineation of the cause of acquired CN III (oculomotor) palsy is important. Distinction must be made between *ischemic* and *compressive* etiologies. Most acquired CN III palsies are *ischemic* and associated with diabetes mellitus, hypertension, or arteriosclerotic disease. Typically, *ischemic* acquired CN III palsies do not include pupillary abnormalities, they may be associated with pain, and they resolve spontaneously with satisfactory levator function within 3 months. If a pupil-sparing CN III palsy fails to resolve spontaneously within 3–6 months, further workup for a compressive lesion is indicated. However, if a patient presents with a CN III palsy involving the pupil, an immediate workup (including neuroimaging) should commence in order to rule out a compressive neoplastic or aneurysmal lesion. Surgical correction of ptosis related to CN III palsy usually requires frontalis suspension and should be reserved for patients in whom strabismus surgery allows single binocular vision in a useful field of gaze.

Temporary neurogenic ptosis can be caused by inadvertent diffusion of botulinum toxin into the levator muscle complex following therapeutic injection in the forehead or orbital region. The resultant ptosis usually resolves after several weeks.

Myasthenia gravis MG is an autoimmune disorder in which autoantibodies attack the acetylcholine receptors of the neuromuscular junction. The disease is most often generalized and systemic. Approximately 10% of patients with generalized MG have an associated thymoma; thus, chest computed tomography (CT) should be considered for all patients with

MG to rule out this lesion. Surgical thymectomy results in clinical improvement in 75% of cases of generalized MG and complete remission in 35% of cases. Early manifestations of MG are often ophthalmic, with ptosis being the most common presenting sign; diplopia is often present as well. When the effects of MG are isolated to the periocular musculature, the condition is called *ocular myasthenia gravis*. Marked variability in the degree of ptosis during the day and complaints of diplopia should suggest ocular MG. Other autoimmune disorders may occur in myasthenic patients.

No single test for MG will detect all cases. Neuro-ophthalmologic consultation is useful in the evaluation and treatment of MG. Surgical treatment of ptosis should be delayed until medical management of MG is maximized. Because of the variability of levator function, frontalis suspension may be considered. See BCSC Section 5, *Neuro-Ophthalmology*, for further discussion.

Gilbert ME, Savino PJ. Ocular myasthenia gravis. *Int Ophthalmol Clin.* 2007;47(4):93–103, ix.

Mechanical ptosis

In mechanical ptosis, the upper eyelid is weighed down by a mass or swelling in the eyelid or orbit. It may be caused by a congenital abnormality, such as a plexiform neurofibroma or hemangioma, or by an acquired neoplasm, such as a large chalazion (Fig 12-16) or skin carcinoma. Postsurgical or posttraumatic edema may also cause temporary mechanical ptosis.

Traumatic ptosis

Trauma to the levator aponeurosis or the levator palpebrae superioris muscle may also cause ptosis through myogenic, aponeurotic, neurogenic, or mechanical defects. An eyelid laceration that exposes preaponeurotic fat indicates that the orbital septum has been violated and suggests possible damage to the levator muscle and/or aponeurosis. Exploration of the levator and repair may be indicated in this situation. Orbital and neurosurgical procedures can also lead to traumatic ptosis. Since such ptosis may resolve or improve spontaneously, the ophthalmologist typically observes the patient for an extended period before considering surgical intervention.

Pseudoptosis

Pseudoptosis, which gives the appearance of a drooping eyelid, should be differentiated from true ptosis. An eyelid may appear to be abnormally low in various conditions, including brow ptosis, hypertropia, enophthalmos, microphthalmia, anophthalmia, phthisis

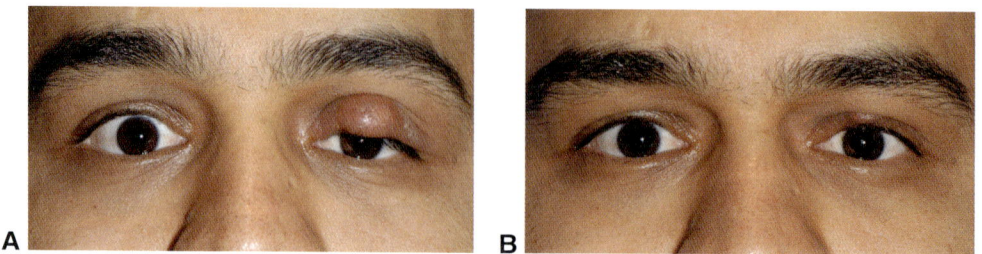

Figure 12-16 Mechanical ptosis. **A,** Chalazion of the left upper eyelid causing mechanical ptosis. **B,** Ptosis is improved after incision and drainage of the chalazion. *(Courtesy of Bobby S. Korn, MD, PhD.)*

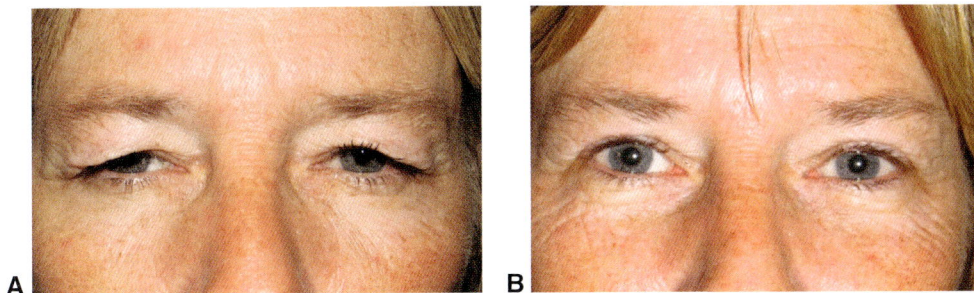

Figure 12-17 Bilateral upper dermatochalasis. **A,** Patient with dermatochalasis and pseudoptosis of both upper eyelids. **B,** Clearance of the visual axis is achieved through blepharoplasty alone. *(Courtesy of Bobby S. Korn, MD, PhD.)*

bulbi, or a superior sulcus defect secondary to trauma or other causes. Contralateral upper eyelid retraction may also simulate ptosis. The term *pseudoptosis* is also sometimes used to describe *dermatochalasis,* the condition in which excess upper eyelid skin overhangs the eyelid margin (Fig 12-17).

Management

Ptosis repair is a challenging and often-debated topic. The patient's ocular, medical, and surgical history help determine whether surgical repair is appropriate. Specifically, the surgeon should be aware of any history of dry eye, thyroid eye disease, previous eye or eyelid surgery, and periorbital trauma.

Ptosis that causes amblyopia, significant superior visual field loss, or difficulty with reading is considered to be a *functional* problem. In other instances, ptosis may be considered a *cosmetic* issue. Because ptosis repair is often an elective surgical procedure, it is particularly important for the surgeon to review the cosmetic and functional consequences of the procedure as well as potential risks.

Ptosis repair surgery should be directed toward correction of the underlying pathologic condition. The 3 categories of surgical procedures most commonly used in ptosis repair are

- external (transcutaneous) levator advancement
- internal (transconjunctival) levator/tarsus/Müller muscle resection approaches
- frontalis muscle suspensions

The amount and type of ptosis and the degree of levator function are the most common determining factors in selecting the type of corrective surgery. Other important considerations are the surgeon's experience and comfort level with various procedures. In patients with good levator function, surgical correction is generally directed toward the levator aponeurosis. However, if levator function is poor or absent, frontalis muscle suspension techniques are preferred.

External (transcutaneous) levator advancement surgery is most commonly used when levator function is normal and the upper eyelid crease is high (Video 12-5). In these patients, the levator muscle itself is normal, but the levator aponeurosis is stretched or

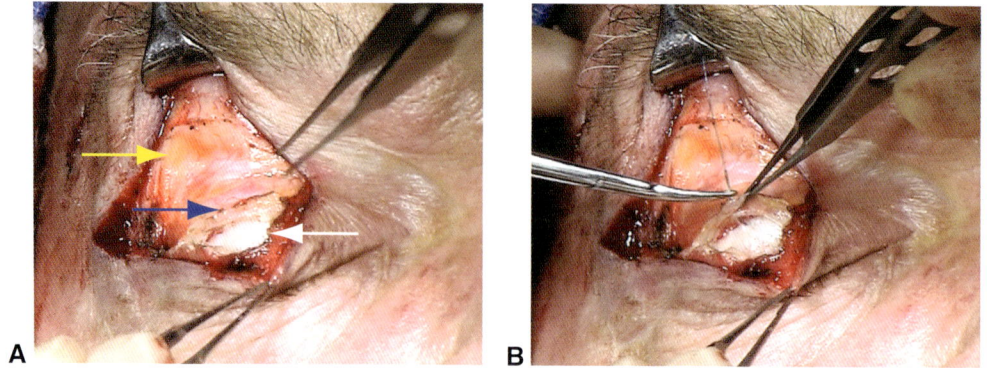

Figure 12-18 External levator advancement surgery. **A,** Intraoperative view shows the preaponeurotic fat *(yellow arrow),* disinserted edge of levator aponeurosis *(blue arrow),* and tarsal plate *(white arrow).* **B,** Advancement of the levator muscle to the tarsal plate. *(Courtesy of Bobby S. Korn, MD, PhD.)*

disinserted, thus requiring advancement (Fig 12-18). The levator aponeurosis is approached externally through an upper eyelid crease incision and is advanced to the superior tarsal border. The patient's cooperation is elicited to open the eyelids to obtain optimal height and contour.

VIDEO 12-5 External levator advancement ptosis repair.
Courtesy of Jill Foster, MD; Dan Straka, MD; and Craig Czyz, DO.

The *internal (transconjunctival)* approach to ptosis repair is directed toward the Müller muscle, the tarsus, or the levator aponeurosis or muscle (Video 12-6). A comparison of MRD_1 before and after the instillation of 2.5% phenylephrine may be performed to identify patients who are candidates for the internal approach (Fig 12-19A, B). The Müller muscle–conjunctival resection procedure (MMCR) was traditionally used for repair of minimal ptosis (2 mm or less). However, recent evidence supports its use in cases of severe ptosis. The procedure is generally considered useful for maintaining the preoperative eyelid contour. The *Fasanella-Servat* ptosis repair procedure, which is used for small amounts of ptosis, includes removal of the superior tarsus with the conjunctiva and Müller muscle.

VIDEO 12-6 Müller muscle–conjunctival resection.
Courtesy of Jill Foster, MD; Dan Straka, MD; and Craig Czyz, DO.

Many patients with significant ptosis use the frontalis muscle in an attempt to raise the eyelid and clear the visual axis. In *frontalis suspension* surgery (Fig 12-20), which is performed when levator function is poor or absent, the eyelid is suspended directly from the frontalis muscle so that movement of the brow is efficiently transmitted to the eyelid. Thus, the patient is able to elevate the eyelid by using the frontalis muscle to lift the brow. Several sling options exist for frontalis suspension; they can be grouped as autogenous, allogenic, or synthetic.

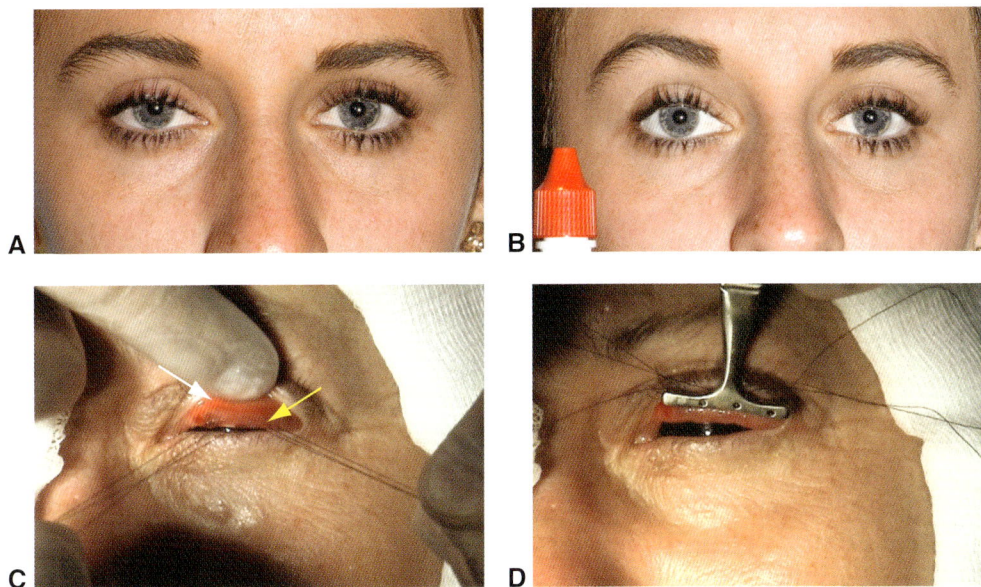

Figure 12-19 Internal approach to ptosis repair. **A,** Patient with ptosis of the right upper eyelid. **B,** Improvement of ptosis after instillation of 2.5% phenylephrine hydrochloride. **C,** Intraoperative photograph showing tarsus *(white arrow)*, conjunctiva, and Müller muscle *(yellow arrow)*. **D,** Ptosis clamp securing conjunctiva and Müller muscle prior to excision. *(Courtesy of Bobby S. Korn, MD, PhD.)*

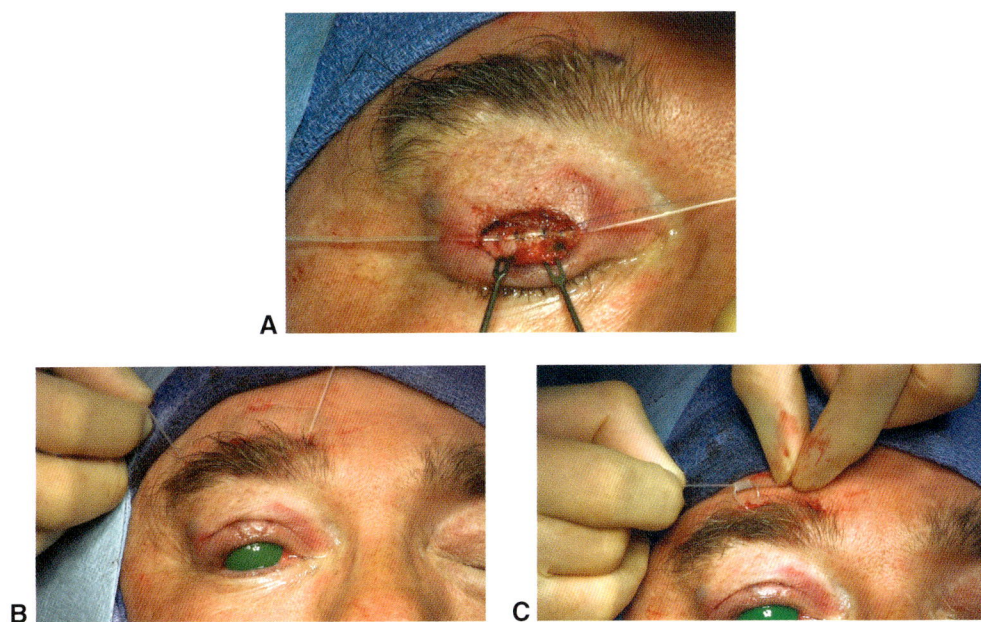

Figure 12-20 Frontalis suspension surgery. **A,** Fixation of silicone rod to tarsal plate. **B,** Passage of silicone rod through nasal and temporal brow incisions. **C,** Fixation of silicone rod through central brow incision over sleeve. *(Courtesy of Bobby S. Korn, MD, PhD.)*

Autogenous tensor fascia lata has shown good long-term results but requires the patient to undergo additional surgery related to tissue harvesting. Generally, autogenous fascia lata can be used in patients who are at least 3 years old or weigh 35 pounds or more. Alternatively, the frontalis muscle can be advanced inferiorly to the eyelid as a flap for eyelid elevation.

Allogenic slings include banked fascia lata, which can be obtained from a variety of sources and spares the patient from harvesting surgery. However, this material may incite inflammation and has the theoretical potential to transmit infectious disease.

Synthetic materials such as silicone rods are commonly used. No tissue harvesting is involved, and this option allows for easier adjustment or removal if necessary.

There is some controversy about whether bilateral frontalis suspension should be performed in patients with unilateral congenital ptosis. A bilateral procedure may improve the patient's symmetry and stimulate the need to utilize the frontalis muscle to lift the eyelids, but it subjects the normal eyelid to surgical risks. The decision of whether to modify a normal eyelid in an attempt to gain symmetry must be discussed by the surgeon and the patient or the patient's caregiver.

Lee MJ, Oh JY, Choung HK, Kim NJ, Sung MS, Khwarg SI. Frontalis sling operation using silicone rod compared with preserved fascia lata for congenital ptosis a three-year follow-up study. *Ophthalmology.* 2009;116(1):123–129.

Patel RM, Aakalu VK, Setabutr P, Putterman AM. Efficacy of Muller's muscle and conjunctival resection with or without tarsectomy for the treatment of severe involutional blepharoptosis. *Ophthalmic Plast Reconstr Surg.* 2017;33(4):273–278.

Complications

Undercorrection is the most common complication of ptosis repair. Astute judgment is required to differentiate this from a mechanical ptosis caused by early postoperative edema. Other potential complications include overcorrection, unsatisfactory eyelid contour, scarring, wound dehiscence, eyelid crease asymmetry, conjunctival prolapse, tarsal eversion, implant extrusion, and lagophthalmos with exposure keratopathy. This latter condition is usually temporary, but it requires treatment with lubricating drops or ointments until it resolves. Achieving symmetry between the 2 eyelids is a difficult aspect of ptosis repair, and some ptosis surgeons use adjustable suture techniques or early adjustment in the office during the first 2 postoperative weeks when indicated.

Eyelid Retraction

Eyelid retraction is the superior displacement of the upper eyelid or the inferior displacement of the lower eyelid (or both), exposing sclera between the limbus and the eyelid margin (Fig 12-21). It can be unilateral or bilateral. Lower eyelid retraction may also be a normal anatomic variant in patients who have shallow orbits or certain genetic orbital or eyelid characteristics. Retraction of the eyelids often leads to lagophthalmos and exposure keratopathy, with consequences ranging from ocular irritation and discomfort to vision-threatening corneal decompensation.

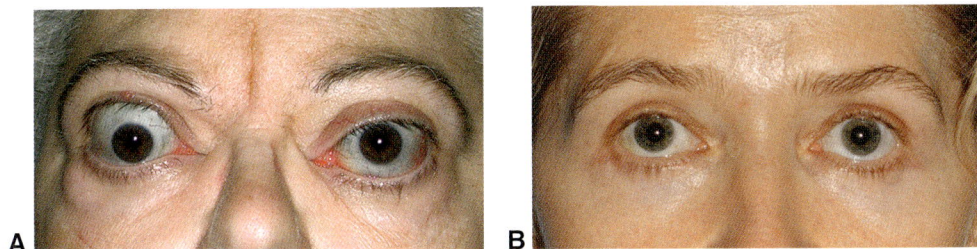

Figure 12-21 Upper and lower eyelid retraction. **A,** Retraction secondary to thyroid eye disease. **B,** Retraction resulting from excessive skin removal and middle lamellar scarring after cosmetic blepharoplasty. *(Part A courtesy of Jill Foster, MD; part B courtesy of Bobby S. Korn, MD, PhD.)*

Causes

Eyelid retraction can have local, systemic, or central nervous system causes. The most common are thyroid eye disease (TED), recession of the vertical rectus muscles, aggressive tissue removal during blepharoplasty, and overcompensation for a contralateral ptosis (Hering's law of equal innervation).

Thyroid eye disease is the most common cause of both upper and lower eyelid retraction, as well as unilateral or bilateral proptosis. Because proptosis commonly coexists with and may mimic eyelid retraction in patients with TED, these conditions are evaluated through eyelid measurements and exophthalmometry. A common finding in TED-related eyelid retraction is *temporal flare*. In this condition, the eyelid retraction is more severe laterally than medially, resulting in an abnormal upper eyelid contour that appears to flare upward along the lateral half of the eyelid margin. See Chapter 4 for a more extensive discussion of TED.

Iatrogenic eyelid retraction may be induced by recession of the vertical rectus muscles, owing to anatomic connections between the superior rectus and the levator palpebrae superioris muscle in the upper eyelid and between the inferior rectus muscle and capsulopalpebral fascia in the lower eyelid. Another iatrogenic cause of eyelid retraction, especially of the lower eyelids, is excessive resection of skin, middle lamellar scarring, and untreated lower eyelid laxity during cosmetic lower blepharoplasty. Correction may require any combination of lower eyelid tightening, midface-lifting, full-thickness skin grafting, or spacer grafting. Conservative excision of skin in lower blepharoplasty, along with concomitant correction of any lower eyelid laxity, minimizes the risk of this problem.

Other etiologies include *Parinaud syndrome,* an example of eyelid retraction caused by a central nervous system lesion. *Congenital* eyelid retraction occurs as a rare, isolated entity.

Management

Treatment of eyelid retraction is based on the severity and underlying etiologic factors. In patients with mild eyelid retraction, artificial tears, lubricants, and ointments may be sufficient to protect the cornea and minimize symptoms. Mild eyelid retraction resulting

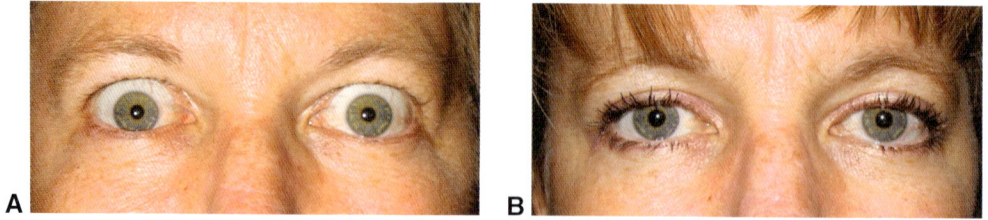

Figure 12-22 Bilateral upper eyelid retraction in thyroid eye disease. **A,** Preoperative appearance. **B,** Same patient after upper eyelid retractor recession. *(Courtesy of Bobby S. Korn, MD, PhD.)*

from lower blepharoplasty or TED may resolve spontaneously over time. A variety of surgical techniques have been developed to correct eyelid retraction that persists or that poses an immediate threat to the eye. Except in cases of severe exposure keratopathy, surgical intervention is undertaken only after serial measurements have established stability of the eyelid position. Upper eyelid retraction can be corrected by excision or recession of the Müller muscle (anterior or posterior approach), recession of the levator aponeurosis with or without hang-back sutures or other spacer (Fig 12-22), measured myotomy of the levator muscle, or full-thickness transverse blepharotomy.

If the patient has lateral flare, a small eyelid-splitting lateral tarsorrhaphy combined with recession of the upper and lower eyelid retractors can improve the upper eyelid contour; however, this technique may limit the patient's lateral visual field.

As with correction of the upper eyelids, treatment of lower eyelid retraction is directed by the underlying etiologic factors. *Anterior lamellar deficiency* (eg, excess skin resection from blepharoplasty) requires recruitment of vertical skin by means of a midface-lift or addition of skin with a full-thickness skin graft. *Middle lamellar deficiency* (eg, posttraumatic septal scarring) requires scar release and possible placement of a spacer graft. *Posterior lamellar deficiency* from congenital scarring or conjunctival shortage (eg, mucous membrane pemphigoid) may require a full-thickness mucous membrane graft.

Severe retraction of the lower eyelids, common in patients with TED, may require a spacer graft between the lower eyelid retractors and the inferior tarsal border. Autogenous auricular cartilage, hard-palate mucosa, free tarsal grafts, acellular dermal matrix, and dermis fat are common spacer materials. It is often necessary to perform some type of horizontal eyelid or lateral canthal tightening or elevation as well. However, because horizontal tightening of the lower eyelid in a patient with proptosis may exacerbate the eyelid retraction, use of this technique requires caution.

Facial Paralysis

Paralytic Ectropion

Paralytic ectropion usually follows CN VII paralysis or palsy. Typically, concomitant upper eyelid lagophthalmos is present secondary to paralytic upper eyelid orbicularis dysfunction. Poor blinking and eyelid closure lead to chronic ocular surface irritation from corneal exposure, as well as inadequate tear film replenishment and distribution. Chronically

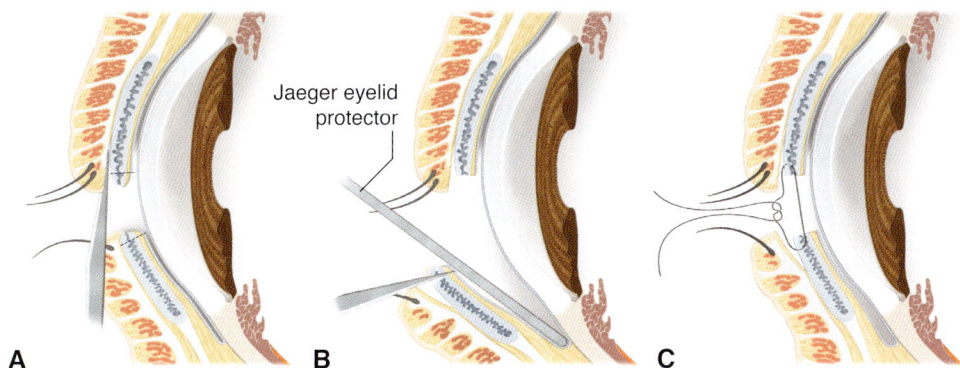

Figure 12-23 Tarsorrhaphy. **A,** The eyelid is split 2–3 mm deep. **B,** Epithelium is carefully removed along the upper and lower eyelid margins; the lash follicles are avoided. **C,** The raw surfaces are then joined with absorbable sutures. *(Illustration by Mark Miller.)*

stimulated reflex tear secretion, atonic eyelids, and lacrimal pump failure account for the frequent reports of tearing in these patients.

Neurologic evaluation may be needed to determine the cause of the CN VII paralysis. In cases resulting from stroke or intracranial surgery, clinical evaluation of corneal sensation is indicated because neurotrophic keratopathy combined with paralytic lagophthalmos increases the risk of corneal decompensation.

Lubricating drops, viscous tear supplementation, ointments, taping of the temporal half of the lower eyelid, or moisture chambers can be used. Such measures may be the only treatment necessary, especially for temporary paralysis. In select patients with long-term or permanent paralysis, tarsorrhaphy, medial or lateral canthoplasty, suspension procedures, and horizontal tightening procedures are useful.

Tarsorrhaphy can be performed either medially or laterally. An adequate temporary tarsorrhaphy (1–3 weeks) can be achieved with placement of nonabsorbable sutures between the upper and lower eyelid margins. A "temporary tarsorrhaphy" can also be created by injection of botulinum toxin into the levator muscle. Permanent tarsorrhaphy involves deepithelialization of the upper and lower eyelid margins, avoiding the lash follicles. Absorbable or nonabsorbable sutures are then placed to unite the raw surfaces of the upper and lower eyelids (Fig 12-23).

Occasionally, a fascia lata or silicone suspension sling of the lower eyelid may be indicated. Vertical elevation of the lower eyelid is useful in reducing exposure of the inferior cornea. This elevation may be accomplished through recession of the lower eyelid retractors, combined with use of a spacer graft. Surgical midface elevation can also play an important role in lower eyelid support.

Upper Eyelid Paralysis

Upper eyelid loading remains the most commonly performed procedure for the treatment of paralytic lagophthalmos. The appropriate weight can be selected through a process of preoperatively taping eyelid weights of different sizes to the upper eyelid skin to determine

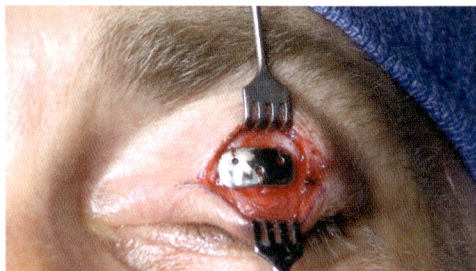

Figure 12-24 Left upper eyelid loading with a platinum weight anterior to the tarsal plate. *(Courtesy of Bobby S. Korn, MD, PhD.)*

which one best achieves adequate relaxed eyelid closure with minimal ptosis in primary gaze. After the weight is selected, it is inserted through an upper eyelid crease incision and is either sutured to the anterior surface of the tarsal plate (Fig 12-24) or placed behind the orbital septum; the latter may avoid thickening of the pretarsal area. If orbicularis function returns, the weight can be removed easily. Weights made of gold and platinum allow for magnetic resonance imaging (3 Tesla or less). Brow ptosis repair and blepharoplasty may be considered after improvement of corneal exposure.

Facial Dystonia

Benign Essential Blepharospasm

Benign essential blepharospasm (BEB) is a bilateral focal dystonia that affects approximately 30 of every 100,000 people. The condition is characterized by increased blinking and involuntary spasms of the periocular protractor muscles (Video 12-7). The spasms generally start as mild twitches and progress over time to forceful contractures. Other muscles of the face may also be involved with blepharospasm. Unlike hemifacial spasm, BEB typically abates during sleep. The involuntary episodes of forced blinking or contracture may severely limit the patient's ability to drive, read, or perform activities of daily living. Women are affected more frequently than men. The age of onset is usually older than 40 years. BEB is a clinical diagnosis, and neuroimaging is rarely indicated in the workup. BEB must be differentiated from *reflex blepharospasm,* which can occur secondary to dry eye syndrome and other medical conditions.

VIDEO 12-7 Benign essential blepharospasm.
Courtesy of Pete Setabutr, MD.

The cause of BEB is unknown; however, it is probably of central origin, in the basal ganglia. BEB can be managed by medical or surgical approaches. Neurotoxin injections are the primary treatment for blepharospasm. (See BCSC Section 5, *Neuro-Ophthalmology.*)

Botulinum toxin injection

Repeated periodic injection of one of the botulinum toxin type A formulations is the treatment of choice for BEB (Fig 12-25). Injection of these agents at therapeutic doses results in chemical denervation and localized muscle paralysis. Botulinum toxin injection is typically effective, but the improvement is temporary. Average onset of action is in 2–3 days, and

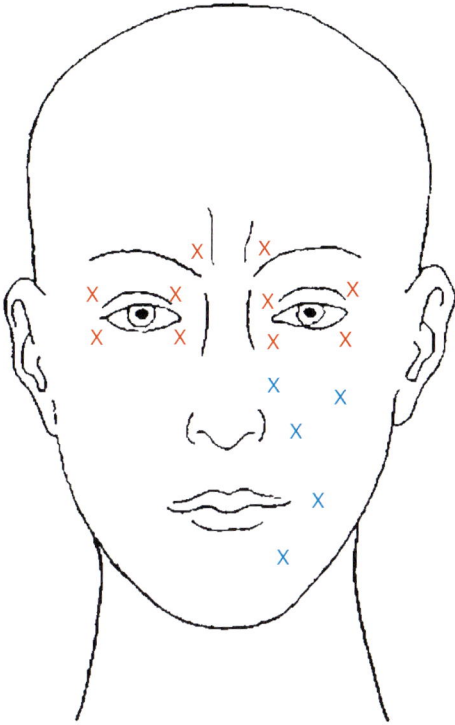

Figure 12-25 Injection patterns of botulinum toxin type A for benign essential blepharospasm *(red)* and hemifacial spasm *(unilateral red sites plus blue)*. *(Modified from Dutton JJ, Fowler AM. Botulinum toxin in ophthalmology.* Focal Points: Clinical Modules for Ophthalmologists. *San Francisco: American Academy of Ophthalmology; 2007, module 3.)*

average peak effect occurs at about 7–10 days following injection. Duration of effect also varies but is typically 3–4 months, at which point recurrence of the spasms and need for reinjection is anticipated. Complications associated with botulinum toxin injection include bruising, blepharoptosis, ectropion, epiphora, diplopia, lagophthalmos, and corneal exposure. These adverse reactions are usually transient and result from spread of the toxin to adjacent muscles.

Dutton JJ, Fowler AM. Botulinum toxin in ophthalmology. *Focal Points: Clinical Modules for Ophthalmologists.* San Francisco: American Academy of Ophthalmology; 2007, module 3.

Surgical myectomy

Treatment with surgical myectomy is reserved for patients with severe spasm who do not respond adequately to botulinum therapy. Meticulous removal of the orbital and palpebral orbicularis muscle in the upper (and sometimes lower) eyelids can be an effective and permanent treatment for blepharospasm. Complications of surgical myectomy include lagophthalmos, chronic lymphedema, and periorbital contour deformities. Limited upper eyelid protractor myectomy is helpful in patients with less severe disease. Recurrence of spasm is not uncommon after myectomy, and treatment with reduced dosage of botulinum toxin is indicated.

Many patients with BEB have an associated dry eye condition that may be aggravated by any treatment modality that decreases eyelid closure. Artificial tears, ointments, punctal plugs or occlusion, moisture chamber shields, and tinted (FL-41) spectacle lenses may help minimize discomfort from ocular surface problems.

Pariseau B, Worley MW, Anderson RL. Myectomy for blepharospasm 2013. *Curr Opin Ophthalmol.* 2013;24(5):488–493.

Surgical ablation of the facial nerve

Though effective in treating BEB, selective facial neurectomy has been largely abandoned. Recurrence rates as high as 30% and frequent hemifacial paralysis from facial nerve dissection limit this treatment's appeal. The results obtained with facial nerve dissection are, therefore, less satisfactory than those of direct orbicularis oculi myectomy. Some surgeons have had greater success with microsurgical ablation of selected branches of the facial nerve.

Muscle relaxants and sedatives

Muscle relaxants and sedatives are rarely effective in the primary treatment of BEB. Oral medications such as orphenadrine, lorazepam, or clonazepam are sometimes effective in suppressing mild cases of BEB, prolonging the interval between botulinum toxin injections, or helping to dampen oromandibular dystonia associated with BEB. Psychotherapy has little or no value for the patient with blepharospasm.

Hirabayashi KE, Vagefi MR. Oral pharmacotherapy for benign essential blepharospasm. *Int Ophthalmol Clin.* 2018;58(1):33–47.

Hemifacial Spasm

Blepharospasm should be differentiated from hemifacial spasm (HFS). HFS is characterized by intermittent synchronous gross contractures of the entire side of the face and is rarely bilateral (Video 12-8). HFS often begins in the periocular region and then progresses to involve the entire half of the face. Unlike BEB, HFS persists during sleep.

HFS is often associated with ipsilateral facial nerve weakness. In most cases, HFS is the result of a vascular compression of the facial nerve root exit zone at the brain stem. Magnetic resonance imaging (MRI) often reveals the ectatic vessel. MRI can also help rule out other cerebellopontine angle lesions that may be the cause in less than 1% of cases. Neurosurgical decompression of the facial nerve may be curative in HFS, but it exposes the patient to the relative risk of neurosurgical intervention. Periodic injection of botulinum toxin is a commonly used, effective treatment option for HFS (see Fig 12-25). Oral medications, including drugs with membrane-stabilizing properties such as carbamazepine and clonazepam, are used less frequently because of their low efficacy.

VIDEO 12-8 Hemifacial spasm.
Courtesy of Pete Setabutr, MD.

Aberrant regeneration after facial nerve palsy may also present with hemifacial contracture and synkinetic facial movements. The history (eg, previous Bell palsy, trauma) and clinical examination are distinctive. Functionally troublesome synkinetic facial movements often respond well to botulinum toxin injection.

Involutional Periorbital Changes

Dermatochalasis

Dermatochalasis refers to redundancy of eyelid skin and is often associated with orbital fat prolapse (see Fig 12-17). Though more common in elderly patients, dermatochalasis also occurs in middle-aged persons, particularly if there is a familial predisposition. It may also accompany true ptosis of the upper eyelids.

Patients with significant dermatochalasis of the upper eyelids may report a heavy feeling around the eyes, brow-ache, eyelashes in the visual axis, and reduction in the superior visual field. Dermatochalasis is often exacerbated by brow ptosis. Lower eyelid dermatochalasis is considered a cosmetic issue unless the excess skin and prolapsed fat are so severe that the patient cannot be fitted with bifocals.

Blepharochalasis

Although blepharochalasis is not an involutional change, it is included in this discussion because it can resemble, and must be differentiated from, dermatochalasis. Blepharochalasis is a rare familial variant of angioneurotic edema. It occurs most commonly in young females and is characterized by idiopathic episodes of inflammatory edema of the eyelids. As a result of recurrent bouts of inflammation and edema, the eyelid skin becomes thin and wrinkled, simulating the appearance of dermatochalasis. In addition, true ptosis, herniation of the orbital lobe of the lacrimal gland, atrophy of the orbital fat pads, and prominent eyelid vascularity may be associated with blepharochalasis. Surgical repair of the eyelid skin changes and ptosis associated with blepharochalasis may be complicated by repeated episodes of inflammation and edema.

Koursh DM, Modjtahedi SP, Selva D, Leibovitch I. The blepharochalasis syndrome. *Surv Ophthalmol.* 2009;54(2):235–244.

Blepharoplasty

Upper Eyelid

Upper blepharoplasty is one of the most commonly performed oculoplastic procedures (Video 12-9). Involutional skin and structural changes often begin in the periorbital area, and they can obstruct the superior visual field. Blepharoplasty is frequently performed to relieve this obstruction. Brow ptosis may also play a role and may need to be addressed. Functional indications for blepharoplasty are documented by means of external photography and visual field testing with and without manual eyelid elevation. Patients undergoing blepharoplasty for cosmetic reasons may have different expectations than those undergoing functional blepharoplasty. Thus, a thorough preoperative discussion of the anticipated results is critical to preoperative planning.

VIDEO 12-9 Upper blepharoplasty.
Courtesy of Jill Foster, MD; Dan Straka, MD; and Craig Czyz, DO.

Lower Eyelid

Lower blepharoplasty is most commonly performed for cosmetic indications. However, some patients undergo this procedure because of functional concerns such as difficulty reading, which can occur when prolapsed orbital fat and skin cover the bifocal spectacle segment. For cosmetic lower eyelid surgery, satisfactory results often require additional skin rejuvenation with skin removal, chemical peels, or laser resurfacing. In the preoperative discussion, the surgeon should clearly describe reasonable expectations for, as well as the risks of, the procedure. Patients should understand that aggressive resection of lower eyelid skin and fat may lead to eyelid retraction, ectropion, or a sunken, aged periorbital appearance.

Preoperative Evaluation

Evaluation of any potential blepharoplasty patient includes the following:

- a complete ocular examination that includes visual acuity testing and documentation
- a history of prior periocular surgery
- identification of amount and areas of excess skin, as well as the amount and contours of prolapsed orbital fat, in the upper and lower eyelids
- presence or absence of lagophthalmos, which can lead to postoperative dryness and exposure keratopathy
- evaluation of tear secretion or the tear film, which may be carried out through Schirmer testing, tear breakup time, or assessment of the adequacy of the tear meniscus
- photographic documentation

Upper blepharoplasty

In addition to the assessments above, the examination before upper blepharoplasty includes the following elements:

- visual field testing to determine the presence and degree of superior visual field defects (if needed for documentation)
- evaluation of the forehead and eyebrows (including brow height and contour) to detect forehead and brow ptosis; the surgeon should make careful observations when the patient's facial and brow musculature is relaxed
- notation of the position of the upper eyelid crease

Lower blepharoplasty

Preoperative examination for lower blepharoplasty further includes

- testing of the elasticity (snapback test) and distractibility of the lower eyelid; the surgeon should be alert to the possible need for horizontal tightening of the lower eyelids along with the blepharoplasty
- notation and discussion of prominent orbital rims, if present; malar hypoplasia or relative exophthalmos may predispose the patient to postoperative scleral show after lower blepharoplasty

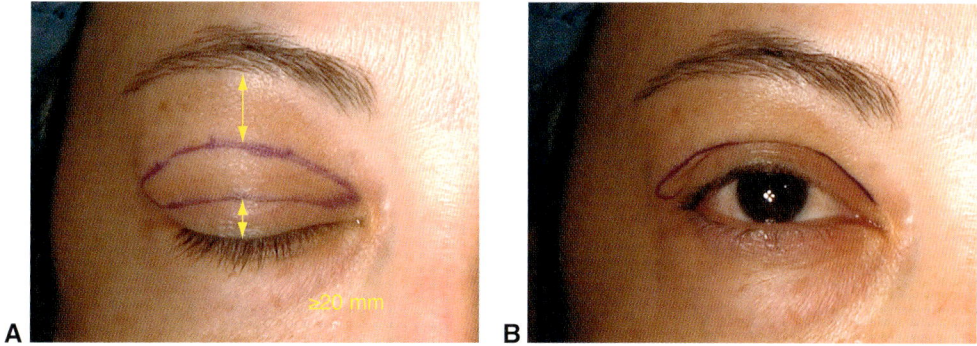

Figure 12-26 Preoperative marking. **A,** Typical skin marking for upper eyelid blepharoplasty. After skin marking, there should be at least 20 mm of remaining upper eyelid skin *(sum of the distance indicated by the arrows).* **B,** The upper and lower markings are superimposed when the eye is open. *(Courtesy of Bobby S. Korn, MD, PhD.)*

Techniques

A thorough working knowledge of periorbital and eyelid anatomy (discussed in Chapter 9) is essential for successful blepharoplasty. In addition, just as the brow and glabellar areas affect the upper eyelids, the midfacial structures influence the position, tone, contour, and function of the lower eyelid and must be considered in surgical planning.

Surgical preparation involves marking excess skin for excision prior to infiltration of local anesthetic. The surgeon can determine the amount of skin to be excised by grasping the upper eyelid skin with toothless forceps and identifying the amount of redundancy *(pinch technique).* To avoid excessive skin removal, the surgeon usually leaves at least 20 mm of skin remaining between the inferior border of the brow and the upper eyelid margin (Fig 12-26).

Upper blepharoplasty

Upper blepharoplasty begins with the surgeon incising along the lines marked on the upper eyelid. The surgeon removes skin and then may selectively remove orbicularis and a conservative amount of orbital fat to reshape the upper eyelid. Adjunctive procedures to re-form the eyelid crease and reposition the lacrimal gland may be necessary.

Lower blepharoplasty

Lower blepharoplasty can be accomplished through a transconjunctival incision or a transcutaneous, infraciliary incision (Video 12-10). The *transconjunctival incision* offers a lower rate of postoperative eyelid retraction and absence of an external postoperative scar (Fig 12-27). The preoperative evaluation defines the location and extent of lower eyelid fat prolapse and thus determines the boundaries of surgical excision. The surgeon should be aware of the location of the inferior oblique muscle, which is between the medial and central fat pads. As in the upper eyelid, the medial fat pad of the lower eyelid is less yellow than the lateral fat pads. The central fat compartment is separated from the lateral fat compartment by the arcuate expansion of the inferior oblique muscle; removal or incision of this arcuate expansion may improve access to the lateral fat pad. The surgeon can remove or reposition

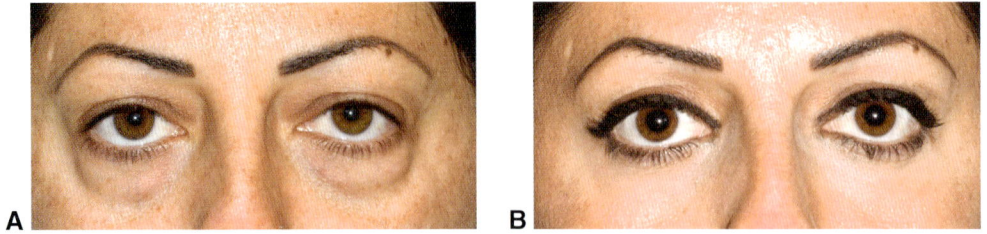

Figure 12-27 Photos taken before **(A)** and after **(B)** lower eyelid blepharoplasty through a transconjunctival approach. *(Courtesy of Bobby S. Korn, MD, PhD.)*

the fat. Horizontal tightening or resuspension (see Fig 12-2) is often performed with lower blepharoplasty.

VIDEO 12-10 Lower blepharoplasty.
Reproduced with permission from Korn BS, Kikkawa DO, eds. Video Atlas of Oculofacial Plastic and Reconstructive Surgery. *Philadelphia: Elsevier/Saunders; 2011.*

After structural alteration of the lower eyelid (eg, fat removal, fat transposition, midface resuspension, horizontal eyelid tightening), skin removal can be performed. When skin resection is necessary, an *infraciliary incision* is used to remove only the skin, while preserving the underlying orbicularis muscle. It is important to note that aggressive skin removal during lower blepharoplasty increases the risk of lower eyelid contour abnormalities, retraction, and ectropion. This risk can be minimized with conservative skin removal and lower eyelid tightening.

Complications

Although it is rare, *loss of vision* is the most dreaded complication of blepharoplasty and is usually associated with *lower* blepharoplasty. Such blindness is typically thought to occur secondary to postoperative retrobulbar hemorrhage, with the increased intraorbital pressure causing ischemic compression of the ciliary arteries supplying the optic nerve. Other mechanisms of injury include ischemia caused by excessive surgical retraction or constriction of retrobulbar blood vessels in response to epinephrine in the local anesthetic. Orbital hemorrhage may result from injury to the deeper orbital blood vessels or from bleeding anteriorly. Risk factors for this complication include hypertension, blood dyscrasias, and anticoagulant use. Postoperative pressure dressings should be avoided: they increase orbital pressure and obscure underlying problems.

Patients should be observed immediately postoperatively to detect possible orbital hemorrhage. Those with significant pain, marked asymmetric swelling, or new proptosis should be evaluated. In addition, visual dimming or darkness, as well as significant or asymmetric blurred vision, following eyelid surgery may indicate orbital hemorrhage and should be assessed and treated immediately (see the discussion of orbital compartment syndrome in Chapter 6 for management).

Diplopia, another serious complication of blepharoplasty, may result from injury to the inferior oblique, inferior rectus, or superior oblique muscle. The inferior oblique muscle originates in the anterior orbital floor lateral to the lacrimal sac and travels posterolaterally within the lower eyelid retractors. It separates the central and medial fat pads of the lower eyelid and, thus, may be injured during removal of fat in lower blepharoplasty. In upper blepharoplasty, the trochlea of the superior oblique muscle may be damaged by deep dissection of orbital fat in the superonasal aspect of the upper eyelid.

Excessive removal of skin is a complication that can lead to lagophthalmos of the upper eyelids, as well as cicatricial ectropion or eyelid retraction. Topical lubricants and massage may be helpful for managing mild postoperative lagophthalmos, retraction, or ectropion, all of which may resolve over time. Injectable steroids or 5-fluorouracil can be used if a deep cicatrix contributes to the retraction. Severe cases require the use of free skin grafts, lateral canthoplasty, or surgical release of scar tissue or eyelid retractors. Even if no skin has been excised, inferior scleral show can occur secondary to septal scarring, orbicularis hematoma, and malar hypoplasia.

Brow Ptosis

Loss of elastic tissues and facial volume, as well as involutional changes of the forehead skin, lead to drooping of the forehead and eyebrows. This condition is known as *brow ptosis*. Severe brow ptosis may also result from facial nerve palsy. Brow ptosis frequently accompanies dermatochalasis and must be recognized as a factor that contributes to the appearance of aging in the periorbital area. If severe, brow ptosis may impinge on the superior visual field (Fig 12-28). The patient often involuntarily compensates for this condition by using the frontalis muscle to elevate the eyebrows. Such chronic contracture of the frontalis muscle often leads to brow-ache, headache, and prominent transverse forehead rhytids.

In most individuals, the brow is located at the level of or above the superior orbital rim. Generally, the female brow is higher and more arched than the typical male brow. The brow is considered ptotic when it falls below the superior orbital rim.

Management

Brow ptosis should be recognized and treated prior to or concomitant with the surgical repair of coexisting dermatochalasis of the eyelids. Because brow elevation reduces the amount of dermatochalasis present, it should be performed or simulated first when

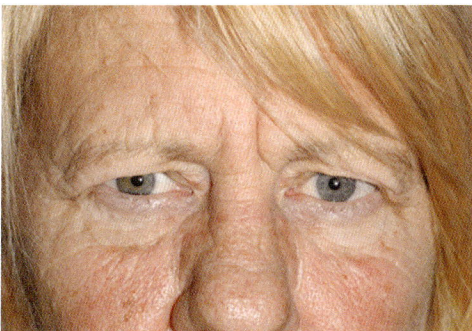

Figure 12-28 Brow ptosis causing functional impairment in the patient's peripheral visual field. *(Courtesy of Bobby S. Korn, MD, PhD.)*

combined with upper blepharoplasty. Aggressive upper blepharoplasty alone in a patient with concomitant brow ptosis leads to further depression of the brow. Brow ptosis may be corrected with browpexy, direct brow elevation, or endoscopic or pretrichial brow- and forehead-lift.

Browpexy

Browpexy is used for treatment of mild brow ptosis and is performed through an upper eyelid blepharoplasty incision. The sub-brow tissues are resuspended with sutures to the frontal bone periosteum above the orbital rim as part of a blepharoplasty. Although this

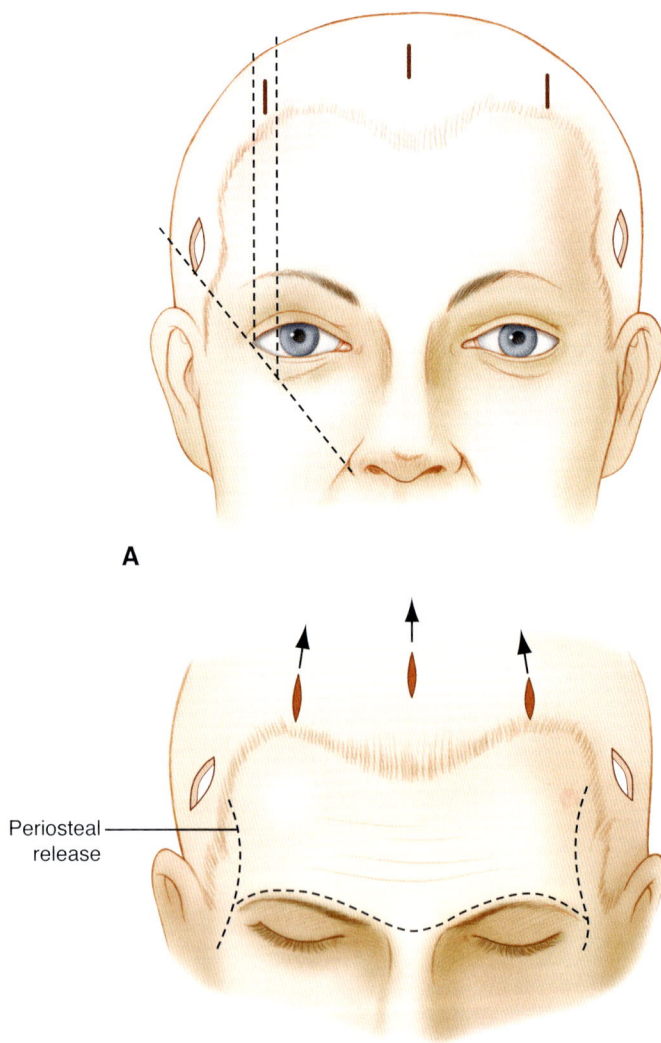

Figure 12-29   Endoscopic forehead-lift. **A,** Location of incisions. **B,** After periosteal release, the scalp is retracted posteriorly and fixated in the 2 paracentral incisions with a fixation screw, drilled bone tunnel, or absorbable implant. *(Illustration by Christine Gralapp.)*

procedure provides minimal improvement in brow position, it can help prevent the retro–orbicularis oculi fat from descending into the eyelid.

Direct brow elevation

The brows can be elevated with incisions placed at the upper edge of the brow hairs. This is an effective technique for treatment of brow ptosis and is particularly useful for men and women with lateral brow ptosis. When direct eyebrow elevation is used across the entire brow, it may result in an arch or displeasing scar. Sensory paresthesias may be an adverse effect of the direct brow procedure.

Endoscopic brow- and forehead-lift

Endoscopic techniques allow the surgeon to raise the brow and rejuvenate the forehead *(foreheadplasty)* through small incisions approximately 1 cm (though incisions may vary) behind the hairline (Fig 12-29). Dissection is accomplished with an endoscopic periosteal elevator and blunt dissectors. Key steps are the incisions, creation of an optical cavity, periosteal release at the orbital rim, and fixation of the elevated flap. The forehead can be fixated using a drilled bone tunnel through the calvarium, resorbable anchors, or fixation screws. The advantages of the endoscopic technique are smaller incisions hidden within the hair, elevation of a lower hairline (short forehead), customized lifting of specific segments of the brow, and faster recovery (relative to pretrichial brow-lift). The disadvantages include the need for endoscopic equipment, risk of damage to the facial nerve, the possibility of alopecia around scalp incisions, and skin changes related to the fixation technique used.

Pretrichial brow- and forehead-lift

The pretrichial approach is used in patients who have a high hairline. Access is gained through a pretrichial incision (Fig 12-30) instead of the small skin incisions used with the

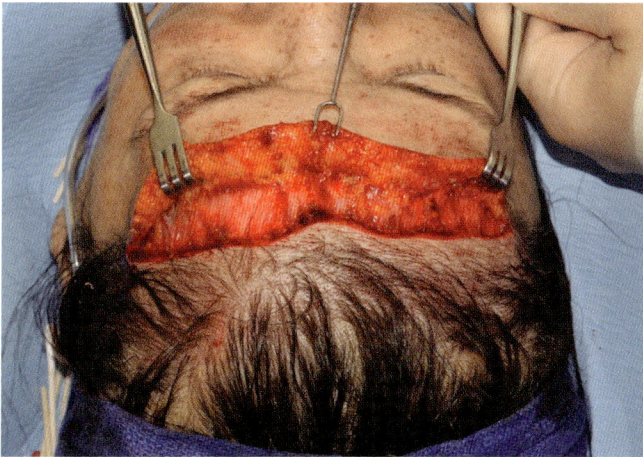

Figure 12-30 Pretrichial incision for forehead and brow elevation. The plane of dissection is the subcutaneous layer. *(Courtesy of Bobby S. Korn, MD, PhD.)*

endoscopic approach. Dissection is performed in the subcutaneous layer. An appropriate amount of forehead skin is resected, and the underlying frontalis and galea are plicated with a subsequent layered closure. The advantages of the pretrichial technique are powerful lifting of the brow without elevation of the hairline and no need for endoscopic equipment. The disadvantages are a relatively high incidence of postoperative sensory paresthesias and visible pretrichial scar line.

CHAPTER 13

Facial Rejuvenation

Highlights

- Facial rejuvenation techniques vary and include both nonsurgical and surgical interventions.
- Laser skin resurfacing is designed to reduce wrinkles and enhance the texture and appearance of the facial and periorbital skin.
- The US Food and Drug Administration (FDA) has approved the use of botulinum toxin to temporarily reduce wrinkles in the glabellar area, the lateral canthal lines (crow's-feet), and the forehead.
- Complications from intravascular injection of facial fillers include regional soft-tissue necrosis and central retinal artery occlusion.
- Rhytidectomy involves surgical management of the jowls and neck, including liposuction with or without platysmaplasty.

Pathogenesis of the Aging Face

An individual's facial contours and appearance are derived from soft tissue draped over underlying bone. The soft-tissue component consists of skin, subcutaneous fat, muscle, deeper fat pads, and fascial layers. The underlying structural element is composed of bone, cartilage, and teeth.

As the face ages, the soft-tissue component descends, and the bone component loses mass. With these changes, relatively more soft tissue hangs from its attachments to the bone. Loss of subcutaneous fat, skin atrophy, and descent of facial fat pads compound this facial sagging. Around the eyes, the lateral brow typically descends more than the medial brow, which leads to temporal hooding. The orbital septum attenuates, allowing fat to prolapse forward. In the lower eyelid, midface descent produces the skeletonization of the infraorbital rim and increases the prominence of the orbital fat. Sagging of the platysma muscle in the neck posterior to the mandibular ligament gives rise to jowling.

Physical Examination of the Aging Face

Much of the surgeon's appraisal of the aging face can be performed through close observation during the introduction and history phase of the initial meeting. The surgeon should observe the patient's hairstyle, including the presence or absence of bangs, hair thickness, and the height of the hairline; the use of the frontalis; the position of the brow; the texture and quality of the facial skin; and the presence and location of rhytids, telangiectasias, pigmentary dyschromia, and expressive furrows.

If chemical peeling or laser skin resurfacing is being considered, the surgeon should also note the patient's Fitzpatrick skin type, which affects the skin's response to these procedures. The Fitzpatrick scale classifies skin into 6 types according to skin color (before sun exposure) and the reaction of the skin to sun exposure. The higher the number is, the greater the amount of skin pigment. Thus, Fitzpatrick type I refers to fair skin with minimal pigmentation, and type VI represents skin with marked pigmentation.

In addition, the surgeon should assess eyelid skin and fat along with eyelid margin position relative to the pupil and cornea, presence or absence of horizontal lower eyelid laxity, midface position, presence of jowling, accumulation of subcutaneous fat in the neck, and chin position, noting any nasal deformities, tip descent, or broadening, as well as thinning of the lips. The surgeon may find a side view of the neck to be particularly helpful in determining the extent of aging. Preoperative photographs should be available in the operating room.

Nonsurgical Facial Rejuvenation

Nonsurgical facial rejuvenation techniques such as laser resurfacing, soft-tissue dermal fillers, neurotoxin injection, chemical peels, and microdermabrasion are used to treat involutional and actinic facial skin changes. These superficial procedures may precede or be combined with surgical procedures that reposition deeper structures. It is important to remember that the upper eyelid appearance is inextricably linked to the position of the eyebrow. Similarly, the lower eyelid appearance is linked to the position of the midface, as well as the lower face and neck. Subunits of the facial cosmetic superstructure should not be viewed or manipulated individually but must be addressed in the context of the entire face and neck.

Laser Skin Resurfacing

Laser skin resurfacing, a technology popularized in the early 1990s, is designed to reduce wrinkles and enhance the texture and appearance of the facial and periorbital skin. A variety of lasers have been developed to perform laser resurfacing; superpulsed or ultrapulsed carbon dioxide (CO_2) and erbium:yttrium-aluminum-garnet (Er:YAG) lasers are the most widely used. The development of superpulsed CO_2 lasers has allowed ablative skin resurfacing without excessive thermal damage. Superpulsed and ultrapulsed CO_2 lasers deliver small pulses of high-energy light to the skin; pauses between these pulses allow cooling of the tissues in the treated area, minimizing the risk of thermal damage. The Er:YAG laser has a nearly pure ablative effect on collagen and water-containing tissues, with a much smaller zone of thermal injury and much less heat transfer into the tissues than the CO_2 lasers.

Laser resurfacing is a useful adjunct to lower blepharoplasty. The skin-shrinking, collagen-tightening effect of laser skin resurfacing often allows the surgeon to avoid making an external incision and removing skin.

Patient selection is vital for successful laser skin resurfacing. Patients with a fair complexion and generally healthy, well-hydrated skin are ideal candidates. Patients with greater degrees of skin pigmentation can be safely treated, but care and caution are needed.

The darker the skin pigmentation is, the greater the risk of postoperative inflammatory hyperpigmentation. Contraindications include inappropriate, unrealistic expectations, the presence of collagen vascular disease such as active systemic lupus erythematosus, and significant uncorrected lower eyelid laxity.

Herpes simplex virus infection after laser resurfacing may lead to scarring; therefore, most surgeons prophylactically treat patients with suppressing doses of antiviral agents against outbreaks of herpes simplex virus. Other complications associated with laser skin resurfacing include a variety of ophthalmic problems such as lagophthalmos, exposure keratitis, corneal injury, ectropion, and lower eyelid retraction.

A desire to improve superficial skin characteristics and facial wrinkling without the prolonged period of healing and erythema seen with ablative laser skin resurfacing has led to the development of devices that use fractionated lasers, intense pulsed light, ultrasound, or radiofrequency to deliver energy to the skin. These modalities can potentially even skin tone, remove cutaneous dyschromias or fine wrinkles, and even lift and smooth facial tissues. Each of these devices has its own risks and limitations but offers some improvement in aspects of facial aging, with fewer risks and shorter recovery times than with ablative laser skin resurfacing.

Aslam A, Alster TS. Evolution of laser skin resurfacing: from scanning to fractional technology. *Dermatol Surg.* 2014;40(11):1163–1172.

Cosmetic Uses of Botulinum Toxin

The use of botulinum toxin in patients with blepharospasm and hemifacial spasm (HFS) led to the observation that botulinum toxin reduces or eliminates some facial wrinkles. The first neurotoxin available for aesthetic indications was onabotulinumtoxinA, which already had a long history of ophthalmic use in the treatment of blepharospasm and HFS. The US FDA approved it to temporarily reduce wrinkles in the glabellar area, the lateral canthal lines (crow's-feet), and the forehead. AbobotulinumtoxinA, the second neurotoxin to become available in the United States, has also been approved for the treatment of wrinkles in the glabellar area. IncobotulinumtoxinA has been approved for both cosmetic and medical applications. A number of non–FDA-approved botulinum toxin products are available worldwide; however, US physicians should recognize the significant risks associated with using a non–FDA-approved substance for injection. Also, unit potency differs among these products, requiring that careful dosing adjustments be made.

Apart from the glabella, the areas most amenable to neuromodulation are the forehead, lateral canthal lines, perioral rhytids, and platysmal bands. The amount of botulinum toxin required and the location of injections vary significantly among patients and should be individualized.

The eyebrow can be chemically lifted when botulinum toxin is injected into the depressors of the eyebrow. The corners of the mouth can be elevated with injection into the depressor anguli oris muscle. The onset of action, peak effect, duration of effect, and complications of botulinum toxin for cosmetic purposes are the same as those noted for botulinum toxin as therapy for benign essential blepharospasm in Chapter 12 of this volume.

Lorenc ZP, Kenkel JM, Fagien S, et al. Consensus panel's assessment and recommendations on the use of 3 botulinum toxin type A products in facial aesthetics. *Aesthet Surg J.* 2013;33(1 Suppl):35S–40S.

Soft-Tissue Dermal Fillers

Many formulations of fillers are available for nonsurgical facial rejuvenation. Bovine collagen was initially approved by the FDA in 1995. However, its use required patch skin testing for possible allergic response. With the increased use of hyaluronic acid fillers derived from bacteria, bovine collagen usage has since declined. Hyaluronic acid fillers do not require allergy testing and have been approved by the FDA for the treatment of facial wrinkles or folds such as the nasolabial folds (Fig 13-1), for lip augmentation, and to correct age-related volume loss in the cheek area. Off-label usage of hyaluronic acid fillers for the periocular region (Fig 13-2) has been described extensively in the literature, but these fillers must be used with care. Complications from intravascular injection,

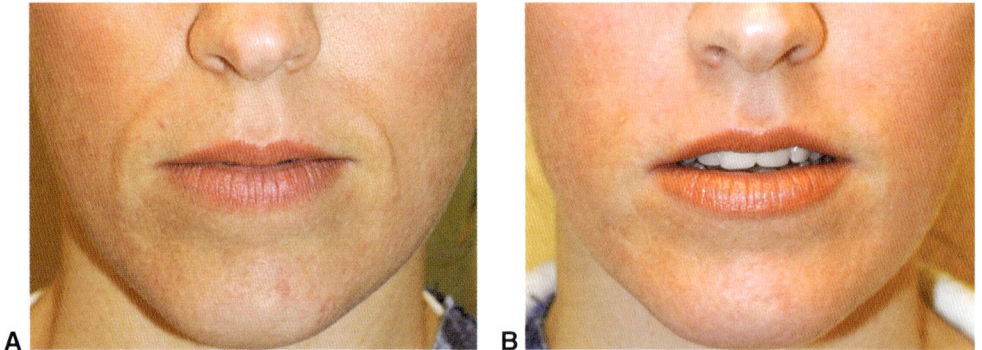

Figure 13-1 Before **(A)** and after **(B)** injection of a hyaluronic acid filler to the nasolabial folds. *(Courtesy of Bobby S. Korn, MD, PhD.)*

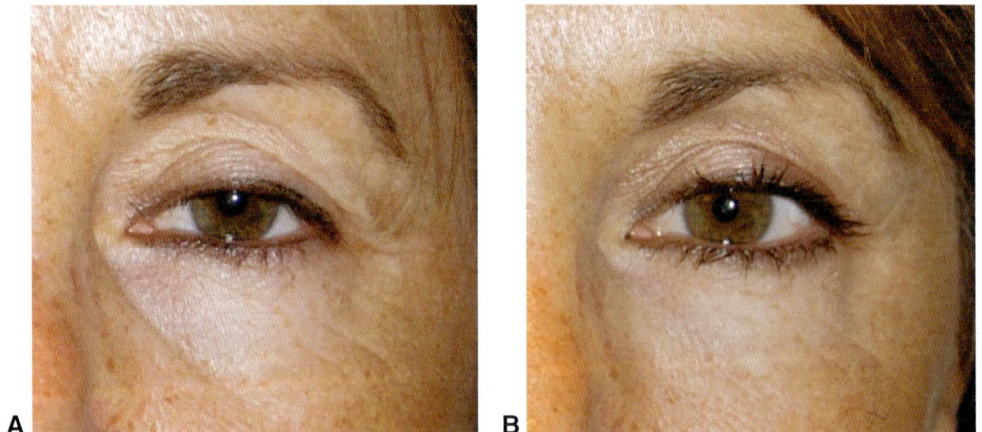

Figure 13-2 Before **(A)** and after **(B)** injection of a hyaluronic acid filler to improve the contour of the lower eyelid (tear trough). *(Courtesy of Bobby S. Korn, MD, PhD.)*

including regional soft-tissue necrosis and central retinal artery occlusion, have been reported. In central retinal artery occlusion, retrograde embolization follows inadvertent high-pressure injection into an artery (see Chapter 9, Fig 9-9).

Goldberg RA, Fiaschetti D. Filling the periorbital hollows with hyaluronic acid gel: initial experience with 244 injections. *Ophthalmic Plast Reconstr Surg.* 2006;22(5):335–341.

Peter S, Mennel S. Retinal branch artery occlusion following injection of hyaluronic acid (Restylane). *Clin Exp Ophthalmol.* 2006;34(4):363–364.

Autologous Fat Grafting

The use of autologous fat transfer was first reported in 1893 by Neuber. With the advent of liposuction and refinements in the technique, this procedure has evolved into a safe and predictable means of restoring facial volume. Its biocompatibility makes fat an ideal filler. Any area treatable with the commercial dermal fillers discussed in the previous section is potentially treatable with fat grafting. These areas include, but are not limited to, the periocular area, temples, forehead, brow, cheeks, midface, lips, nasolabial fold, jawline, submental crease, and chin. As with commercial dermal filler injection, fat grafting carries the risk of intravascular injection. Additionally, fat grafts can exhibit variable growth, resorption, or palpability if injected too superficially.

Coleman SR. Facial augmentation with structural fat grafting. *Clin Plast Surg.* 2006,33(4):567–577.

Surgical Facial Rejuvenation

Facial and eyelid surgery should be approached with care. Adequate preoperative preparation includes properly informing the patient of the proposed benefits as well as the potential complications of the procedure. Significant complications—including facial nerve paralysis, skin flap necrosis, and vision loss—are potential risks.

Rejuvenation of the aging face requires a multitude of techniques. Chemical peeling, laser resurfacing, dermabrasion, and liposculpting can enhance the results of surgery, or, at times, may be preferred to incisional surgery.

Lower Blepharoplasty

Lower eyelid rejuvenation is considered an aesthetic operation and is discussed in Chapter 12 in this volume.

Forehead Rejuvenation

Many options are available for forehead rejuvenation (see the section Brow Ptosis in Chapter 12).

Midface Rejuvenation

The entire midface should be evaluated in a patient presenting for lower eyelid blepharoplasty. With age, cheek tissue descends, and orbital fat herniates, creating a double-convexity

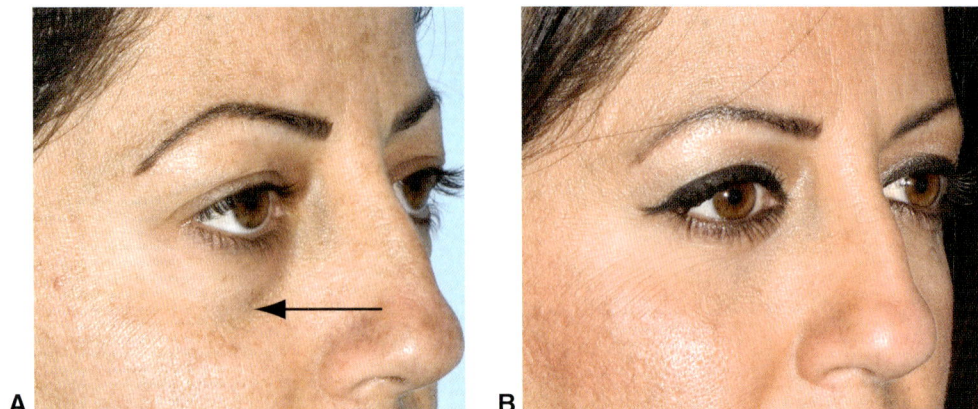

Figure 13-3 Lower eyelid blepharoplasty with orbital fat redraping. **A,** Image taken before surgery demonstrates the double convexity deformity with orbital fat prolapse and unmasking of the inferior orbital rim *(arrow).* **B,** Image taken after surgery shows resolution of the double-convexity deformity and a smooth eyelid and cheek junction. *(Courtesy of Bobby S. Korn, MD, PhD.)*

deformity (Fig 13-3). Attenuation of the orbitomalar, masseteric cutaneous, and zygomatic ligaments are the pathologic changes that occur with midfacial ptosis. Elevation of the suborbicularis oculi fat (SOOF) and midface, combined with conservative fat removal or redistribution, can restore the youthful anterior projection of the midface.

Midface elevation can be achieved through a preperiosteal or subperiosteal approach. The preperiosteal plane can be accessed through the lower eyelid, with or without release of the lateral canthal tendon, or by using the temporal scalp incision employed in an endoscopic brow-lift (endobrow). The subperiosteal midface can also be accessed through these incisions or through a superior gingival sulcus incision (Fig 13-4). The goal of these procedures is to provide release of the midface tissues, followed by elevation and resuspension. Midface elevation is commonly combined with additional procedures such as a brow-lift, lower face-lift, or volume augmentation.

Lucarelli MJ, Khwarg SI, Lemke BN, Kozel JS, Dortzbach RK. The anatomy of midfacial ptosis. *Ophthalmic Plast Reconstr Surg.* 2000;16(1):7–22.

Williams EF III, Lam SM. Midfacial rejuvenation via an endoscopic browlift approach: a review of technique. *Facial Plast Surg.* 2003;19(2):147–156.

Lower Face and Neck Rejuvenation

During preoperative evaluation, the face and neck should be considered as a single cosmetic unit. Correction of the cosmetic subunits of the upper face and midface without addressing the lower face and neck can create an unbalanced appearance. At the very least, these concerns must be discussed with the patient preoperatively, along with surgical options.

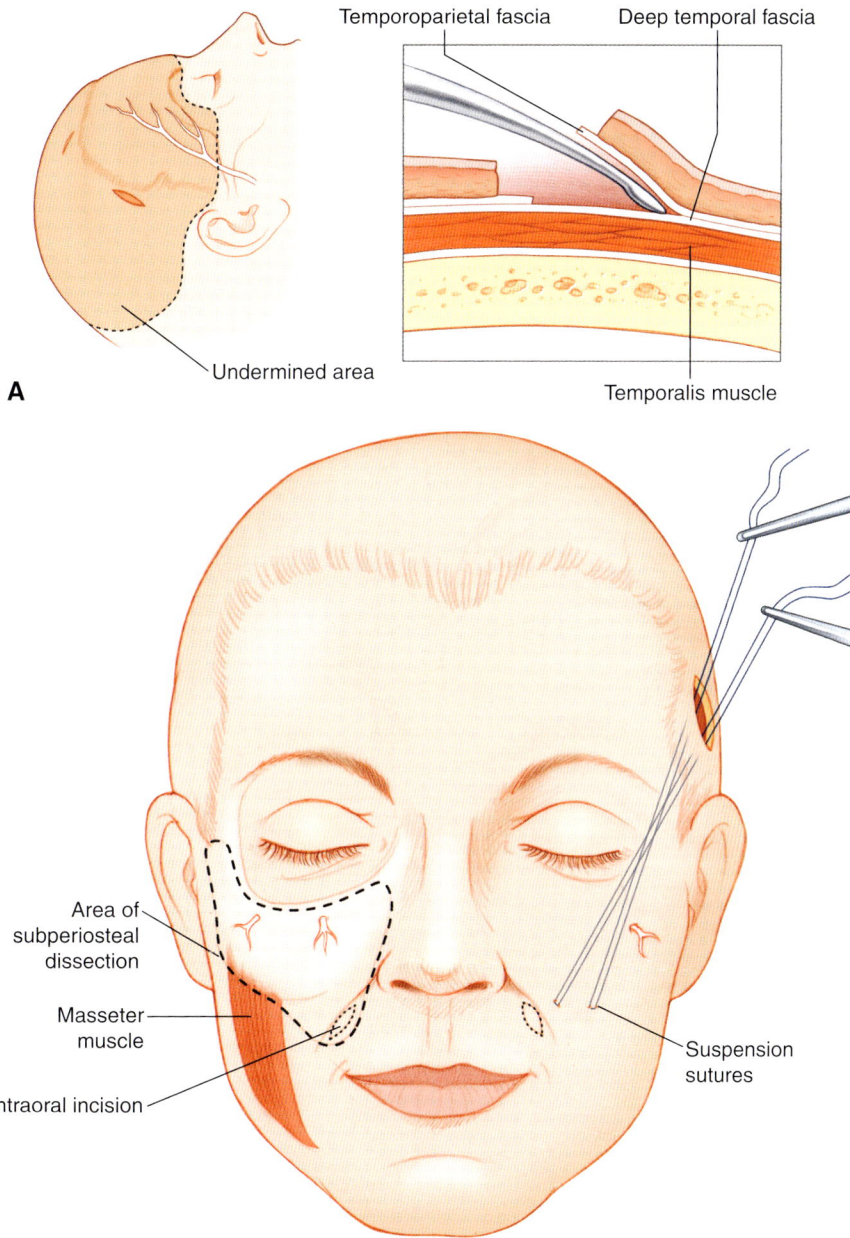

Figure 13-4 Endoscopic approach to subperiosteal midface-lift. **A,** Undermining between the temporoparietal fascia and the deep temporal fascia to approach the anterior face of the maxilla. **B,** Midface subperiosteal dissection and suture fixation. *(Illustration by Christine Gralapp.)*

Rhytidectomy

The most commonly performed procedures include the vintage (subcutaneous) rhytidectomy, the rhytidectomy with superficial elevation and refixation of the superficial musculoaponeurotic system (SMAS) (Fig 13-5), and the deep-plane rhytidectomy. Rhytidectomies

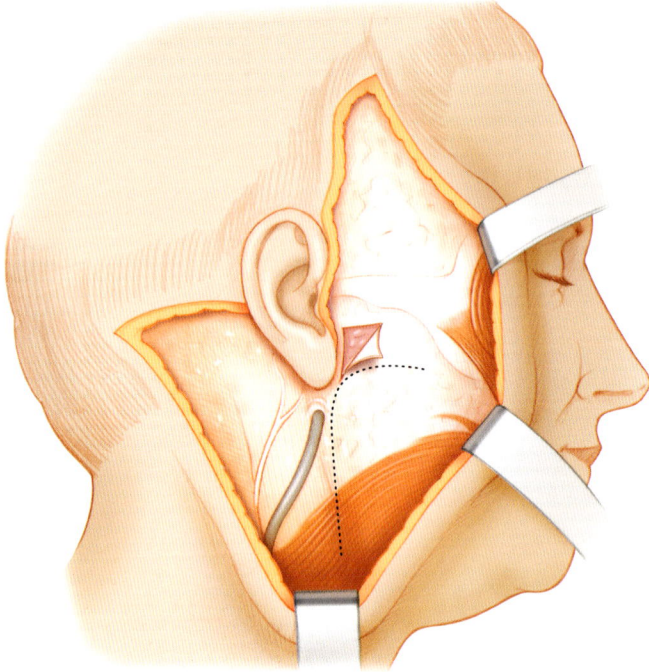

Figure 13-5 The common goal of rhytidectomy procedures is modification of the superficial musculoaponeurotic system (SMAS) that translates to changes in the overlying anatomy. After release of the SMAS *(dotted line),* the SMAS is pulled laterally and superiorly for elevation of the jowls and lower face. *(Illustration by Christine Gralapp.)*

typically include surgical management of the jowls and neck, including liposuction with or without platysmaplasty (Fig 13-6). The 3 rhytidectomy procedures mentioned differ mainly in the location and extent of dissection. Although the more superficial procedures are less likely to cause facial nerve damage, they may produce shorter-lasting results. The more extensive procedures have greater risks (eg, facial nerve injury), but the likelihood that they will produce dramatic, longer-lasting improvement is also greater.

Complications of rhytidectomy are directly related to the extent of subcutaneous undermining; they include hematoma, seroma, skin necrosis, hair loss, paresthesias, motor deficits, incisional scarring, asymmetry, earlobe distraction (pixie-ear deformity), and contour irregularities. Hematoma is the leading surgical face-lift complication, but patient dissatisfaction may be the most common issue postoperatively.

Neck liposuction

Neck liposuction enhances the neckline and is often done in conjunction with other cosmetic procedures. Stab incisions, or *adits,* are made just posterior to the earlobe on each side and along the submental incision line; if liposuction is performed as a stand-alone procedure, they are made just anterior to the submental crease. Small liposuction cannulas are used for fat removal. A layer of fat is left on the dermis, and the liposuction cannula openings are always oriented away from the dermis to avoid injury to the

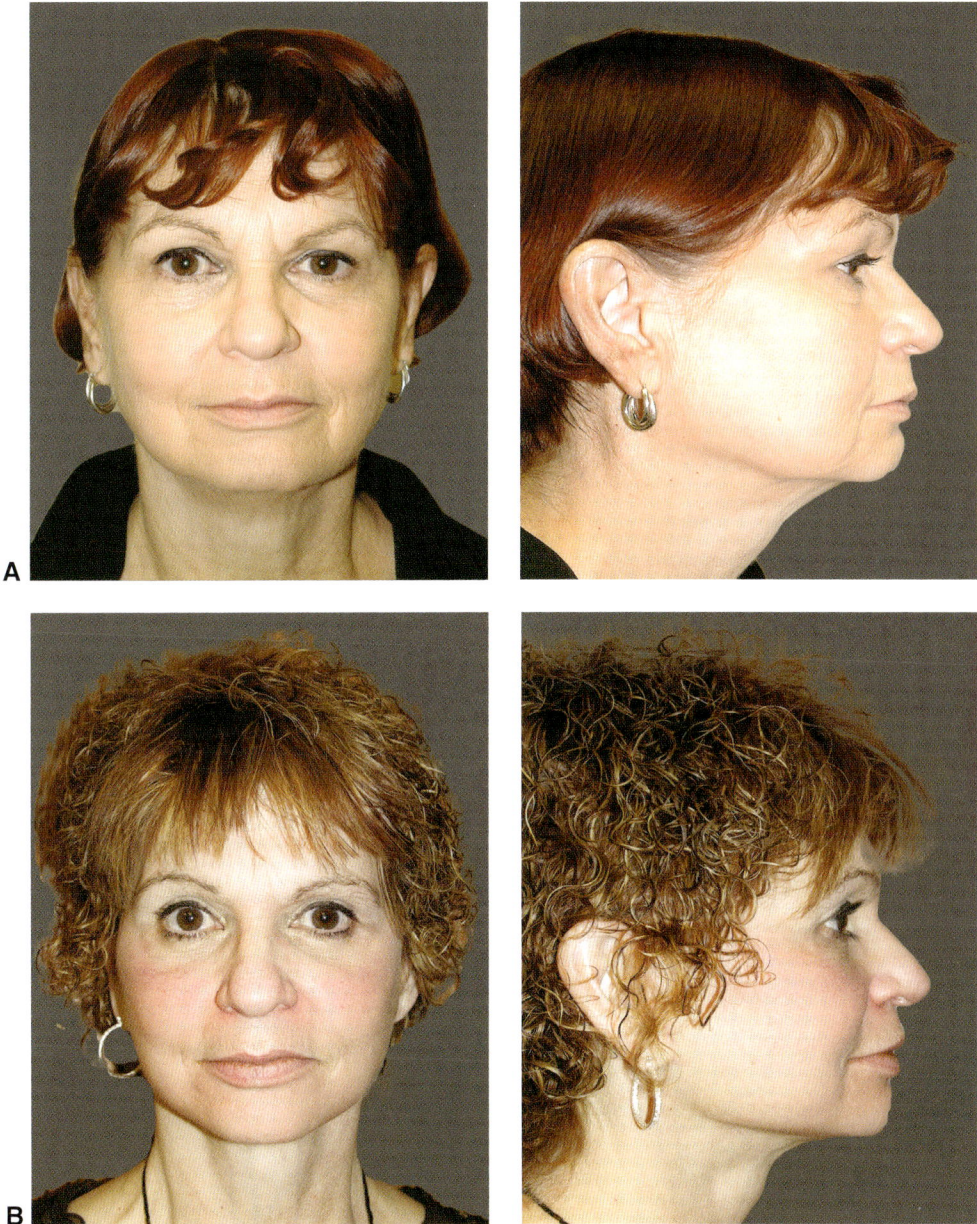

Figure 13-6 Photographs of a patient who underwent rhytidectomy with submental liposuction. **A,** Images taken prior to surgery. **B,** Images taken after the procedure. Note the improvement in the jowls and sharpening of the cervicomental angle. *(Courtesy of Robert G. Fante, MD.)*

vascular plexus deep to the dermis. In addition to abnormalities in skin quality, damage in this area can lead to unsightly scarring of the dermis of the underlying neck musculature. The adits are left open or sutured, and a compression bandage is worn for 1 week after the procedure.

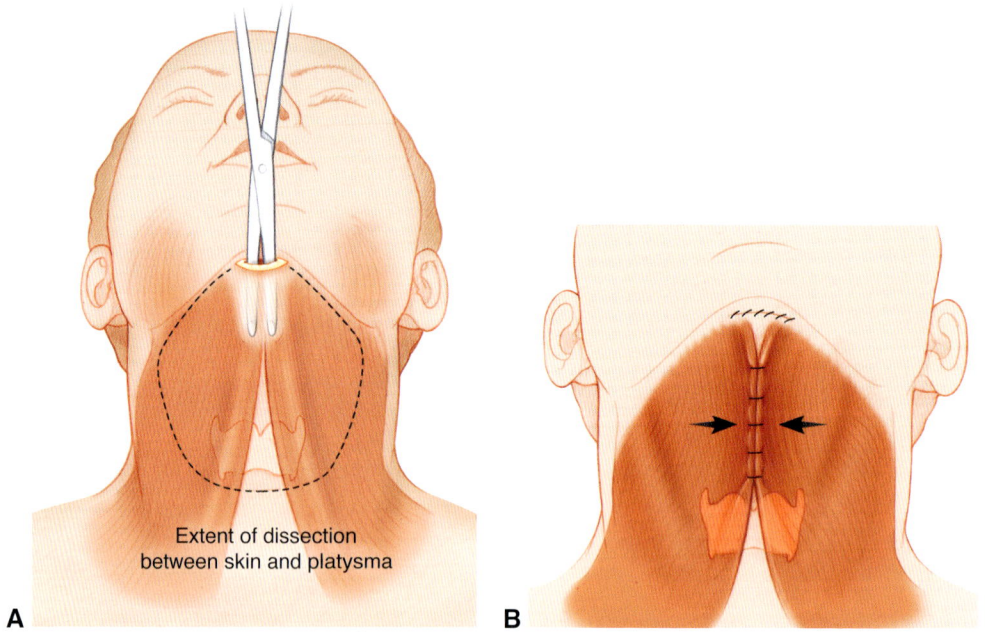

Figure 13-7 Cervicoplasty. **A,** Undermining of the skin. **B,** Platysmaplasty. *(Illustrations by Christine Gralapp.)*

Platysmaplasty

Platysmaplasty is performed to correct platysmal bands and is typically done in conjunction with a lower face-lift. A subcutaneous dissection is carried out in the preplatysmal plane centrally under the chin to the level of the thyroid cartilage (Fig 13-7A). Lateral platysmal undermining and suspension may be performed as part of a rhytidectomy. Midline platysma resection and reconstruction (Fig 13-7B) are performed if midline neck support is needed. A drain and a light compression dressing are placed. Postoperatively, the cervicomental angle is more acute, yielding a more youthful look.

Dailey RA, Jones LT. Rejuvenation of the aging face. *Focal Points: Clinical Modules for Ophthalmologists.* San Francisco: American Academy of Ophthalmology; 2004, module 2.

PART III

Lacrimal System

CHAPTER **14**

Anatomy, Development, and Physiology of the Lacrimal Secretory and Drainage Systems

▶ *This chapter includes a related video, which can be accessed by scanning the QR code provided in the text or going to www.aao.org/bcscvideo_section07.*

Highlights

- Biopsy of the lacrimal gland is preferentially performed on the orbital lobe to avoid damage to the secretory ductules.
- Congenital nasolacrimal duct obstruction (NLDO) may not be apparent until tearing function commences at approximately 6 weeks of age.
- The tear pump actively drains tears during the blink cycle.

See Chapters 1 and 4 in BCSC Section 2, *Fundamentals and Principles of Ophthalmology,* for additional discussion, including illustrations, of some of the topics covered in this chapter.

Anatomy

Secretory System

The lacrimal gland is an exocrine gland located in the superolateral orbit within the fossa for the lacrimal gland. Embryologic development of the lateral horn of the levator aponeurosis indents the lacrimal gland, dividing it into orbital and palpebral lobes (see Chapter 1, Fig 1-7) as it traverses laterally to insert on the Whitnall tubercle. The superior transverse ligament (Whitnall ligament) forms septa through the stroma of the gland, with some fibers also projecting onto the lateral orbital wall several millimeters above Whitnall tubercle, as noted in Chapter 1 of this volume.

Between 8 and 12 major lacrimal ducts empty into the superior cul-de-sac approximately 5 mm above the lateral tarsal border after passing posterior to the levator aponeurosis, and through the Müller muscle and conjunctiva. Because the lacrimal excretory ducts pass through the palpebral portion of the gland, removal of the palpebral lobe may reduce

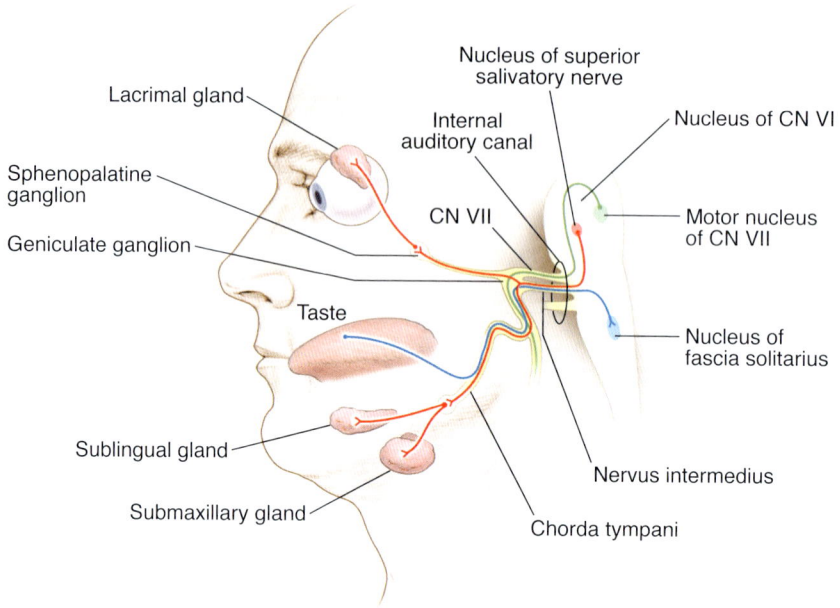

Figure 14-1 Nonmotor pathways of cranial nerve (CN) VII, including the efferent pathway to the lacrimal gland. *(Illustration by Christine Gralapp.)*

secretion from the entire gland. Therefore, biopsy of the lacrimal gland is preferentially performed on the orbital lobe.

Ocular surface irritation activates tear production from the lacrimal gland. The ophthalmic branch of the trigeminal nerve, cranial nerve (CN) V, provides the sensory *(afferent)* pathway in this reflex tear arc. The *efferent* pathway is more complicated. Parasympathetic fibers, originating in the superior salivatory nucleus of the pons, exit the brainstem with the facial nerve, CN VII (Fig 14-1). Lacrimal fibers leave CN VII as the greater superficial petrosal nerve and pass into the sphenopalatine ganglion. From there, they are believed to enter the lacrimal gland via the superior branch of the zygomatic nerve, through an anastomosis between the zygomaticotemporal nerve and the lacrimal nerve. It is unclear whether this anastomosis is uniformly present. The role of the sympathetic nervous system in lacrimation is not well understood.

The *accessory glands of Krause* and *Wolfring* are exocrine glands located deep within the superior fornix and just above the superior border of the tarsus, respectively. Aqueous lacrimal secretion has traditionally been divided into basal secretion and reflex secretion. Previously, it was thought that the accessory glands predominate in basal tear secretion, and that the lacrimal gland predominates in reflex tearing. It is now believed that all lacrimal glands respond as a unit.

The tear film is an extremely complex composition of mucin, aqueous, and oily layers of variable osmolality with components including lysozyme, lactoferrin, immunoglobulins, and prostaglandins (see BCSC Section 2, *Fundamentals and Principles of Ophthalmology,* for a more detailed discussion of the tear film).

Saleh GM, Hussain B, Woodruff SA, Sharma A, Litwin AS. Tear film osmolarity in epiphora. *Ophthalmic Plast Reconstr Surg.* 2012;28(5):338–340.

Drainage System

Tears enter the lacrimal drainage system through *puncta* located medially on the margin of the upper and lower eyelids (Fig 14-2). Each punctum appears at the apex of a fleshy papilla that protrudes slightly above the eyelid margin and is slightly inverted and apposed to the globe to rest within the tear lake. The inferior punctum is slightly more lateral than the superior. The puncta are approximately 0.3 mm in diameter and lead to a vertical segment of the *lacrimal canaliculi* known as the ampulla. The canaliculi then turn 90°, continuing 8–10 mm medially to join at the common canaliculus and connect

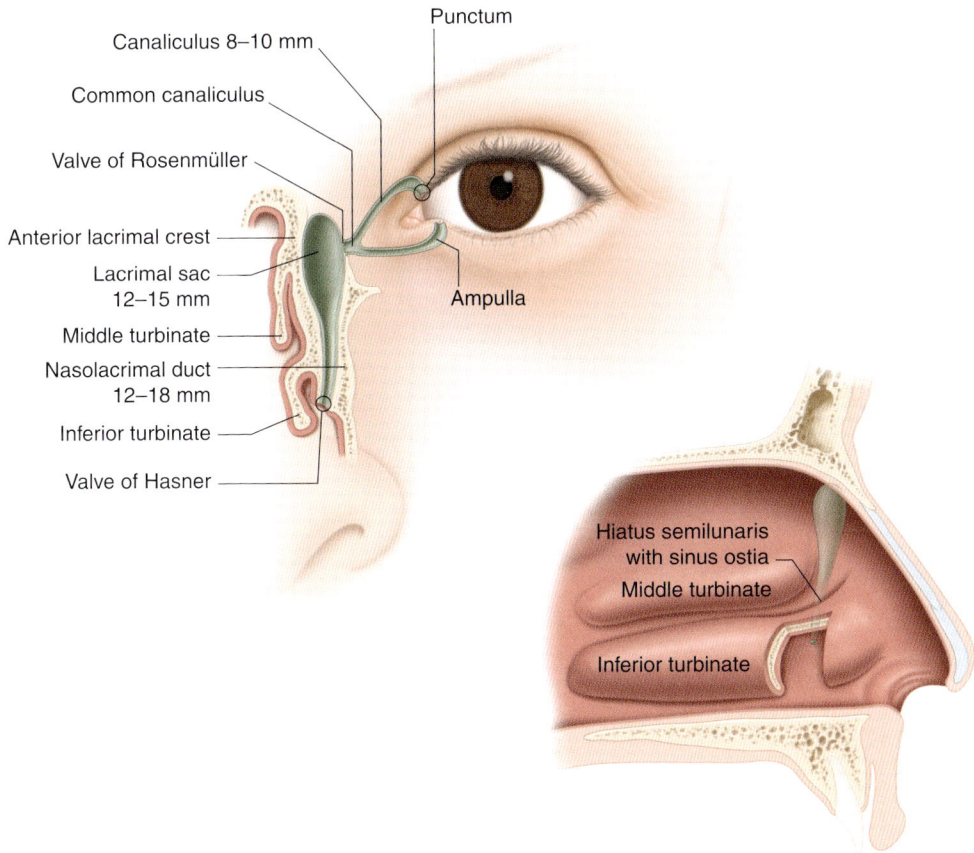

Figure 14-2 Normal anatomy of the lacrimal drainage system. The measurements given are for adults. *(Illustration by Mark Miller.)*

with the *lacrimal sac* through the valve of Rosenmüller. Less commonly, the canaliculi connect directly to the lacrimal sac without a common portion. The canaliculi are lined with nonkeratinized, non–mucin-producing stratified squamous epithelium. This epithelium transitions to a stratified columnar epithelium in the distal portion of the canaliculi, which continues through the lacrimal sac and *nasolacrimal duct (NLD)*. For reasons that are not completely understood, the Na^+/I (sodium/iodide) symporter (NIS) is present in this epithelium, which can lead to stenosis during treatment with high-dose radioactive iodine for thyroid cancer.

The *valve of Rosenmüller* (see Fig 14-2) is a fold of mucosal tissue that has traditionally been described as the structure that prevents reflux of tears from the sac into the canaliculi. However, studies suggest that the common canaliculus consistently bends from posterior to anterior behind the medial canthal tendon before entering the lacrimal sac at an acute angle. This bend, in conjunction with the fold of mucosa, may play a role in blocking reflux.

The lacrimal sac lies within a bony fossa bordered by the anterior and posterior lacrimal crests (see BCSC Section 2, *Fundamentals and Principles of Ophthalmology,* Fig 1-1, for an illustration of this fossa). Wrapping around the anterior and posterior aspects of the lacrimal sac, the medial canthal tendon is a complex structure composed of anterior and posterior crura. The superficial head attaches to the anterior lacrimal crest; the deep head (with the Horner muscle), to the posterior lacrimal crest. The medial wall of the fossa is composed of the lacrimal bone posteriorly and the frontal process of the maxillary bone anteriorly. Medial to the fossa is the middle meatus of the nose, sometimes with intervening ethmoid air cells. From an intranasal view, the location of the lacrimal sac corresponds to the lateral nasal wall just anterior to the middle turbinate (Fig 14-3). The fundus of the sac, which is more fibrous than the rest of the sac, extends several millimeters above the medial canthal tendon. Inferiorly, the lacrimal sac transitions into the NLD. When performing an external dacryocystorhinostomy, the surgeon may encounter the angular artery and vein medial to the medial canthal angle, which may cause bleeding. Additionally, distal fibers of the zygomatic and buccal branches of the facial nerve may be affected, resulting in temporary lagophthalmos.

In adults, the NLD measures 12–18 mm in length. The intraosseous portion of the duct is typically 12 mm long, and the meatal duct extends 5–6 mm inferior to the bony

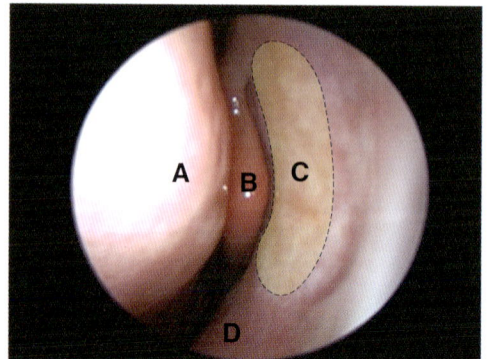

Figure 14-3 Endoscopic intranasal anatomy *(left side).* Note the septum **(A),** middle turbinate **(B),** and area of mucosa and bone to be removed to expose the lacrimal sac **(C).** The superior portion of the inferior turbinate is visible at the bottom **(D).** *(Courtesy of Eric A. Steele, MD.)*

ostium. The NLD travels through bone within the nasolacrimal canal, which initially curves in an inferior and slightly lateral and posterior direction from the lacrimal sac. The NLD opens into the nose through an ostium under the inferior turbinate (the inferior meatus), which is usually partially covered by a mucosal fold (the valve of Hasner; see Fig 14-2). The mucosal ostium in adults is typically located 30–35 mm from the external naris.

Morgenstern KE, Vadysirisack DD, Zhang Z, et al. Expression of sodium iodide symporter in the lacrimal drainage system: implication for the mechanism underlying nasolacrimal duct obstruction in I[131]-treated patients. *Ophthalmic Plast Reconstr Surg.* 2005;21(5):337–344.

Development

Secretory System

The lacrimal gland develops from multiple solid ectodermal buds in the anterior superolateral orbit. These buds branch, canalize, and form ducts and alveoli. The lacrimal glands are small and do not function fully until approximately 6 weeks after birth. Thus, newborn infants do not produce tears when crying.

Drainage System

By the end of the fifth week of gestation, the nasolacrimal groove forms as a furrow lying between the nasal and maxillary prominences. In the floor of this groove, the NLD develops from a linear thickening of the ectoderm. A solid cord separates from adjacent ectoderm and sinks into the mesenchyme. The cord canalizes, forming the NLD and the lacrimal sac at its cranial end. The canalicular system is an outgrowth of the lacrimal sac. Caudally, the developing duct extends intranasally, exiting within the inferior meatus. The central tissue of this cord eventually breaks down, forming a lumen. Canalization of the NLD is usually complete around the time of birth. Incomplete development of the distal aspect of the duct with obstruction at the valve of Hasner represents the most common cause of congenital NLD obstruction (NLDO); it is symptomatic in approximately 5% of infants at birth. Patency usually occurs spontaneously within the first few months of life. As noted earlier, lacrimation does not function normally until around age 6 weeks; therefore, excessive tearing, which is often associated with this obstruction, may not be immediately obvious even if an obstruction exists.

Physiology

Evaporation accounts for approximately 10% of tear elimination in the young and for 20% or more in elderly persons. Most of the tear flow is actively pumped from the tear lake by the actions of the orbicularis oculi muscle. Blinking pushes the tears from lateral to nasal on the eyelid margin. When the eyelids open, negative pressure pulls the tears into the sac; when the eyelids close, the action of the orbicularis muscle creates positive pressure that forces those tears through the NLD (Fig 14-4, Video 14-1). A weakened blink interferes with the

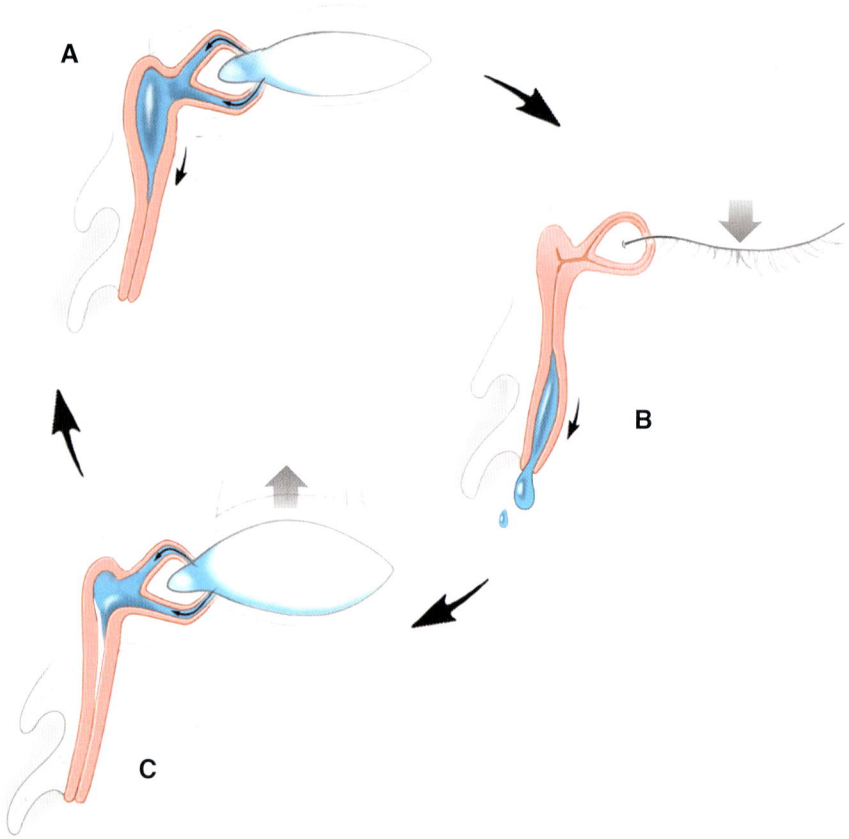

Figure 14-4 Lacrimal pump mechanism. **A,** In the relaxed state, the puncta lie in the tear lake, and the lacrimal sac is filled with tears. **B,** With eyelid closure, contraction of the pretarsal orbicularis closes the puncta and canaliculi. The preseptal orbicularis fibers, which insert onto the sac, also compress the sac, creating positive pressure that propels tears through the duct. **C,** With eyelid opening, the orbicularis relaxes, and the puncta and sac open, creating negative pressure that draws tears into the canaliculi and lacrimal sac. As the eyelids close, the cycle repeats. *(Original illustration by Christine Gralapp; revision based on an illustration by Cat N. Burkat, MD.)*

normal pumping mechanism and contributes to epiphora in patients with eyelid laxity or CN VII palsy.

Doane MG. Blinking and the mechanics of the lacrimal drainage system. *Ophthalmology.* 1981;88(8):844–851.

VIDEO 14-1 Lacrimal pump mechanism.
Courtesy of Cat N. Burkat, MD; illustration by Christine Gralapp.
Access all Section 7 videos at www.aao.org/bcscvideo_section07.

CHAPTER 15

Abnormalities of the Lacrimal Secretory and Drainage Systems

▶ *This chapter includes related videos, which can be accessed by scanning the QR codes provided in the text or going to www.aao.org/bcscvideo_section07.*

Highlights

- Congenital defects in the lacrimal system can be isolated or associated with other abnormalities.
- Management of congenital nasolacrimal obstruction includes conservative and surgical techniques.
- Tearing can be due to a wide variety of conditions.
- Canalicular injuries are commonly encountered with eyelid trauma.

Developmental Abnormalities

Lacrimal Secretory System

Congenital abnormalities of the lacrimal gland are rare. Hypoplasia and agenesis of the lacrimal gland can occur in isolation or in conjunction with congenital abnormalities of the salivary glands. Both are usually sporadic but have been reported in an apparent autosomal dominant pattern. Ectopic lacrimal gland tissue can be present within the orbit and eyelids, and lacrimal gland prolapse is sometimes seen in patients with craniosynostosis syndromes.

Occasionally, children are born with an aberrant ductule that exits externally through the eyelid overlying the lacrimal gland; this was previously referred to as a *lacrimal gland fistula*. These aberrant ductules exit laterally several millimeters above the eyelash line and are usually accompanied by an adjacent cluster of eyelashes. Tears produced from the aberrant ductules can mimic epiphora. These ductules can be successfully managed with simple excision.

Lacrimal Drainage System

Developmental abnormalities of the lacrimal drainage system include

- errors in the genesis of the proximal system
  - multiple puncta
  - lacrimal–cutaneous fistula

- incomplete patency
  - punctal or canalicular hypoplasia or aplasia
  - nasolacrimal duct (NLD) obstruction

Duplication

In rare cases, multiple puncta and additional canaliculi develop (Fig 15-1). When the extra opening is on the eyelid margin, it may be asymptomatic and requires no treatment. The term *congenital lacrimal–cutaneous fistula* has been used to describe uncommon fistulas that exit through the skin, typically infranasal to the medial canthus (Fig 15-2). These anlage ducts or fistulas from an otherwise normal canalicular system or lacrimal sac are sometimes asymptomatic, or they may be associated with tears that appear on the skin. Approximately one-third of patients have an underlying NLD obstruction (NLDO); in these cases, chronic mucoid discharge from the affected nasolacrimal sac may be present.

In symptomatic patients, direct surgical excision of the epithelium-lined fistulous tract with direct suture closure is indicated. In patients with underlying NLDO and chronic dacryocystitis, lacrimal intubation or dacryocystorhinostomy may also be required. (See the management subsection in the section Acquired Nasolacrimal Duct Obstruction later in this chapter.)

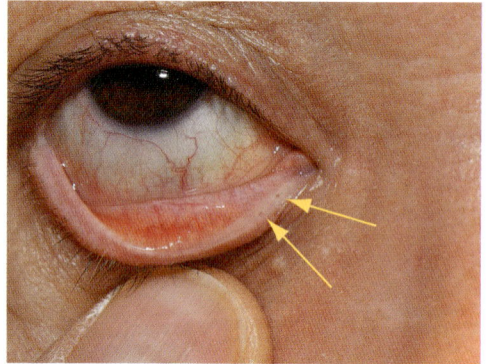

Figure 15-1 Congenital accessory canaliculi *(arrows)* of the right lower eyelid. *(Courtesy of Bobby S. Korn, MD, PhD.)*

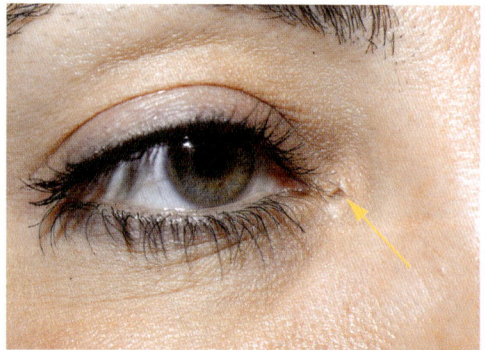

Figure 15-2 Congenital lacrimal–cutaneous fistula *(arrow)*. *(Courtesy of Bobby S. Korn, MD, PhD.)*

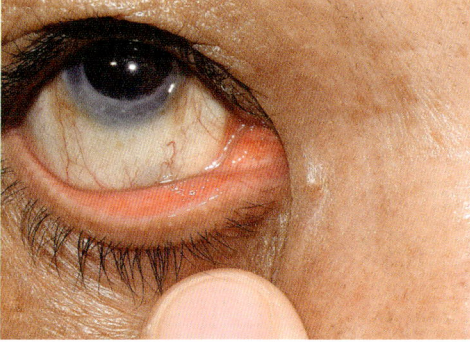

Figure 15-3 Congenital punctal aplasia. *(Courtesy of Bobby S. Korn, MD, PhD.)*

Aplasia and hypoplasia

Punctal hypoplasia or stenosis is encountered more frequently than true aplasia (Fig 15-3). Management of punctal stenosis, membranes, and aplasia is discussed later in this chapter.

Nasolacrimal duct obstruction

Congenital NLDO is typically due to failure of the duct to fully canalize but can be associated with more severe abnormalities. For example, major facial cleft deformities can pass through or be adjacent to the nasolacrimal drainage pathways and can result in outflow disorders.

Treatment of lacrimal drainage obstruction differs according to the cause and location of the obstruction. Obstruction may involve the puncta, canaliculi, lacrimal sac, or NLD. Because the pathophysiology and management of congenital and acquired lacrimal drainage abnormalities differ, these disorders are addressed separately.

Congenital Lacrimal Drainage Obstruction

Evaluation

The evaluation of a patient with congenital tearing is usually straightforward. The patient's parents report a history of tearing, mucopurulent discharge, or both, beginning shortly after birth. In rare cases, visible distention of the lacrimal sac is present, suggesting a congenital dacryocystocele. Otherwise, distinction should be made among the following:

- constant tearing with minimal mucopurulence, suggesting blockage of the upper system (puncta, canaliculi, and common canaliculus) caused by punctal or canalicular dysgenesis
- constant tearing with frequent mucopurulence and mattering of the eyelashes, suggesting complete obstruction of the NLD
- intermittent tearing with mucopurulence, suggesting intermittent obstruction of the NLD

Office examination includes inspection of the eyelid margins for proper apposition and patent puncta and evaluation for extrinsic causes of reflex hypersecretion, such as

- ocular surface irritation
- infectious conjunctivitis
- entropion
- epiblepharon
- trichiasis
- congenital glaucoma

Additional aspects of the examination include inspection of the medial canthal region to assess for a distended lacrimal sac (below the tendon), inflammation, or congenital defects such as an encephalocele (above the tendon). The single most important maneuver is application of digital pressure over the tear sac. If mucoid reflux is present, complete obstruction at the level of the NLD becomes the working diagnosis.

Punctal and Canalicular Agenesis and Dysgenesis

The medial eyelid margin is inspected for the presence of elevated lacrimal papillae and puncta. Close inspection may reveal a punctum with a membranous occlusion, which can usually be opened with a sharp probe. Temporary intubation (discussed in the subsection Congenital Nasolacrimal Duct Obstruction) or placement of a silicone plug may help prevent recurrence. If the punctum is truly absent, the surgeon may cut down through the eyelid margin medial to the expected punctum location to try to identify the canaliculus. Alternatively, retrograde probing through an open lacrimal sac with direct visualization of the common canalicular opening (common internal punctum) may identify the canaliculus. Occasionally, these maneuvers reveal a relatively mature canalicular system with a patent nasolacrimal sac and duct, in which case intubation may be performed. Symptomatic patients with a single punctum may require surgery to relieve NLDO rather than canalicular obstruction. Symptomatic patients with complete absence of the puncta and the canalicular system require a conjunctivodacryocystorhinostomy (CDCR). This is performed when the patient is old enough to allow proper care of the Jones tube. (CDCR is discussed in the section Canalicular Obstruction later in this chapter.)

Congenital Nasolacrimal Duct Obstruction

Congenital obstruction of the lacrimal drainage system is usually caused by a membrane blocking the valve of Hasner at the nasal end of the NLD. Many newborns are born with imperforate NLDs, but most obstructions open spontaneously within the first few months of life. Such an obstruction becomes clinically evident in only 2%–6% of full-term infants at 3–4 weeks of age. Of these, one-third have bilateral involvement.

Management can be divided into conservative (nonsurgical) and surgical options. Conservative options include observation, digital compression over the lacrimal sac, and topical or even oral antibiotics. The long-term use of topical antibiotics may be necessary to suppress chronic mucoid discharge with mattering of the lashes.

When the obstruction fails to resolve with conservative measures, more invasive intervention may be required. Most often, this consists of probing of the NLD to rupture the membrane occluding the duct at the valve of Hasner (discussed in detail later in this chapter). Opinions differ regarding the optimal time to initiate probing, as approximately 90% of all symptomatic congenital NLD obstructions resolve in the first year of life. Prompt treatment may be required in cases with dacryocystitis or airway obstruction secondary to nasal occlusion by an enlarged lacrimal sac.

Most surgeons perform probing if symptoms persist at 1 year of age. Some advocate earlier probing for those with significant recurrent infections, and several reports have suggested that delaying probing past 13 months of age may be associated with a decreased success rate.

Children aged 1 year or older usually require general anesthesia during probing. Topical anesthesia is safe in well-trained hands, but it limits the acquisition of information about the nature of the obstruction and the physician's intervention choices at the time of the procedure.

In some instances of congenital NLDO, dacryocystitis manifests as an acutely inflamed lacrimal sac with cellulitis of the overlying skin. Treatment with systemic antibiotics should be started promptly. Management of the pediatric patient is similar to that of the adult patient (discussed in detail later). Following resolution of the acute infectious process, elective probing is performed promptly to prevent recurrence of dacryocystitis.

Miller AM, Chandler DL, Repka MX, et al. Office probing for treatment of nasolacrimal duct obstruction in infants. *J AAPOS*. 2014;18(1):26–30.

Dacryocystocele

Mucoceles may form within the lacrimal sac or within the nasal cavity as a consequence of congenital NLDO. The type of mucocele involved in lacrimal sac distention has been termed a *dacryocystocele,* and it may be present at birth or may develop within 1 to 4 weeks after birth. It occurs when mucus (secreted by lacrimal sac goblet cells) is trapped in the tear sac because of a functional block above the sac (valve of Rosenmüller) and obstruction at the distal end (valve of Hasner) of the NLD. The dacryocystocele is initially sterile and may respond to conservative management with prophylactic topical antibiotics and digital compression of the lacrimal sac. When there is minimal improvement or infection develops, probing of the lacrimal drainage system may be necessary to address the disorder. Extension of the dacryocystocele cyst into the nasal cavity at the level of an occluded valve of Hasner may also occur. The intranasal cystic portion often extends inferiorly under the inferior turbinate, where it can be observed during nasal examination (Fig 15-4). Intranasal examination and urgent treatment are needed if the condition is bilateral and causes airway obstruction, as infants are obligate nasal breathers.

In most patients, dacryocystoceles demonstrate expansion inferior to the medial canthal tendon. Congenital swelling above the medial canthal tendon suggests alternative etiologies, such as a dermoid cyst or meningoencephalocele. Computed tomography (CT) or magnetic resonance imaging (MRI) is useful in evaluating the patient for these more complex diagnoses.

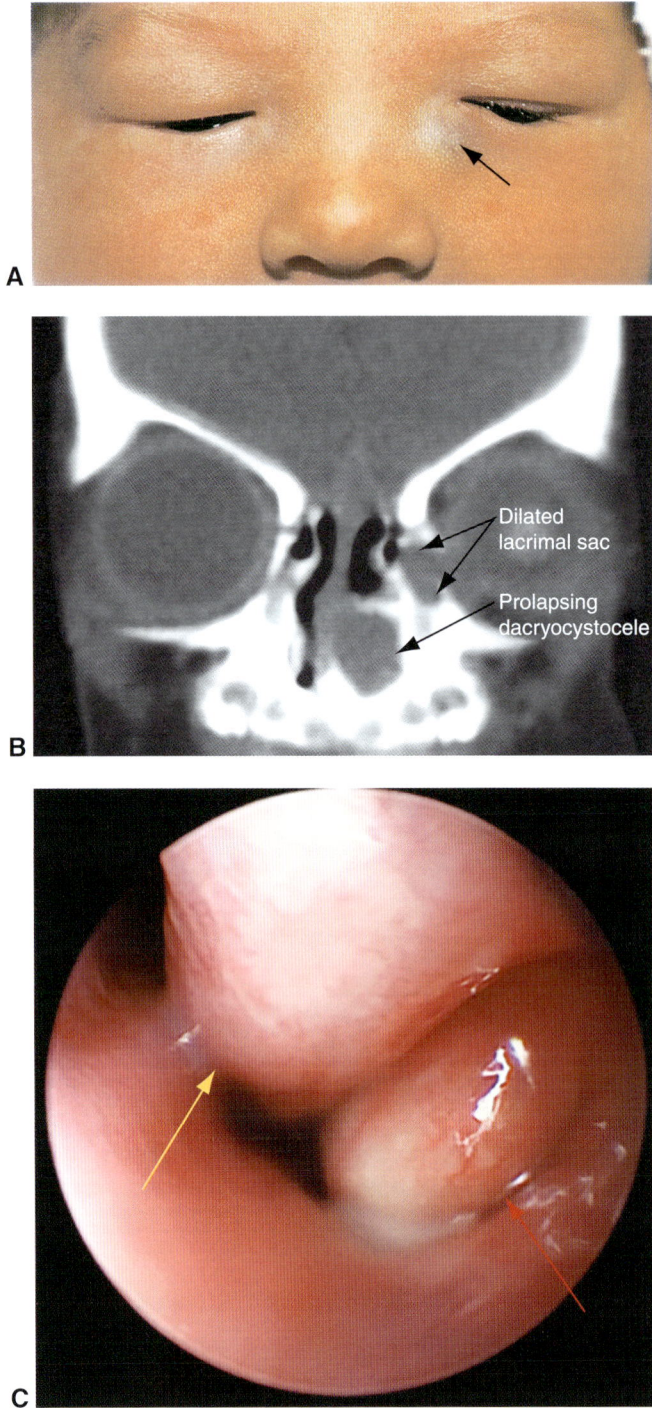

Figure 15-4 Congenital dacryocystocele. **A,** Left congenital dacryocystocele *(arrow)* 1 week postpartum. **B,** Computed tomography (CT) scan of a congenital dacryocystocele. **C,** Endoscopic view of a left dacryocystocele *(red arrow)* prolapsing under the inferior turbinate *(yellow arrow)*. *(Parts A and B courtesy of Pierre Arcand, MD; part C courtesy of Pete Setabutr, MD.)*

Probing and irrigation

Probing is a delicate procedure that is facilitated by immobilization of the pediatric patient and by constriction of the nasal mucosa with a topical vasoconstrictor, usually oxymetazoline hydrochloride. Punctal dilation is often needed to safely introduce a size 00 Bowman lacrimal probe. The probe is initially inserted into the punctum perpendicular to the eyelid margin and then turned parallel to the eyelid margin as it is advanced down the canalicular system, toward the medial canthal tendon (Fig 15-5). Manual lateral traction of the eyelid with the opposite hand straightens the canaliculus, decreasing the risks of damage to the canalicular mucosa and creation of a false passage.

Resistance to passage of the probe—along with medial movement of the eyelid soft tissue ("soft stop"), causing wrinkling of the overlying skin—may signify canalicular obstruction. More commonly, resistance is simply due to a kink in the canaliculus created by bunching of the soft tissues in front of the probe tip. If kinking is encountered, the probe is withdrawn and reinserted while lateral horizontal traction is maintained (Fig 15-6). If the probe advances successfully through the common canalicular system and across the lacrimal sac, the medial wall of the lacrimal sac and adjacent lacrimal bone will be encountered, resulting in a tactile "hard stop."

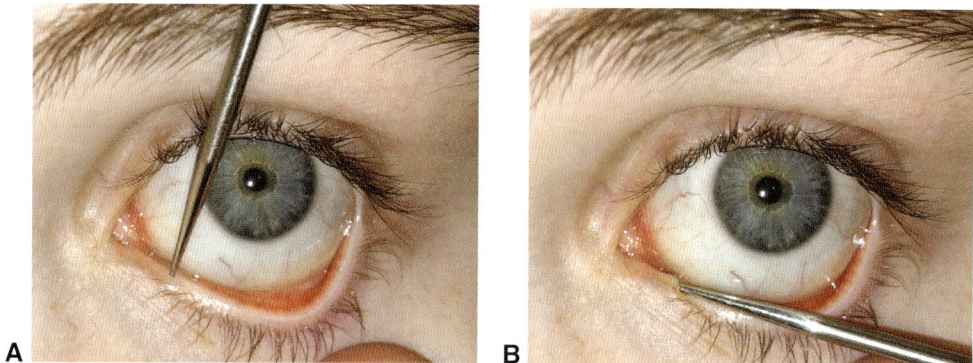

A   **B**

Figure 15-5   Punctal dilatation. **A,** Initial insertion of the punctal dilator is perpendicular to the eyelid margin. **B,** Next, with lateral countertraction on the eyelid, the dilator is directed horizontally into the canaliculus. *(Courtesy of Eric A. Steele, MD.)*

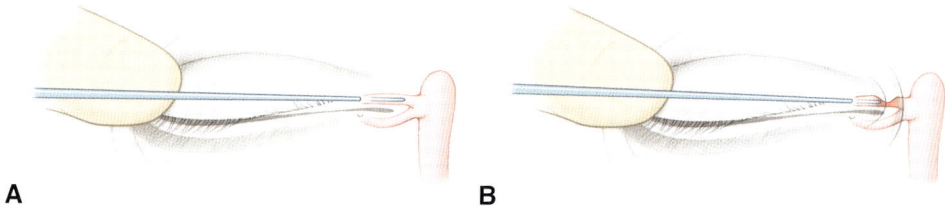

A   **B**

Figure 15-6   Proper technique for canalicular probing. **A,** Bowman probe in the right upper horizontal canaliculus with lateral traction on the eyelid. **B,** When canalicular obstruction is present or when the probe is not in the correct position, resistance to passage of the probe ("soft stop") with wrinkling of the overlying skin is encountered. *(Illustration by Christine Gralapp.)*

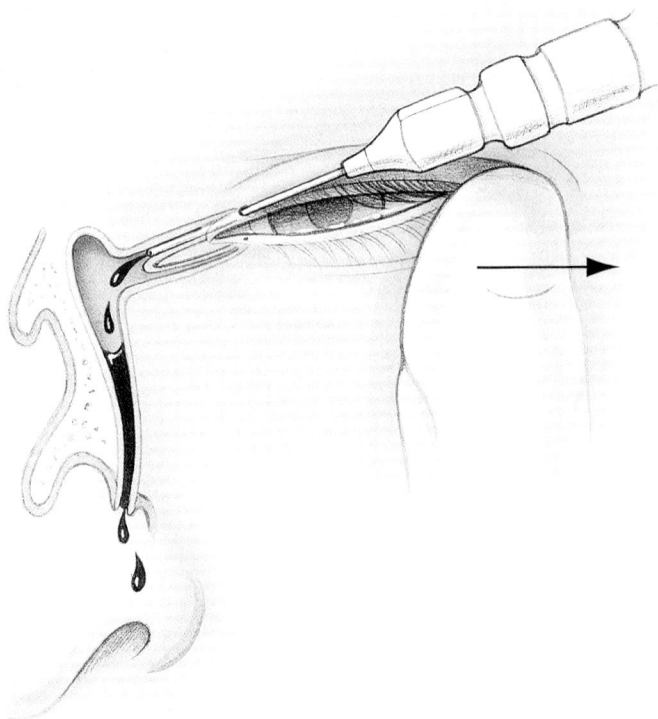

Figure 15-7 Irrigation of the nasolacrimal system. Dye is injected from the syringe, and patency of the system is confirmed by suctioning the dye from the inferior meatus of the nose. *(Illustration by Christine Gralapp.)*

The probe is then rotated 90° superiorly toward the brow until it lies adjacent to the supraorbital notch. The probe is directed posteriorly and slightly laterally as it is advanced down the NLD. Creation of a false passage makes it difficult to redirect the probe back into the native lacrimal system. Therefore, if resistance is encountered and the surgeon is uncertain whether the probe is in the natural pathway, the probe is repositioned and passage attempted again. At some points of narrowing, particularly at the distal end of the NLD, gentle pressure may be necessary to push through the blockage. The probe tip can be visualized along the lateral wall of the nose under the inferior turbinate, approximately 2 cm back from the nostril, using an endoscope or a nasal speculum with a fiber-optic headlight. Alternatively, patency of the duct can be confirmed by metal-on-metal contact with another probe inserted through the naris or by irrigation with saline mixed with fluorescein (Fig 15-7). The fluorescein can be retrieved from the inferior meatus and visualized with a transparent suction catheter. A single lacrimal probing successfully resolves congenital NLDO in 90% of patients who are 13 months or younger.

Intubation

Intubation with a lacrimal stent is indicated for children who have recurrent epiphora following nasolacrimal system probing and for older children in whom initial probing reveals

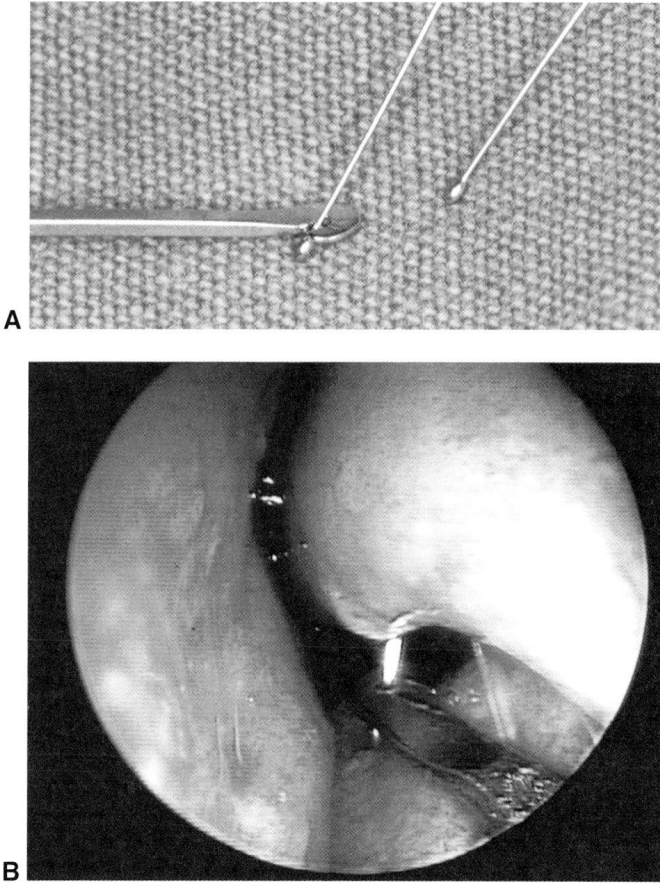

Figure 15-8 Crawford stent and hook. **A,** Hook engaging the "olive tip" of the stent. **B,** Intranasal view of the engaged hook retrieving the stent. *(Reproduced with permission from Nerad JA. Oculoplastic Surgery: The Requisites in Ophthalmology. Philadelphia: Mosby; 2001:233.)*

significant stenosis or scarring. Intubation is also useful for the treatment of upper-system abnormalities such as canalicular stenosis, trauma, and agenesis of the puncta. Nasolacrimal intubation after failed probing has a reported success rate greater than 70%.

There are many intubation techniques and types of intubation sets. Figure 15-8 illustrates one of the more commonly used stents (ie, the Crawford stent). Keys to successful intubation include shrinkage of the nasal mucosa with a topical vasoconstrictor and adequate lighting with a fiber-optic headlight. In more difficult cases, an endoscope can be used, and medialization of the inferior turbinate is sometimes performed. The lacrimal stent can be secured with a simple square knot, which allows removal of the stent through the canalicular system in a retrograde fashion. Alternatively, the lacrimal stent may be directly sutured to the lateral wall of the nose (without tension), or the limbs of the stent can be secured by passing them through either a silicone band or a sponge in the inferior meatus of the nose.

A self-retaining bicanalicular lacrimal stent comes preloaded with a rigid inserter and does not require intranasal retrieval or fixation (Fig 15-9A). Alternatively, a monocanalicular

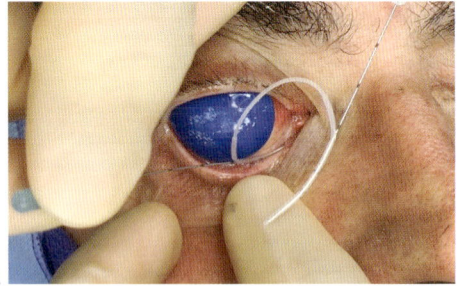

Figure 15-9 Lacrimal intubation stents. **A,** Self-retaining bicanalicular lacrimal stent with a rigid insertion device. **B,** Monocanalicular stent with a soft barb and collarette, which secure the stent within the punctum. *(Part A courtesy of Bobby S. Korn, MD, PhD; part B courtesy of Roberta Gausas, MD).*

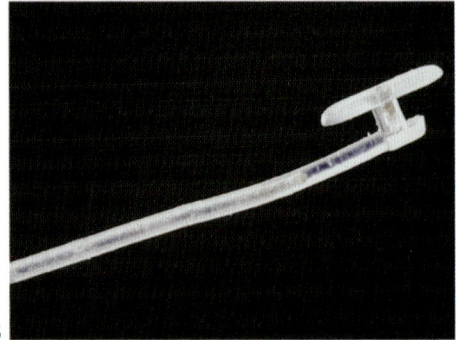

stent is useful for patients with only one patent canaliculus (Fig 15-9B). This type of stent is passed through a single punctum to the nasal cavity, where the end of the stent is allowed to retract loosely into the nose. The proximal end has a punctal plug and is self-secured at the punctum.

Balloon dacryoplasty

Balloon catheter dilation of the nasolacrimal canal has been used successfully in patients with congenital nasolacrimal obstruction. A collapsed balloon catheter is placed in a manner similar to probing and is inflated inside the duct. The role of this modality remains undefined, in part because the necessary catheter equipment is expensive, and because simple probing has a high success rate, obviating the need for further procedures.

> American Academy of Ophthalmology OTAC Oculoplastics and Orbit Panel, Hoskins Center for Quality Eye Care. *Balloon Dacryoplasty for Congenital Nasolacrimal Duct Obstruction.* Ophthalmic Technology Assessment. San Francisco: American Academy of Ophthalmology; 2018.

Turbinate infracture

If the inferior turbinate appears to be lateralized against the NLD at the time of probing and irrigation, medial infracture of the inferior turbinate should be performed. The blunt end of a periosteal elevator is placed within the inferior meatus along the lateral surface of the inferior turbinate. The inferior turbinate is then rotated medially toward the septum. Fracturing the turbinate at its base significantly enlarges the inferior meatus and permits direct visualization of the lacrimal probe tip.

Dacryocystorhinostomy

Dacryocystorhinostomy (DCR) is usually reserved for children who have persistent epiphora following intubation and/or balloon dacryoplasty, children who experience recurrent dacryocystitis, and patients with extensive developmental abnormalities of the nasolacrimal drainage system that prevent probing and intubation. DCR is more fully discussed later in this chapter in the section Acquired Nasolacrimal Duct Obstruction.

Acquired Lacrimal Drainage Obstruction

Evaluation

History

Patients with acquired tearing can be loosely divided into 2 groups: those with hypersecretion of tears (lacrimation) and those with impairment of drainage (epiphora). The initial step in evaluating the tearing patient is differentiating between the 2 conditions. The following list aids in the assessment of the patient with acquired tearing:

- constant versus intermittent tearing
- periods of remission versus no remission
- unilateral versus bilateral condition
- subjective ocular surface discomfort
- history of allergies
- use of topical medications such as glaucoma drops
- history of probing during childhood
- prior ocular surface infections such as conjunctivitis or herpes simplex
- prior sinus disease or surgery, midfacial trauma, or nasal fracture
- previous episodes of lacrimal sac inflammation
- clear tears versus tears with discharge or blood (hemolacrima; blood in the tear meniscus may indicate malignancy; Fig 15-10)

Examination

Systematic examination helps pinpoint the cause of acquired tearing. The initial step of the examination is to distinguish patients with obstruction of the lacrimal drainage system from those with secondary hypersecretion.

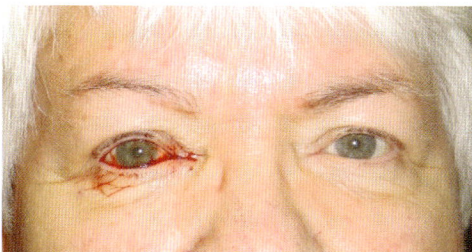

Figure 15-10 Right hemolacrima in a patient with lacrimal sac neoplasm. *(Courtesy of Eric A. Steele, MD.)*

Pseudoepiphora evaluation *Epiphora* is defined as overflow tearing. Some patients feel like their eyes have too many tears, but they do not exhibit frank epiphora. These sensations are often caused by other ocular or eyelid abnormalities. For example, patients with dry eye may perceive foreign-body sensation or increased mucus production as excess tearing, but they do not exhibit true overflow of tears over the eyelid margin or down the cheek. An assessment for pseudoepiphora includes the following considerations:

- *Tear meniscus.* The size and asymmetry of the lacrimal lake and presence of precipitated proteins and stringy mucus may indicate an abnormal tear film or outflow obstruction.
- *Tear breakup time.* To determine tear breakup time, fluorescein dye is instilled, and the patient is asked to refrain from blinking. The tear film is examined using a broad beam of a slit lamp with a cobalt blue filter. A tear-film breakup time of less than 10 seconds may indicate poor function of the mucin or meibomian layer despite a sufficient amount of tears.
- *Evaluation of corneal and conjunctival epithelium.* Topical rose bengal and lissamine green dyes can aid in the detection of subtle ocular surface abnormalities by staining devitalized conjunctival and corneal epithelium. Fluorescein staining indicates more severe tear film malfunction with epithelial loss.
- *Basal tear secretion.* Basal tear secretion can be measured with Schirmer testing. See also BCSC Section 8, *External Disease and Cornea,* for further discussion of tear film tests and tear film abnormalities.
- *Corneal irritation.* Irritation of the ocular surface is a common cause of secondary hypersecretion. This can be seen in individuals with misdirected eyelashes (trichiasis, distichiasis) or eyelid malposition (entropion). Other ocular irritants include allergy, chronic infection (eg, chlamydia or molluscum), and giant papillary conjunctivitis from contact lens wear. Careful examination of the palpebral conjunctiva can aid in the identification of such disorders.

Lacrimal outflow examination

Examination of a patient with abnormal lacrimal outflow begins with an observation of the eyelid and puncta positions during the blink cycle. Facial nerve dysfunction can result in a weakened blink and poor lacrimal pump function (Fig 15-11). An enlarged caruncle or conjunctivochalasis (Fig 15-12) can also mechanically block the aperture of the puncta and lead to tearing. Punctal stenosis, occlusion, or aplasia may be present.

Palpation of the lacrimal sac may cause reflux of mucoid or mucopurulent material through the canalicular system, confirming complete NLDO. No further diagnostic tests are needed if a lacrimal sac tumor is not suspected.

Nasal examination may uncover an unsuspected cause of the epiphora, such as an intranasal tumor or polyp, turbinate impaction, deviated septum, or chronic allergic rhinitis. These conditions may occlude the nasal end of the NLD.

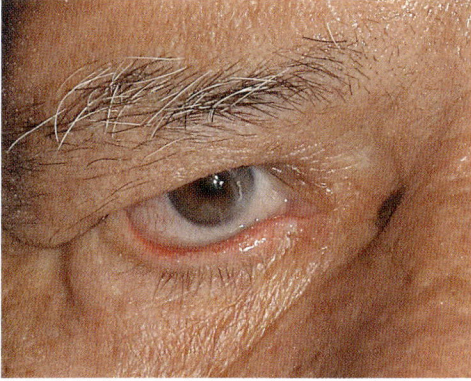

Figure 15-11 Right facial nerve palsy resulting in paralytic ectropion and absent lacrimal pump function. *(Courtesy of Bobby S. Korn, MD, PhD.)*

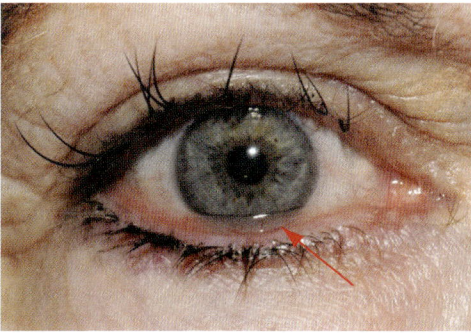

Figure 15-12 Right conjunctivochalasis *(arrow)* obstructing lacrimal outflow through the inferior punctum. *(Courtesy of Bobby S. Korn, MD, PhD.)*

Diagnostic tests

As originally outlined by Lester Jones, the clinical evaluation of the lacrimal drainage system historically comprised a *dye disappearance test (DDT)* followed by the Jones I test (swabbing the inferior meatus to see if dye passes through physiologically) and the Jones II test (irrigating with saline and assessing the passage of fluid and presence or absence of dye). Although some clinicians continue to rely on formal Jones testing, most use a simplified approach involving only the DDT and lacrimal irrigation.

The DDT is useful for assessing the presence or absence of adequate lacrimal outflow, especially in unilateral cases. It is more heavily relied upon for children, in whom lacrimal irrigation is impossible without deep sedation. Fluorescein is instilled in both eyes, and the tear film is observed with the cobalt blue filter of a slit lamp or direct ophthalmoscope. Persistence of significant dye over a 5-minute period implies decreased outflow. Asymmetry in dye clearance during the DDT can be a particularly helpful diagnostic clue (Fig 15-13). If the DDT result is normal, severe lacrimal drainage dysfunction is unlikely. However, intermittent causes of tearing, such as an allergy, dacryolith, or intranasal obstruction, cannot be ruled out.

Lacrimal drainage system irrigation is most frequently performed immediately after the DDT to determine the level of lacrimal drainage system occlusion (Video 15-1). After instillation of topical anesthesia, the lower eyelid punctum is dilated, and any punctal stenosis is

Figure 15-13 Physiologic evaluation of tearing with the dye disappearance test. On the right side, normal lacrimal outflow is present, whereas on the left side, drainage is impaired. *(Courtesy of Eric A. Steele, MD.)*

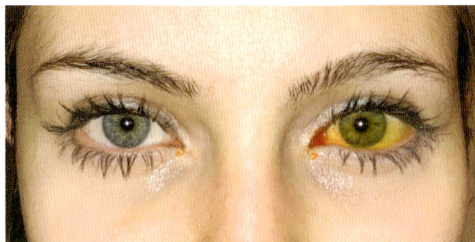

noted. The irrigating cannula is placed in the canalicular system. To prevent canalicular kinking and difficulty in advancing the irrigating cannula, the clinician maintains lateral traction of the lower eyelid (see Fig 15-6). Canalicular stenosis or occlusion should be recorded and confirmed by subsequent diagnostic probing. Once the irrigating cannula has been advanced into the horizontal canaliculus, clear saline is injected and the results are noted. Careful observation and interpretation determine the area of obstruction without additional testing.

VIDEO 15-1 Lacrimal dilation and irrigation.
Courtesy of Eric A. Steele, MD.
Access all Section 7 videos at www.aao.org/bcscvideo_section07.

Difficulty advancing the irrigating cannula and an inability to irrigate fluid suggest *total canalicular obstruction*. If saline can be irrigated successfully but it refluxes through the upper canalicular system and no distention of the lacrimal sac is observed on palpation, *complete blockage of the common canaliculus* is probable (Figs 15-14, 15-15). Subsequent probing determines whether the common canalicular stenosis is total or whether it can be dilated. If mucoid material or saline refluxes through the opposite punctum and lacrimal sac distention is palpable, the diagnosis is *complete NLDO* (Video 15-2). If saline irrigation is not associated with canalicular reflux or fluid passing down the NLD, the lacrimal sac will become distended, causing patient discomfort. This result confirms a complete NLDO with a functional valve of Rosenmüller, preventing reflux through the canalicular system. A combination of simultaneous saline reflux through the opposite canaliculus and saline irrigation through the NLD into the nose may indicate a *partial NLD stenosis*.

VIDEO 15-2 Lacrimal irrigation showing a complete nasolacrimal duct obstruction.
Courtesy of Bobby S. Korn, MD, PhD.

If saline irrigation passes freely into the nose with no reflux through the canalicular system, an anatomically *patent nasolacrimal drainage system* is present. However, it is important to note that even though this irrigation is successful under increased hydrostatic pressure from the irrigating saline, a *functional obstruction* may still be present. A dacryolith may also impair tear flow without blocking irrigation.

Diagnostic probing of the upper system (puncta, canaliculi, and lacrimal sac) is useful in confirming the level of obstruction. In adults, this procedure can easily be performed with topical anesthesia. A small probe is used initially to detect any canalicular obstruction. If an obstruction is encountered, the probe is clamped at the punctum before withdrawal, thereby measuring the distance to the obstruction. A larger probe may be useful to

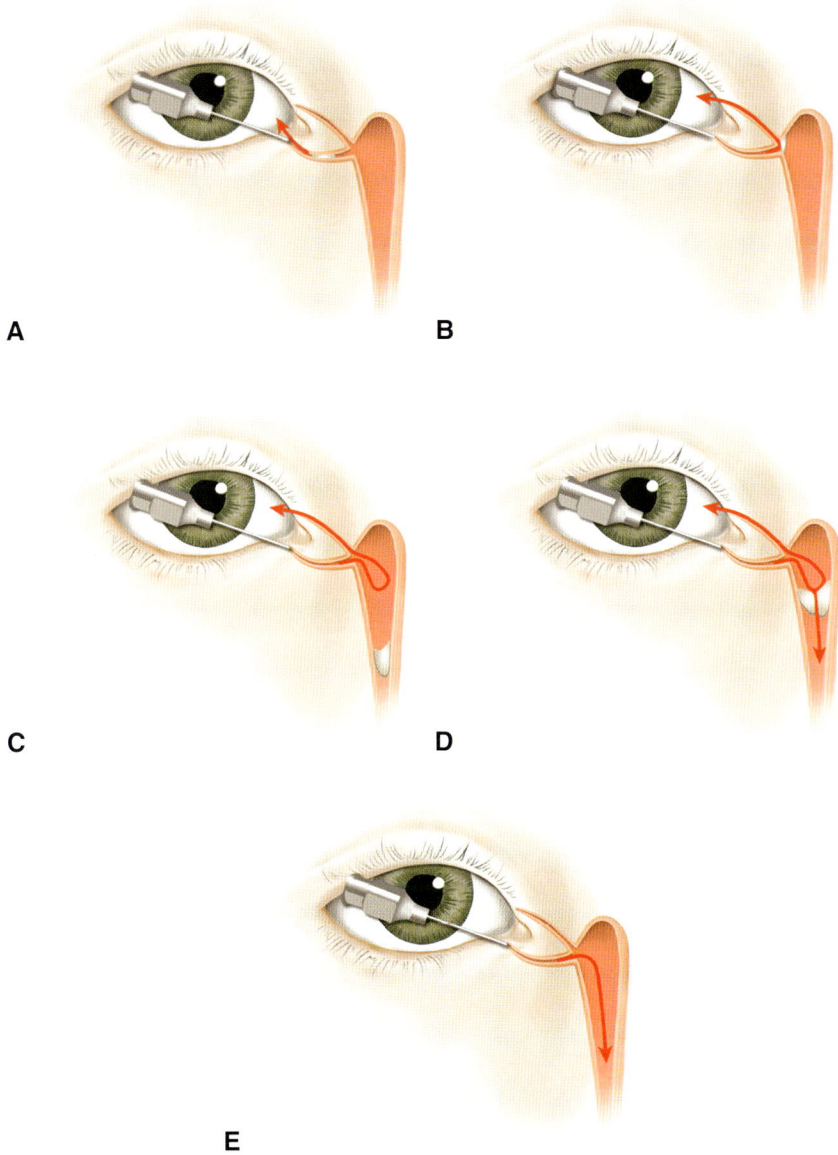

Figure 15-14 Lacrimal drainage system irrigation. **A,** Complete canalicular obstruction. The cannula is advanced with difficulty, and irrigation fluid refluxes from the same canaliculus. **B,** Complete common canalicular obstruction. A "soft stop" is encountered at the level of the common canaliculus, and irrigated fluid refluxes through the opposite punctum and sometimes partially from the same canaliculus as well. **C,** Complete nasolacrimal duct obstruction (NLDO). The cannula is easily advanced to the medial wall of the lacrimal sac; then a "hard stop" is felt, and irrigation fluid refluxes through the opposite punctum. Often, the refluxed fluid contains mucus and/or pus. With a tight valve of Rosenmüller, lacrimal sac distention without reflux of irrigation fluid may occur. **D,** Partial NLDO. The cannula is easily placed, and irrigation fluid passes into the nose as well as refluxing through the opposite punctum. **E,** Patent lacrimal drainage system. The cannula is placed with ease, and most of the irrigation fluid passes into the nose. *(Illustration by Cyndie C. H. Wooley.)*

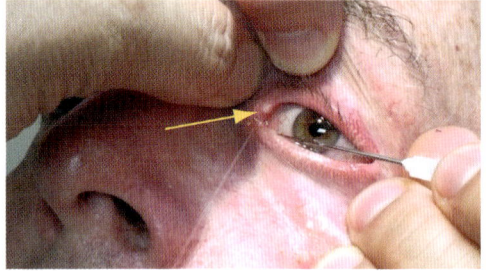

Figure 15-15 Lacrimal irrigation through the inferior canaliculus shows complete reflux through the superior canaliculus *(arrow)*, indicative of a complete NLDO (hard stop is noted along the medial wall of the lacrimal fossa). *(Courtesy of Bobby S. Korn, MD, PhD.)*

determine the extent of a partial obstruction, but the probe should not be forced through any area of resistance.

Diagnostic probing of the NLD is not used in adults because there are other means of diagnosing NLDO. In addition, probing in adults has limited therapeutic value, rarely producing lasting patency. In contrast, probing in infants is a useful and largely successful procedure. This reflects the differing pathophysiologies of congenital NLDO and acquired NLDO: The former often results from occlusion of the NLD by a thin membrane and the latter from more extensive fibrosis of the duct itself.

Intranasal examination is performed with a nasal speculum and light source. Diagnostic nasal endoscopy can be helpful in the evaluation of the nasal anatomy and in the identification of disease processes.

Contrast dacryocystography and *dacryoscintigraphy* are alternative methods of evaluation. Contrast dacryocystography, which involves injection of dye into the lacrimal system followed by computerized digital subtraction imaging, provides anatomical information of any obstructed sites. In dacryoscintigraphy, a physiologic picture of lacrimal outflow is obtained by using radionucleotide eyedrops to follow tear flow on a scintigram.

CT and *MRI* are useful in the evaluation of craniofacial injury, congenital craniofacial deformities, or suspected neoplasia. CT is superior for the evaluation of suspected bony abnormalities, such as fractures. MRI is superior for the evaluation of suspected soft-tissue disease, such as malignancy. Either CT or MRI may be helpful in evaluating concomitant sinus or nasal disease that may contribute to excess tearing.

Kashkouli MB, Mirzajani H, Jamshidian-Tehrani M, Pakdel F, Nojomi M, Aghaei GH. Reliability of fluorescein dye disappearance test in assessment of adults with nasolacrimal duct obstruction. *Ophthalmic Plast Reconstr Surg.* 2013;29(3):167–169.

Punctal Disorders

Several punctal abnormalities can result in epiphora. Puncta may be stenotic, too large (usually iatrogenic), malpositioned, or occluded by adjacent structures.

Punctal stenosis and occlusion can be due to numerous causes, including

- congenital conditions
- inflammatory diseases
  - Stevens-Johnson syndrome
  - mucous membrane pemphigoid (ocular cicatricial pemphigoid)

- infectious diseases (eg, herpes)
- iatrogenic causes
  - glaucoma medications
  - deliberate occlusion in the treatment of dry eye disease (plugs, cautery)

Punctal stenosis may be associated with punctal ectropion or atrophy in the absence of tear flow. It may be treated with dilation, punctoplasty, or stenting. Most often, the benefits of dilation are short-lived, and punctoplasty is required. This is usually accomplished with a snip procedure, in which a small portion of the ampulla is excised. If stenosis recurs, stenting may be required during healing to prevent contraction. Treatment of complete occlusion consists of surgical canalization and, in most cases, stenting.

Abnormally large puncta can also cause epiphora due to disruption of the lacrimal pump (Fig 15-16). The expanded opening prevents formation of an adequate seal when the eyes are closed, interfering with the usual development of negative pressure needed to drain the tears. Punctal enlargement is typically iatrogenic in nature and can occur from "cheese-wiring" of a stent secured too tight intranasally (Fig 15-17), punctoplasty, excision of adjacent lesions, or even from rough dilation and probing that cause damage to the normal fibrous ring around the punctum. Damage to the puncta may be difficult to correct.

If the punctum is not in the tear lake, the anatomical abnormality (most commonly ectropion) must be corrected by a medial spindle conjunctivoplasty or horizontal eyelid tightening (see Chapter 12 in this volume for more on both of these topics). Punctal

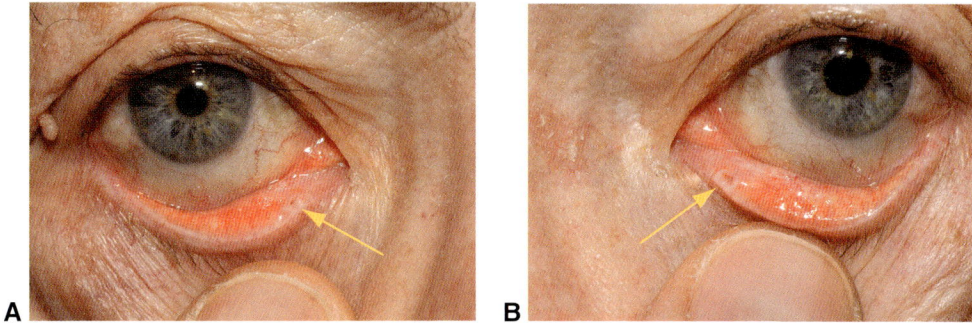

A   **B**

Figure 15-16 Inferior puncta. Punctum with normal caliber *(arrow)* on the right **(A)**, and an abnormally large punctum *(arrow)* on the left **(B)**. *(Courtesy of Bobby S. Korn, MD, PhD.)*

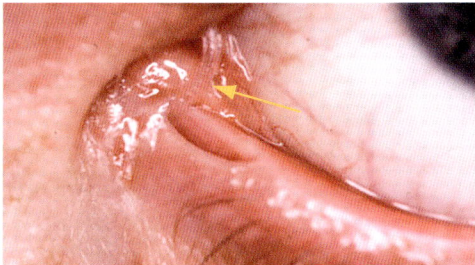

Figure 15-17 Slit inferior punctum caused by tight intranasal fixation of a bicanalicular lacrimal stent *(arrow)*. *(Courtesy of Don O. Kikkawa, MD.)*

stenosis may require punctoplasty. Puncta may also become obstructed by adjacent structures, such as a hypertrophied caruncle or conjunctivochalasis (see Fig 15-12), which can be corrected by reducing the excess tissue.

Canalicular Obstruction

Evaluation

Obstruction can occur within the upper, lower, or common canaliculus. The location of the obstruction is detected by a tactile soft stop during diagnostic probing (typically, the probe would reach a hard stop in the fossa of the lacrimal sac). *Total common canalicular obstruction* is characterized by high-velocity reflux from the opposite canaliculus (see Figs 15-14, 15-15, and Video 15-2), with no flow into the lacrimal sac during lacrimal system irrigation. *Partial obstruction* may be discovered during lacrimal system irrigation when there is partial fluid flow into the nose and partial reflux around the cannula or through the opposite punctum. In some instances, a partial obstruction may represent a *total functional occlusion* due to weakness of the lacrimal pump or inability of tears to pass through the partial obstruction under normal physiologic conditions (as opposed to the high hydrostatic pressure from irrigation).

Etiology

Lacrimal plugs Punctal and canalicular plugs used in the treatment of dry eye disease come in various shapes and sizes. Punctal plugs that are too small may migrate within the canaliculus and result in obstruction, with associated inflammation or infection. The permanent intracanalicular plug also often leads to infection. Even temporary or absorbable plugs have been known to cause a local inflammatory response and canalicular constriction. Canalicular probing is used to identify the location of the problematic plug, which is then surgically excised. Often, excision of a short segment of scarred canaliculus is required, which is then repaired with a technique similar to reconstruction following trauma or after injury of the canaliculus during excision of a neoplasm.

Marcet MM, Shtein RM, Bradley EA, et al. Safety and efficacy of lacrimal drainage system plugs for dry eye syndrome: a report by the American Academy of Ophthalmology. *Ophthalmology*. 2015;122(8):1681–1687.

Medication Medications occasionally cause canalicular obstruction. This is often encountered with the use of idoxuridine and chemotherapeutic agents such as 5-fluorouracil and docetaxel. These drugs are secreted in the tears, leading to inflammation and scarring of the canaliculi. Use of topical steroid drops and artificial tears during chemotherapy may prevent scarring. If this condition is identified early—before the obstruction is complete—stents can be placed to prevent progression while the patient completes the course of chemotherapy. A special canalicular-only stent is available for these cases. Less commonly, canalicular obstruction has been reported following the use of topical medication (eg, phospholine iodide, eserine).

Infection Numerous infections can cause canalicular obstruction. Most frequently, obstruction occurs concurrently with diffuse conjunctival infection (eg, vaccinia virus, herpes simplex virus). Isolated canalicular infection (canaliculitis; discussed later in this chapter) can also result in obstruction.

Inflammatory disease Inflammatory conditions such as mucous membrane pemphigoid (ocular cicatricial pemphigoid), Stevens-Johnson syndrome, and graft-vs-host disease often cause loss of the puncta and/or canaliculi. However, because of concurrent loss of tear secretion, patients often do not experience epiphora.

Trauma Traumatic injury to the canaliculi can result in permanent damage if the injury is not managed in a timely, appropriate manner.

Neoplasm When a neoplasm is present in the medial canthal area, complete resection may include removal of the puncta and canaliculi. Complete tumor excision must be confirmed by histologic examination of excised tissue before connection of the lacrimal drainage system with the middle meatus is considered. When the distal lacrimal drainage system remains intact, the remaining portion of the canaliculi may be marsupialized to the conjunctival surface with or without intubation.

Management

Canalicular stenting *Intubation* or *stenting* of the lacrimal drainage system should be considered as a first-line therapy whenever possible. Intubation of the nasolacrimal drainage system can usually be performed successfully when the patient has symptomatic canalicular constriction but not complete occlusion. For canalicular scarring, the use of a balloon catheter alone is usually not sufficient to correct the condition.

Reconstruction Reconstruction of an obstructed canaliculus is often successful when only a few millimeters are involved. If a limited area of total occlusion is discovered near the punctum, the occluded canaliculus can be resected and the cut ends of the canaliculus anastomosed over a stent. For distal obstructions, including the common canaliculus, trephination with lacrimal stenting can be useful. This is most successful for distal monocanalicular obstructions, followed by distal bicanalicular, common, and proximal obstructions.

> Khoubian JF, Kikkawa DO, Gonnering RS. Trephination and silicone stent intubation for the treatment of canalicular obstruction: effect of the level of obstruction. *Ophthalmic Plast Reconstr Surg.* 2006;22(4):248–252.

Canaliculodacryocystorhinostomy If the common canaliculus is totally obstructed or the lacrimal sac is sclerotic, a canaliculodacryocystorhinostomy or canaliculorhinostomy may be performed. In these procedures, the area of total common canalicular obstruction is removed, and the remaining patent canalicular system is directly anastomosed to the lacrimal sac mucosa or the lateral nasal wall mucosa with placement of a lacrimal stent.

> Lee JH, Young SM, Kim YD, Woo KI, Yum JH. Canaliculorhinostomy—indications and surgical results. *Am J Ophthalmol.* 2017;181:134–139.

Conjunctivodacryocystorhinostomy When 1 or both canaliculi are severely obstructed, a CDCR may be required. This procedure creates a complete bypass of the lacrimal drainage system. The beginning of this surgical technique is similar to a DCR (described later in this chapter) and is followed by placement of a Jones tube through a tract created from the caruncle into the middle nasal meatus. The surgeon should have tubes of different lengths available at the time of surgery to ensure implantation of a tube that emerges clearly in the nose without abutting the nasal septum (Fig 15-18).

Postoperative care and complications can be troublesome. Patients with obstructive sleep apnea may be bothered by air reflux from their continuous positive airway pressure machine. This can sometimes be alleviated by switching to a full-face mask, but it may be so bothersome that the patient requests removal of the tube. Periodic removal, cleaning, and replacement of the Jones tube in the office is required to maintain its proper function and to avoid buildup of debris that can lead to chronic inflammation and even pyogenic granuloma formation. Between in-office cleanings, a daily routine including nasal lavage with saline

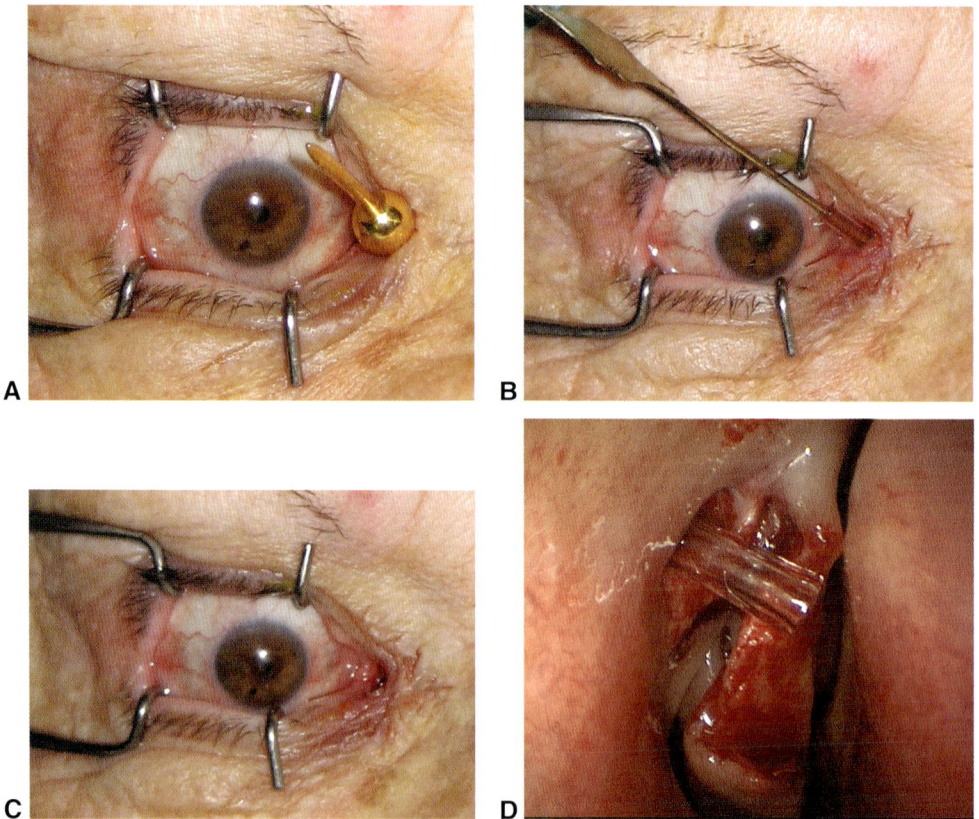

Figure 15-18 Conjunctivodacryocystorhinostomy. **A,** The surgical tract is enlarged with a gold dilator. **B,** The Jones tube is introduced into the tract using a Bowman probe as a guide. **C,** External view of well-positioned Jones tube. **D,** Endoscopic view of well-positioned Jones tube. *(Parts A–C courtesy of Morris Hartstein; part D courtesy of Eric A. Steele, MD.)*

solution and "snuffing" of artificial tears through the tube can help clear mucous debris and prevent obstruction.

Because the tube must be easily removable for cleaning and maintenance, extrusion and migration of the tube can occur, requiring prompt replacement to avoid contracture of the CDCR tract. Various tube modifications have been proposed to help with extrusion, but there is no clear advantage of these modifications over the original Jones tube, particularly because some of the modified tubes prevent easy removal for required periodic cleaning. Despite these drawbacks, conjunctivodacryocystorhinostomy helps many patients with otherwise intractable epiphora.

Steele EA. Conjunctivodacryocystorhinostomy with Jones tube: a history and update. *Curr Opin Ophthalmol.* 2016;27(5):439–442.

Acquired Nasolacrimal Duct Obstruction

An NLDO can usually be diagnosed with irrigation. Clinicians tend to assume that NLDO is a relatively benign condition and proceed directly to a discussion of surgery. Although most cases are benign, alternative causes of NLDO merit consideration.

Etiology

Involutional stenosis Involutional stenosis is probably the most common cause of NLDO in older persons. It affects women twice as frequently as men. Although the inciting event in this process is unknown, clinicopathologic study suggests that inflammatory infiltrates and edema cause compression of the lumen of the NLD. This may be the result of anatomical predisposition, unidentified infection, or possibly autoimmune disease. Management almost always consists of DCR.

Dacryolith Dacryoliths, or concretions formed within the lacrimal sac (Fig 15-19), can also obstruct the NLD. Dacryoliths consist of shed epithelial cells, lipids, and amorphous debris with or without calcium. In most cases, no inciting event or abnormality is identified. Occasionally, infection with *Actinomyces israelii* or *Candida* species or long-term administration of topical medications such as epinephrine can lead to the formation of concretions. Depending on their position, they can sometimes result in intermittent NLDO symptoms,

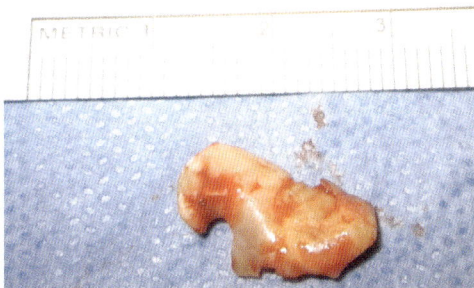

Figure 15-19 Lacrimal sac dacryolith associated with NLDO. *(Courtesy of Eric A. Steele, MD.)*

and acute impaction of a dacryolith in the NLD can produce lacrimal sac distention and pain. Dacryoliths are easily removed during DCR.

Repp DJ, Burkat CN, Lucarelli MJ. Lacrimal excretory system concretions: canalicular and lacrimal sac. *Ophthalmology.* 2009;116(11):2230–2235.

Sinus and nasal disease Sinus disease often occurs in conjunction with, and may contribute to, the development of NLDO. Clinicians should inquire about previous sinus surgery, as the NLD is sometimes inadvertently damaged during sinus procedures. Similarly, nasal conditions such as polyps, chronic congestion, a deviated septum, and prior nasal surgery can also contribute to NLDO.

Trauma Naso-orbital fractures may involve the NLD. Early treatment with fracture reduction and stenting of the entire lacrimal drainage system should be considered. However, such injuries are often not recognized or are initially neglected while more serious injuries are managed. In such cases, late treatment of persistent epiphora usually requires DCR. Injuries may also occur during rhinoplasty or endoscopic sinus surgery; the management of these injuries is similar to the treatment of injuries associated with fractures.

Inflammatory disease Granulomatous disease, including sarcoidosis, granulomatosis with polyangiitis (Fig 15-20), and ulcerating midline lymphoma, may also lead to NLDO. When systemic disease is suspected, a biopsy of the lacrimal sac or the NLD performed at the time of DCR may provide additional diagnostic input.

Lacrimal plugs Dislodged punctal and canalicular plugs can migrate and occlude the NLD. As with most forms of NLDO, treatment consists of DCR. Retained segments of an incompletely removed lacrimal stent may also cause NLDO.

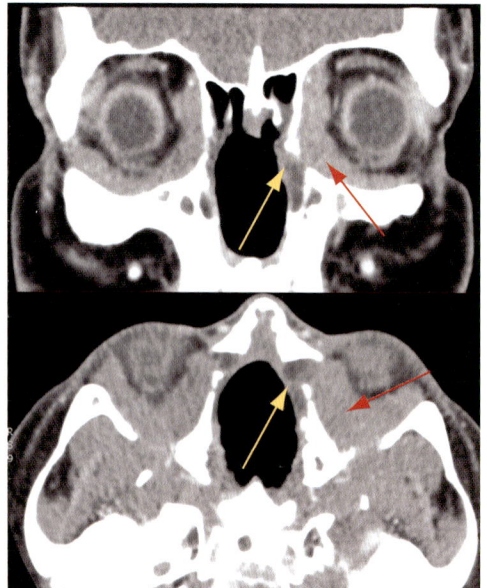

Figure 15-20 CT scans of a patient with granulomatosis with polyangiitis with bilateral orbital involvement *(red arrows)* and secondary nasolacrimal duct obstruction *(yellow arrows). (Courtesy of Bobby S. Korn, MD, PhD.)*

Radioactive iodine Therapeutic radioactive iodine for the treatment of thyroid cancer may also lead to closure of the lacrimal apparatus as a result of the Na^+/I (sodium/iodide) symporter (NIS) in the mucosa of the sac and duct. This is not seen with the lower dosages used to treat the thyroid gland in patients with Graves hyperthyroidism.

Neoplasm Neoplasm should be considered as a possible etiology in any patient presenting with NLDO. In patients with an atypical presentation, including younger age and male sex, further workup should be considered. Bloody punctal discharge (see Fig 15-10) or lacrimal sac distention above the medial canthal tendon is also suggestive of neoplasm. A history of malignancy, especially of sinus or nasopharyngeal origin, warrants further investigation. When malignancy is suspected, appropriate imaging studies (CT or MRI) should be obtained. Preoperative endoscopy can be performed to evaluate for intranasal neoplasm. In addition, if an unexpected mass or other abnormality suggestive of neoplasm is encountered during surgery, a biopsy specimen should be obtained.

When a neoplasm is found to contribute to NLDO, initial treatment focuses on the tumor. In patients with a benign tumor, a DCR or CDCR can then be performed. In patients with a malignant tumor, the surgical correction of the nasolacrimal drainage system should be postponed until there is certainty of clear margins or freedom from recurrence, after which a DCR or CDCR may be undertaken. Tumors of the lacrimal sac and NLD are discussed in further detail later in this chapter, in the section titled Neoplasm.

Management

Intubation and stenting Partial stenosis of the NLD with symptomatic epiphora may respond to surgical intubation of the entire lacrimal drainage system. This procedure should be performed only if the tubes can be passed easily. In cases of complete NLDO, intubation alone is not effective, and a DCR should be considered.

Dacryocystorhinostomy A DCR is the treatment of choice for most patients with acquired NLDO. Surgical indications include recurrent dacryocystitis, chronic mucoid reflux, painful distention of the lacrimal sac, and bothersome epiphora. For patients with dacryocystitis, active infection should be treated, if possible, before DCR is performed.

Although there are many variations in surgical techniques, all of them create an anastomosis between the lacrimal sac and the nasal cavity through a bony ostium. One significant distinction between techniques is whether the surgeon uses an internal (intranasal) approach or the more traditional external (transcutaneous) approach. In both approaches, bicanalicular lacrimal stenting is usually performed at the end of the procedure.

Recent data indicate similar success rates for the 2 approaches. The advantages of an *internal (endonasal) DCR* include lack of a visible scar, a shorter recovery period, and less discomfort. An *external DCR* may allow better exposure for management of canalicular stenosis, unexpected neoplasm, or dacryoliths.

DCR can be performed under general anesthesia or local anesthesia with intravenous sedation. Intraoperative hemostasis can be enhanced by preoperative injection of lidocaine with epinephrine into the medial canthal soft tissues and by the use of intranasally injected anesthetic and nasal packing with vasoconstrictive agents (eg, oxymetazoline hydrochloride, phenylephrine, epinephrine, or cocaine hydrochloride). In external DCR (Fig 15-21), the skin incision should be made so as to avoid the angular blood vessels and prevent wound contractures leading to epicanthal folds. The osteotomy adjacent to the medial wall of the lacrimal sac can be created with a hemostat, rongeur, trephine, or drill. An anterior ethmoidal air cell may require removal to properly drain into the nasal cavity. A large osteotomy site facilitates the formation of posterior and anterior mucosal flaps from both the lacrimal sac and the nasal mucosa. Minimizing trauma to the common internal ostium of the canaliculi into the sac is important when creating the lacrimal sac flaps, to avoid scarring and subsequent failure of the surgery. Suturing of the corresponding posterior flaps and anterior flaps is common, but sometimes only anterior flaps are anastomosed.

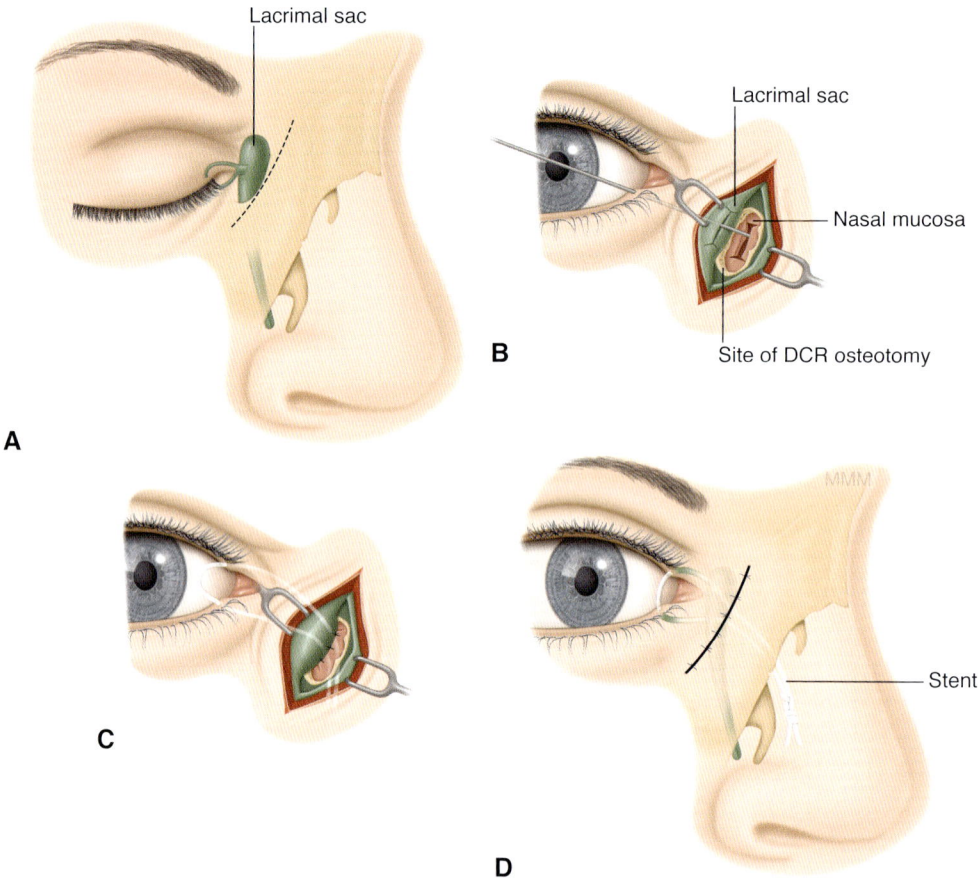

Figure 15-21 External dacryocystorhinostomy (DCR). **A,** The incision is marked 10 mm from the medial canthus, starting just above the medial canthal tendon and extending inferiorly. **B,** Bone from the lacrimal fossa and anterior lacrimal crest has been resected. Flaps have been fashioned in the nasal mucosa. A lacrimal probe extends through an incision in the lacrimal sac. **C,** The anterior lacrimal sac flap is sutured to the anterior nasal mucosal flap after a stent is placed. **D,** Final position of the stent following closure of the skin incision. *(Illustration by Mark Miller.)*

Endonasal DCR consists of removal of the nasal mucosa over the area corresponding to the nasolacrimal sac and duct (Fig 15-22), followed by an osteotomy to remove the frontal process of the maxillary bone and the lacrimal bone covering the lacrimal sac (Video 15-3). To allow proper exposure of the lacrimal sac, the surgeon may also need to remove the uncinate process or an anteriorly located ethmoidal air cell. The lacrimal sac is then opened, and the medial wall of the sac is removed, marsupializing the sac into the nose. Careful selection of patients with an adequate nasal cavity is crucial for success, and the surgeon should be prepared to modify the nasal anatomy for better exposure and access (eg, by performing nasal septoplasty). Several variations of endonasal DCR exist, including direct visualization or visualization with the use of an endoscope *(endoscopic DCR)*. Some surgeons use a fiber-optic probe passed through a canaliculus to transilluminate the lacrimal sac.

VIDEO 15-3 Endonasal dacryocystorhinostomy.
Courtesy of Bobby S. Korn, MD, PhD.

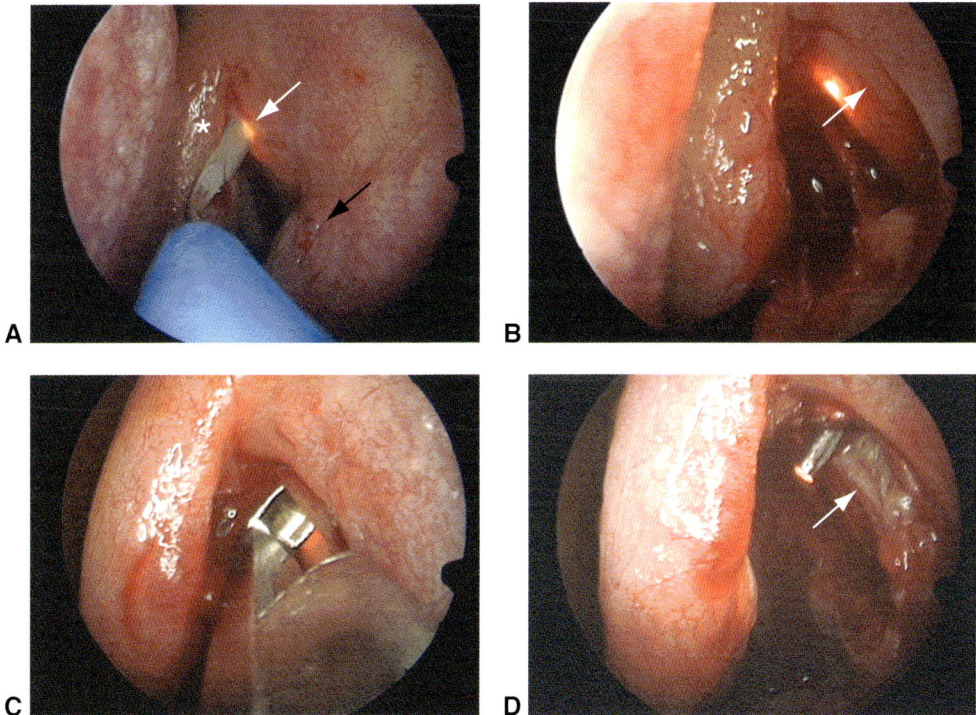

Figure 15-22 Endonasal DCR. **A,** Posterior incision behind the intracanalicular transilluminator *(white arrow),* above the inferior turbinate *(black arrow),* and just anterior to the insertion of the middle turbinate *(asterisk).* **B,** Frontal process of the maxilla after removal of nasal mucosa *(arrow).* **C,** Removal of the frontal process of the maxilla with rongeurs. **D,** The lacrimal sac has been opened *(arrow),* and the transilluminator can be seen in the nose. *(Courtesy of François Codère, MD.)*

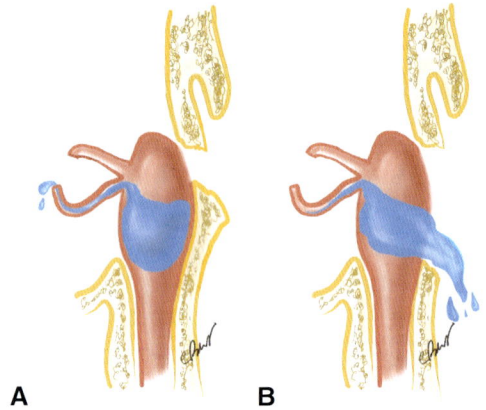

Figure 15-23 Sump syndrome. **A,** Sump syndrome resulting from inadequate superior bone removal during dacryocystorhinostomy. **B,** Treatment involves removing additional bone inferiorly. *(Illustration by Cat N. Burkat, MD.)*

Although DCRs are successful in most patients, failures do occur. DCR failures may be caused by fibrosis and occlusion of the osteotomy, common canalicular obstruction, incomplete opening of the inferior lacrimal sac causing a sump syndrome (Fig 15-23A), or inappropriate placement or size of the bony ostium. Another cause of failure is iatrogenic: If the mucosa of the nasal septum is damaged during surgery, a bridge forms between the ostium and the scar of the septum. Treatment is aimed toward removal of this residual inferior bone through an external or endonasal approach (Fig 15-23B). The outcome of the DCR is also influenced by other factors, including the patient's history of trauma, coexisting autoimmune inflammatory disease, the presence of active dacryocystitis, the development of postoperative infection, or hypersensitivity or foreign body reactions to the stent. When an initial DCR fails, some surgeons apply topical mitomycin to the surgical site during reoperation. This potent antiproliferative alkylating agent helps prevent fibrosis at the osteotomy site.

Endoscopic lacrimal duct recanalization The use of a microendoscope allows for exploration and direct visualization of NLDOs, as well as focal excision and reconstruction of the obstruction, and has had success rates as high as those for DCR. The use of this technology is not widespread, and further study will help define its role in the treatment of NLDO.

Javate RM, Pamintuan FG, Cruz RT. Efficacy of endoscopic lacrimal duct recanalization using microendoscope. *Ophthalmic Plast Reconstr Surg.* 2010;26(5):330–333.

Therapeutic Closure of the Lacrimal Drainage System

In cases of severe dry eye disease, occlusion of the lacrimal puncta may be helpful. Dissolvable collagen plugs may be used on a trial basis, or permanent silicone plugs may be used. Permanent intracanalicular plugs are not recommended. Although punctal plugs are usually well tolerated, complications are occasionally encountered. Minor problems include ocular surface irritation and a foreign-body reaction. Pyogenic granulomas may develop, requiring removal of the plug. In most cases, the pyogenic granuloma regresses once the plug is removed, but surgical excision is needed on occasion. More serious complications usually relate to plug displacement.

Plug extrusion or *migration* is not uncommon. The ophthalmologist can best avoid these complications by using a plug that is the appropriate size. An instrument that measures punctal diameter is available. When appropriately fitted, punctal plugs usually stay in place. In most cases, a plug that is too small will simply be extruded. However, if the plug migrates within the lacrimal drainage system, obstruction of either the canaliculus or the NLD can result. *Canaliculitis* may result from canalicular plugs or from punctal plugs that have migrated to the canaliculus.

When occlusion with plugs is not successful, the clinician may consider surgical occlusion. Surgery is typically reserved for severe cases and must be performed with caution. If a patient experiences subsequent epiphora, no simple solution is available; most cases require a CDCR. To avoid this complication, all patients should undergo a trial of temporary closure before permanent closure.

Once the decision has been made to proceed with surgical occlusion, the puncta are closed in a stepwise fashion, one punctum at a time. Complete loss of lacrimal outflow can result in epiphora, even in patients with fairly severe dry eye disease.

There are numerous surgical techniques for occluding the lacrimal drainage system. *Thermal obliteration* of the puncta and adjacent canaliculi can be performed with a handheld cautery unit or a needle-tip unipolar cautery unit. *Ampullectomy* can be performed with either direct closure or placement of an overlying conjunctival graft. Often, despite aggressive attempts, the puncta persist or reform. In these recalcitrant cases, the punctal and adjacent canalicular epithelia can be completely excised, or the canaliculus can be transected and reconstructed with the severed ends offset from one another.

Trauma

Canaliculus

Traumatic injuries to the canaliculi occur either by direct laceration or by avulsion, when sudden lateral displacement of the eyelid tears the medial canthal tendon and associated canaliculus. Because it lacks tarsal support, the canaliculus lies within the weakest part of the eyelid and is often the first structure to yield. Therefore, when such an injury is suspected in cases of trauma, careful inspection of this area is mandatory, including diagnostic canalicular probing and irrigation. Because the success rate of primary repair is much higher than that of secondary reconstruction, most surgeons recommend repair of all canalicular lacerations.

The first step of the repair is locating the severed ends of the canalicular system. General anesthesia and magnification with optimal illumination facilitate the search. A thorough understanding of the medial canthal anatomy guides the surgeon to the appropriate area to begin exploration for the medial end of the severed canaliculus. Laterally, the canaliculus is located near the eyelid margin, but for lacerations close to the lacrimal sac, the canaliculus is deep to the anterior limb of the medial canthal tendon (See Chapter 11 in this volume, Fig 11-4). Irrigation using air, fluorescein, or yellow viscoelastic material through an intact adjacent canaliculus may be helpful. The use of methylene blue dye should be avoided, as it tends to stain the entire operative field. In difficult cases, the careful use of a smooth-tipped pigtail probe may help identify the medial cut end. The probe is introduced through the opposite, uninvolved punctum; passed through the common canaliculus; and finally passed through the medial cut end.

Stenting of the injured canaliculus is performed to help prevent postoperative canalicular strictures. By putting the stent on traction, the surgeon draws together the severed canalicular ends and other soft-tissue structures, putting them back in their normal anatomical positions. Direct anastomosis of the canaliculus over the lacrimal stent can be accomplished with closure of the pericanalicular tissues, and the medial canthal tendon and eyelid margin can be reconstructed as necessary.

Traditionally, bicanalicular stents have been used, but monocanalicular stents are also available. One type of monocanalicular stent is attached distally to a metal guiding probe that is retrieved intranasally. Another type is inserted into the punctum and threaded directly into the lacerated canaliculus to bridge the laceration but does not extend into the nose. This allows the procedure to be performed under local anesthesia in the office or the emergency department.

Stents are typically left in place for 3 months or longer. However, cheese-wiring, ocular irritation, infection, local inflammation, or pyogenic granuloma formation may necessitate early removal. Bicanalicular stents are usually cut at the medial canthus and retrieved from the nose. Monocanalicular stents are simply retrieved from the punctum.

Lacrimal Sac and Nasolacrimal Duct

The lacrimal sac and NLD may be injured by direct laceration or by fracture of the surrounding bones. Injuries of the lacrimal sac or NLD may also occur during rhinoplasty or endoscopic sinus surgery when the physiologic maxillary sinus ostium is being enlarged anteriorly. Early treatment of the lacrimal sac and NLD is appropriate and consists of fracture reduction, soft-tissue repair, and lacrimal intubation of the entire drainage system. Late treatment of persistent epiphora may require DCR.

Infection

Dacryoadenitis

Acute inflammation of the lacrimal gland *(dacryoadenitis)* is most often seen in association with inflammatory disease and occasionally is the consequence of malignancy, such as lymphoproliferative disease. Noninfectious disease of the lacrimal gland is covered in Chapter 4. Infectious dacryoadenitis is unusual, and gross purulence and abscess formation are uncommon. However, with the emergence of community-acquired methicillin-resistant *Staphylococcus aureus (MRSA),* this condition is seen more frequently. Most cases are the result of bacterial infection, which may develop secondary to an adjacent infection, after trauma, or hematogenously. Alternatively, MRSA infection may appear without preexisting risk factors. Given the rare occurrence of these infections, large case series are lacking, as are a precise breakdown of causative organisms and suggestions for management. Presumably, most cases are due to gram-positive bacteria, but cases due to gram-negative bacteria have been documented. There are case reports of dacryoadenitis related to tuberculosis, involving the formation of discrete tuberculomas in several cases. Epstein-Barr virus is the most frequently reported viral pathogen. Many nonsuppurative cases are treated empirically, without isolation of the alleged pathogen; coverage for MRSA infection should be considered.

Mathias MT, Horsley MB, Mawn LA, et al. Atypical presentations of orbital cellulitis caused by methicillin-resistant *Staphylococcus aureus. Ophthalmology.* 2012;119(6): 1238–1243.

Canaliculitis

Canaliculitis presents with persistent weeping and discharge, sometimes accompanied by a follicular conjunctivitis centered in the medial canthus. The punctum is often erythematous and dilated, or "pouting." A cotton-tipped applicator can be used to apply pressure to the canaliculus ("milking"). The expression of purulent discharge confirms the diagnosis (Fig 15-24). A variety of bacteria, viruses, and mycotic organisms can cause infection within the canaliculus, most commonly *A israelii.*

Canaliculitis can be difficult to eradicate. Conservative management consists of warm compresses, digital compression, and topical and sometimes oral antibiotic therapy. Culture of the discharge may be useful in identifying the cause of the infection. Many patients require more aggressive treatment, particularly those with the formation of concretions (dacryoliths) or a retained intracanalicular plug, which protects the organisms from lethal antibiotic concentrations. Curettage through the punctum is sometimes successful at removing multiple stones, but often a canaliculotomy is required to completely remove all particulate matter. Drainage can be facilitated by an incision through the puncta or through the canaliculus (Video 15-4). The incision is left open to heal by second intention and does not usually require stenting. Some surgeons irrigate or paint the canaliculus with povidone-iodine or irrigate with specially formulated penicillin-fortified drops perioperatively.

VIDEO 15-4 Treatment of canaliculitis.
Courtesy of Bobby S. Korn, MD, PhD.

Dacryocystitis

Inflammation of the lacrimal sac *(acute dacryocystitis)* is usually due to complete NLDO, which prevents normal drainage from the lacrimal sac into the nose. Chronic tear retention and stasis lead to secondary infection. Clinical findings include edema and erythema

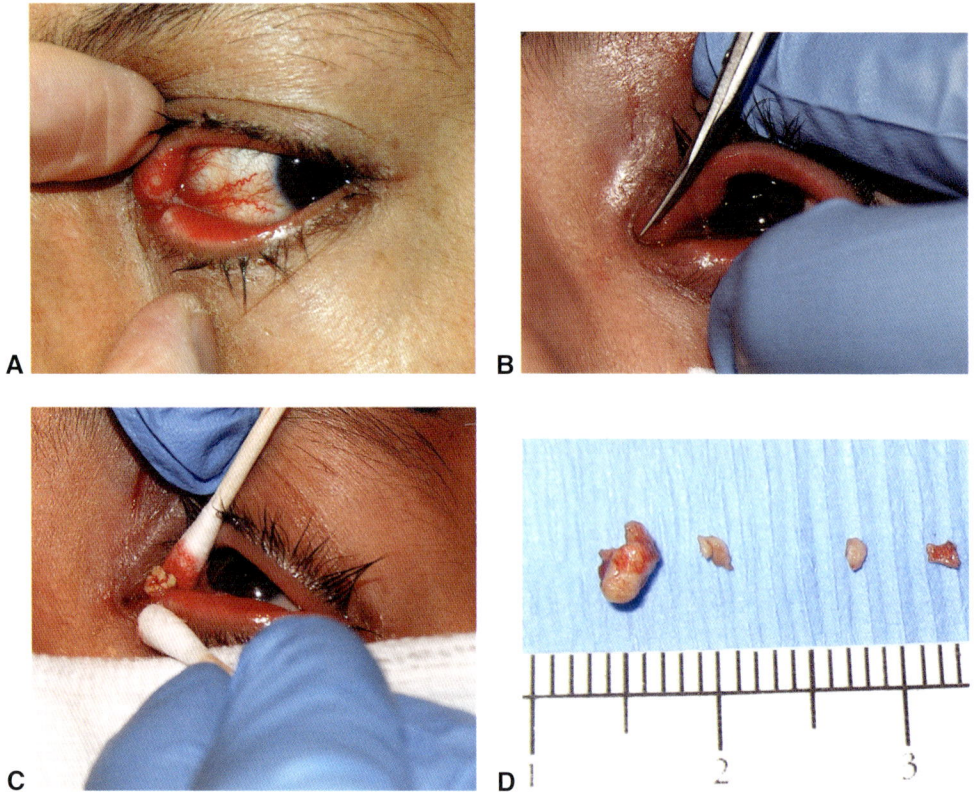

Figure 15-24 Chronic canaliculitis. **A,** Superior and inferior pouting puncta. **B,** Vertical canaliculotomy. **C,** Expression of canaliculi with cotton-tip applicators. **D,** Sulfur granules expressed from canaliculi seen with *Actinomyces israelii.* *(Parts A–C courtesy of Bobby S. Korn, MD, PhD; part D courtesy of Eric A. Steele, MD.)*

with distention of the lacrimal sac (Fig 15-25). The degree of discomfort ranges from none to severe pain. Complications include dacryocystocele formation, chronic conjunctivitis, and spread to adjacent structures (orbital or facial cellulitis).

The following steps may be used in the treatment of acute dacryocystitis:

- Irrigation or probing of the canalicular system should be avoided until the infection subsides. In most cases, irrigation is not needed to establish the diagnosis, and it is extremely painful for patients with active infection.
- Probing of the NLD is not indicated in adults with acute dacryocystitis.
- Topical antibiotics are of limited value. They do not reach the site of the infection because of stasis within the lacrimal drainage system. They also do not penetrate sufficiently within the adjacent soft tissue.
- Oral antibiotics are effective for most infections. Gram-positive bacteria are the most common cause of acute dacryocystitis. However, the clinician should suspect gram-negative organisms in patients who have diabetes mellitus or are

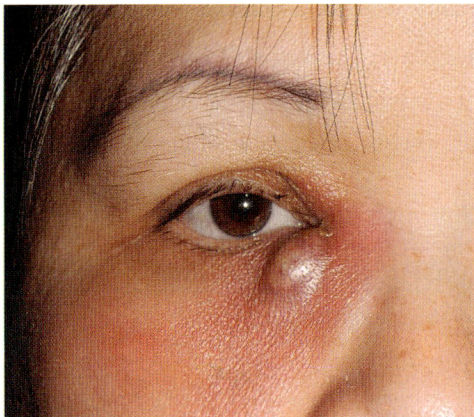

Figure 15-25 Acute dacryocystitis of the right side associated with NLDO. *(Courtesy of Bobby S. Korn, MD, PhD.)*

immunocompromised and in those who have been exposed to atypical pathogens (eg, individuals residing in nursing homes).

- Parenteral antibiotics may be necessary for the treatment of severe cases, especially if cellulitis or orbital extension is present.
- Aspiration of the lacrimal sac may be performed if a pyocele or mucocele is localized and approaching the skin. Smears and cultures of the aspirate may inform the selection of systemic antibiotic therapy.
- A localized abscess involving the lacrimal sac and adjacent soft tissues may require incision and drainage but should be reserved for cases that do not respond to more conservative measures or for patients in severe discomfort.

Dacryocystitis indicating total NLDO requires a DCR in most cases because of inevitable persistent epiphora and recurrence. In general, external surgery is deferred until the acute inflammation is resolved. However, endonasal DCR can be safely performed for acute infection. Some patients, however, continue to have a subacute infection until definitive drainage surgery is performed.

Chronic dacryocystitis, a smoldering low-grade infection, may develop in some individuals. It may result in distention of the lacrimal sac, and massage may reflux mucoid material through the canalicular system onto the surface of the eye. If a tumor is not suspected, no further diagnostic evaluation is indicated to confirm the diagnosis of total NLDO. Chronic dacryocystitis is treated before elective intraocular surgery.

Meireles MN, Viveiros MM, Meneghin RL, Galindo-Ferreiro A, Marques ME, Schellini SA. Dacryocystorhinostomy as a treatment of chronic dacryocystitis in the elderly. *Orbit.* 2017;36(6):419–421.

Neoplasm

Lacrimal Gland

Neoplasms of the lacrimal gland are discussed in Chapter 5.

Lacrimal Drainage System

Neoplastic causes of acquired obstruction of the lacrimal drainage system may be classified into the following groups:

- primary lacrimal drainage system tumors (most commonly papilloma and squamous cell carcinoma; Fig 15-26)
- primary tumors of tissues surrounding the lacrimal drainage system that secondarily invade or compromise lacrimal system structures (most commonly basal and squamous cell carcinoma of the eyelid skin; others include adenoid cystic carcinoma, infantile [capillary] hemangioma, inverted papilloma, epidermoid carcinoma, osteoma, and lymphoma)
- tumors metastatic to the nasolacrimal region

Primary lacrimal sac tumors are rare and should be considered for any mass that presents above the medial canthal tendon. They may be associated with epiphora or chronic dacryocystitis. Some patients report spontaneous bleeding, or blood may reflux from the punctum on irrigation. Tumors that invade the skin may produce ulceration with telangiectasia over the lacrimal sac. Metastasis to regional lymph nodes may also occur. CT and MRI have replaced dacryocystography as the way to identify neoplasms and

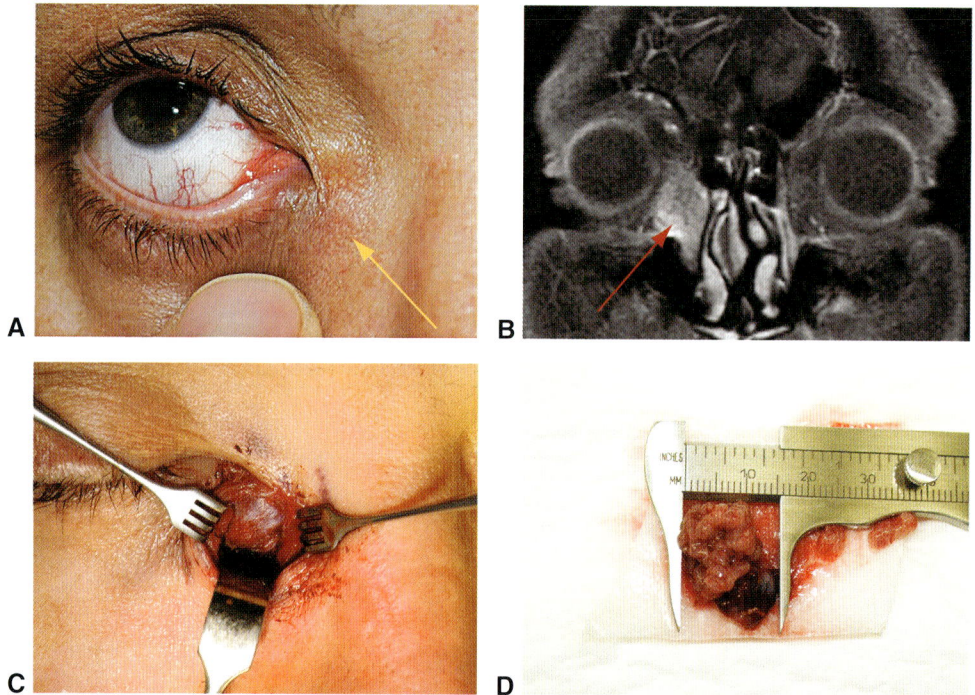

Figure 15-26 Papillary squamous cell carcinoma of the right lacrimal sac. **A,** Palpable mass over the right lacrimal sac *(arrow)*. **B,** Magnetic resonance imaging scan shows a mass within the right lacrimal sac *(arrow)*. **C,** Incisional biopsy through an external approach. **D,** Lacrimal sac biopsy reveals papillary squamous cell carcinoma. *(Courtesy of Bobby S. Korn, MD, PhD.)*

determine disease extent. CT also has the advantage of facilitating the assessment of bone erosion.

On histologic examination, approximately 45% of lacrimal sac tumors are benign and 55% are malignant. Squamous cell papillomas and carcinomas are the most common tumors of the sac. Many papillomas initially grow in an inverted pattern and into the lacrimal sac wall; consequently, their excision is often incomplete. With recurrence, malignant degeneration may occur.

Treatment of benign lacrimal sac tumors commonly requires a *dacryocystectomy*. Malignant tumors may require a dacryocystectomy combined with a lateral rhinotomy and medial maxillectomy, sometimes performed in concert with an otolaryngologist. *Exenteration,* including bone removal in the medial canthal area, is necessary if a malignant epithelial tumor involves bone and the soft tissues of the orbit (see Chapter 8). *Radiation* is useful for treatment of lymphomatous lesions, as an adjuvant after removal of malignant lesions, or as a palliative measure for unresectable lesions.

Basic Texts

Oculofacial Plastic and Orbital Surgery

Albert DM, Lucarelli MJ, eds. *Clinical Atlas of Procedures in Ophthalmic and Oculofacial Surgery*. 2nd ed. New York: Oxford University Press; 2012.

Azizzadeh B, Murphy MR, Johnson CM, Massry GG, Fitzgerald R, eds. *Master Techniques in Facial Rejuvenation*. 2nd ed. Philadelphia: Elsevier; 2017.

Baker SR. *Local Flaps in Facial Reconstruction*. 3rd ed. Philadelphia: Elsevier/Saunders; 2014.

Black EH, Nesi FA, Calvano CJ, Gladstone GJ, Levine MR, eds. *Smith and Nesi's Ophthalmic Plastic and Reconstructive Surgery*. 3rd ed. New York: Springer; 2012.

Bron AJ, Tripathi RC, Tripathi BJ. *Wolff's Anatomy of the Eye and Orbit*. 8th ed. Philadelphia: A Hodder Arnold Publication; 1997.

Chen WP. *Asian Blepharoplasty and the Eyelid Crease*. 3rd ed. Philadelphia: Elsevier; 2016.

Codner MA, McCord CD Jr, eds. *Eyelid and Periorbital Surgery*. 2nd ed. New York: Thieme; 2016.

Dutton JJ. *Atlas of Clinical and Surgical Orbital Anatomy*. 2nd ed. Philadelphia: Elsevier/Saunders; 2011.

Dutton JJ. *Atlas of Oculoplastic and Orbital Surgery*. 2nd ed. Philadelphia: Wolters Kluwer/Lippincott Williams & Wilkins; 2018.

Dutton JJ. *Radiology of the Orbit and Visual Pathways*. Philadelphia: Elsevier/Saunders; 2010.

Ellis E, Zide MF. *Surgical Approaches to the Facial Skeleton*. 3rd ed. Philadelphia: Wolters Kluwer/Lippincott Williams & Wilkins; 2018.

Fagien S. *Putterman's Cosmetic Oculoplastic Surgery*. 4th ed. Philadelphia: Elsevier/Saunders; 2008.

Fay A, Dolman PJ, eds. *Diseases and Disorders of the Orbit and Ocular Adnexa*. Philadelphia: Elsevier; 2016.

Holck DEE. *Evaluation and Treatment of Orbital Fractures: A Multidisciplinary Approach*. Philadelphia: Elsevier/Saunders; 2005.

Katowitz JA, Katowitz WR, eds. *Pediatric Oculoplastic Surgery*. 2nd ed. Cham, Switzerland: Springer International Publishing; 2018.

Korn BS, Kikkawa DO, eds. *Video Atlas of Oculofacial Plastic and Reconstructive Surgery*. 2nd ed. Philadelphia: Elsevier; 2017.

Lemke BN, Della Rocca RC, eds. *Surgery of the Eyelids and Orbit: An Anatomical Approach*. East Norwalk, CT: Appleton & Lange; 1992.

Levine MR, Allen RC, eds. *Manual of Oculoplastic Surgery*. 5th ed. Cham, Switzerland: Springer International Publishing; 2018.

Massry GG, Murphy MR, Azizzadeh B, eds. *Master Techniques in Blepharoplasty and Periorbital Rejuvenation*. New York: Springer-Verlag; 2011.

Nerad JA. *Techniques in Ophthalmic Plastic Surgery: A Personal Tutorial.* Philadelphia: Elsevier/Saunders; 2009.

Rootman J, ed. *Diseases of the Orbit: A Multidisciplinary Approach.* 2nd ed. Philadelphia: Wolters Kluwer/Lippincott Williams & Wilkins; 2002.

Rootman J, ed. *Orbital Surgery: A Conceptual Approach.* 2nd ed. Philadelphia: Wolters Kluwer/Lippincott Williams & Wilkins; 2013.

Shields JA, Shields CL. *Eyelid, Conjunctival, and Orbital Tumors: An Atlas and Textbook.* 3rd ed. Philadelphia: Wolters Kluwer/Lippincott Williams & Wilkins; 2016.

Spencer WH, ed. *Ophthalmic Pathology: An Atlas and Textbook.* 4th ed. Philadelphia: WB Saunders; 1996.

Sundar G, ed. *Orbital Fractures: Principles, Concepts & Management.* New York: Imaging Science Today; 2018.

Tse DT. *Color Atlas of Oculoplastic Surgery.* 2nd ed. Philadelphia: Wolters Kluwer/Lippincott Williams & Wilkins; 2011.

Tyers AG, Collin JRO. *Colour Atlas of Ophthalmic Plastic Surgery.* 4th ed. London: Elsevier; 2018.

Yen MT, ed. *Surgery of the Eyelids, Lacrimal System, and Orbit.* 2nd ed. Ophthalmology Monographs 8. New York: Oxford University Press; 2012.

Zide BM. *Surgical Anatomy Around the Orbit: The System of Zones.* Philadelphia: Wolters Kluwer/Lippincott Williams & Wilkins; 2006.

Related Academy Materials

The American Academy of Ophthalmology is dedicated to providing a wealth of high-quality clinical education resources for ophthalmologists.

Print Publications and Electronic Products

For a complete listing of Academy products related to topics covered in this BCSC Section, visit our online store at https://store.aao.org/clinical-education/topic/oculoplastics -orbit.html. Or call Customer Service at 866.561.8558 (toll free, US only) or +1 415.561.8540, Monday through Friday, between 8:00 am and 5:00 pm (PST).

Online Resources

Visit the Ophthalmic News and Education (ONE®) Network at aao.org/onenetwork to find relevant videos, online courses, journal articles, practice guidelines, self-assessment quizzes, images and more. The ONE Network is a free Academy-member benefit.

Access free, trusted articles and content with the Academy's collaborative online encyclopedia, EyeWiki, at aao.org/eyewiki.

Requesting Continuing Medical Education Credit

The American Academy of Ophthalmology is accredited by the Accreditation Council for Continuing Medical Education (ACCME) to provide continuing medical education for physicians.

The American Academy of Ophthalmology designates this enduring material for a maximum of 10 *AMA PRA Category 1 Credits™*. Physicians should claim only the credit commensurate with the extent of their participation in the activity.

To claim *AMA PRA Category 1 Credits™* upon completion of this activity, learners must demonstrate appropriate knowledge and participation in the activity by taking the posttest for Section 7 and achieving a score of 80% or higher.

This Section of the BCSC has been approved as a Maintenance of Certification Part II self-assessment CME activity.

To take the posttest and request CME credit online:

1. Go to www.aao.org/cme-central and log in.
2. Click on "Claim CME Credit and View My CME Transcript" and then "Report AAO Credits."
3. Select the appropriate media type and then the Academy activity. You will be directed to the posttest.
4. Once you have passed the test with a score of 80% or higher, you will be directed to your transcript. *If you are not an Academy member, you will be able to print out a certificate of participation once you have passed the test.*

CME expiration date: June 1, 2022. *AMA PRA Category 1 Credits™* may be claimed only once between June 1, 2019, and the expiration date.

For assistance, contact the Academy's Customer Service department at 866-561-8558 (US only) or +1 415-561-8540 between 8:00 am and 5:00 pm (PST), Monday through Friday, or send an e-mail to customer_service@aao.org.

Study Questions

Please note that these questions are not part of your CME reporting process. They are provided here for your own educational use and identification of any professional practice gaps. The required CME posttest is available online (see "Requesting CME Credit"). Following the questions are a blank answer sheet and answers with discussions. Although a concerted effort has been made to avoid ambiguity and redundancy in these questions, the authors recognize that differences of opinion may occur regarding the "best" answer. The discussions are provided to demonstrate the rationale used to derive the answer. They may also be helpful in confirming that your approach to the problem was correct or, if necessary, in fixing the principle in your memory. The Section 7 faculty thanks the Self-Assessment Committee for developing these self-assessment questions.

1. While playing baseball, a 22-year-old man was struck in the right eye with a ball. His visual acuity is 20/20 in both eyes. Intraocular pressure and fundus examinations are normal. A computed tomography (CT) scan shows a fracture of the right socket that extends to approximately two-thirds of the orbital floor. What is the most likely clinical finding?

   a. epistaxis

   b. cerebrospinal fluid rhinorrhea

   c. horizontal diplopia

   d. cranial nerve (CN) V_2 hypoesthesia

2. What is the main role of checkpoint inhibitors?

   a. They target the CTLA-4 protein against melanoma.

   b. They allow for T-cell activation for tumor destruction.

   c. They block the sonic hedgehog signaling pathway of basal cell carcinoma.

   d. They treat recurrent multiple myeloma.

3. A patient with diffuse actinic changes and a history of renal transplantation presents with progressive external ophthalmoplegia and forehead numbness that has progressed over several months. What is the most likely diagnosis?

   a. perineural spread of cutaneous squamous cell carcinoma

   b. orbital spread of a bacterial sinusitis

   c. Tolosa-Hunt syndrome

   d. microvascular cranial neuropathy

4. A physician is asked to treat a child who has received a dog bite to the face. What should the antibiotic coverage for this child include?

   a. anaerobic organisms, including bacteroides

   b. *Pasteurella canis*

   c. mixed organism flora

   d. *Neisseria* species

5. A physician is asked to examine a patient with periorbital trauma. What would be the best way to determine whether there has been an avulsion of the medial or lateral canthal tendon?

   a. pulling the eyelid and palpating the insertions of the tendon

   b. observing the contour of the eyelids and the position of the puncta

   c. reviewing the medical history and the mechanism of the trauma

   d. probing and irrigating the lacrimal outflow

6. A 20-year-old man is examined for ptosis of the right upper eyelid. His margin–reflex distance 1 (MRD_1) is 2 mm greater when in downgaze than in primary gaze, and in upgaze the eyelid covers the pupil almost completely. There is decreased retropulsion of the right globe. What is the most likely etiology of his ptosis?

   a. congenital ptosis

   b. superior orbital mass

   c. ocular myasthenia

   d. dehiscence of the aponeurosis

7. While hospitalized for a presumed exacerbation of asthma, a 50-year-old man is noted to have moderate right upper eyelid ptosis. The ptosis has been intermittently present for several months. The ophthalmologist discusses management of the patient with the gastroenterologist, who was called to evaluate dysphagia. What is the optimal next step in this patient's management?

   a. external levator resection, performed while in the hospital

   b. electromyography and edrophonium (Tensilon) testing

   c. internal ptosis repair as an outpatient

   d. anti-acetylcholine receptor antibody testing

8. A patient is referred for an ocular examination for unilateral blurred vision and discomfort that she has experienced since undergoing surgery. The surgical procedures included face-lift, rhytidectomy, upper eyelid blepharoplasty, brow-lift, and injections of dermal filler in both lower eyelids. A decade previously, she had laser in situ keratomileusis (LASIK). What is the most likely etiology to inquire about when speaking to the referring plastic surgeon?

   a. central retinal artery occlusion (CRAO) resulting from intravascular injection of filler

   b. facial nerve paralysis from the face-lift

   c. lower eyelid soft tissue necrosis from injection of filler

   d. lagophthalmos from the brow-lift and blepharoplasty

9. What is the most concerning complication associated with laser skin resurfacing?

   a. herpes simplex virus reactivation

   b. entropion

   c. residual fat prolapse

   d. skin pigmentation irregularities

10. A mother is concerned that her newborn baby does not produce tears when he cries. The ophthalmologist reassures her and explains that the lacrimal gland is not yet fully developed. At approximately what age will the baby's lacrimal gland be fully developed?

 a. 2 weeks

 b. 4 weeks

 c. 6 weeks

 d. 8 weeks

11. What procedure is used to treat tearing following chemotherapy with docetaxel?

 a. frequent irrigation and probing

 b. dacryocystorhinostomy

 c. punctal plugs

 d. conjunctivodacryocystorhinostomy

12. A 58-year-old woman presents for evaluation of right upper eyelid ptosis. The clinical assessment shows that she has an MRD_1 of 2.5 mm on the right and 3.0 mm on the left. The ophthalmologist notices that the right superior sulcus is deeper compared to the left. Hertel exophthalmometry measurements demonstrate 4 mm of right enophthalmos. There is no history of trauma. What is the most likely radiographic finding?

 a. metastatic prostate carcinoma

 b. meningioma

 c. metastatic breast carcinoma

 d. maxillary sinus tumor

13. Following blunt orbital trauma, what imaging modality is most appropriate?

 a. computed tomography (CT) scan with contrast

 b. magnetic resonance imaging (MRI)

 c. CT scan without contrast

 d. MRI with contrast

14. Following excision of a large dermolipoma, a patient reports experiencing severe dry eye. What structure is most likely to have been injured during the procedure?

 a. lacrimal gland ductules

 b. meibomian glands

 c. glands of Zeis

 d. glands of Wolfring

15. A 47-year-old woman presents with unilateral right proptosis and eyelid retraction. Her visual acuity is 20/40 in the right eye, which has limitation in right abduction and upgaze. There is moderate staining of her ocular surface on the right side. What is the most appropriate next step in management?

    a. eyelid retraction repair

    b. orbital decompression

    c. thyroid lab testing

    d. strabismus surgery

16. A 57-year-old nonsmoking woman presents with right orbital inflammation and tenderness along the superior lateral orbital rim. Visual acuity, ocular examination, and motility are normal. Her medical history includes chronic asthma and ulcerative colitis. A CT scan shows a right enlarged lacrimal gland. Pathology shows nonspecific inflammation. A test for what other inflammatory marker should be requested?

    a. interleukin-2 (IL-2)

    b. tumor necrosis factor alpha (TNF-α)

    c. immunoglobulin E (IgE)

    d. immunoglobulin G4 (IgG4)

17. A 41-year-old man presents at a clinic with spontaneous right eye enophthalmos, a deep superior sulcus, and mild upper eyelid retraction that occurred 1 week ago. He has just returned from vacation in Australia, where he went scuba diving for the first time. Since his return, he has had intermittent diplopia in upgaze. On examination, he is alert, oriented, and afebrile; all cranial nerves are intact. He is somewhat tender over the right maxillary sinus with percussion. What is the most likely cause of the spontaneous enophthalmos?

    a. osteoma

    b. neurofibromatosis with plexiform infiltration

    c. new cranial nerve palsy from progression of pseudotumor cerebri

    d. silent sinus syndrome

18. An ophthalmologist receives a call from an emergency department regarding a patient who has a posttraumatic orbital compartment syndrome (OCS) and an orbital floor fracture noted on CT scan. The ophthalmologist is over 90 minutes away from the emergency department. What is the best management for the patient until the ophthalmologist arrives?

    a. intravenous fluids and pain control

    b. lateral canthotomy and cantholysis performed by the emergency department physician

    c. obtain CT to confirm an OCS

    d. medically clear the patient for an urgent bony orbital decompression

19. What distinction makes wooden orbital foreign bodies difficult to manage?
    a. They appear radiopaque on CT.
    b. They often splinter upon entry into the orbit.
    c. They frequently harbor fungal pathogens.
    d. They usually have concomitant intracranial involvement.

20. Because of what anatomic finding are orbital roof fractures more likely to happen in young children than in adults?
    a. larger frontal sinuses in young children
    b. over-projection of the midface in young children
    c. larger cranial vault-to-face ratio in young children
    d. underdeveloped frontal lobe in young children

21. A transnasal endoscopic orbitotomy would be most effective in what procedure?
    a. removal of a lateral orbital apical lesion
    b. removal of the lamina papyracea
    c. excision of a superomedial dermoid cyst
    d. biopsy of a ciliary ganglion tumor

22. What postoperative care should be taken following orbitotomy?
    a. admission for overnight observation
    b. systemic corticosteroids to decrease edema
    c. pressure patching the orbit for 24 to 48 hours
    d. placement of a drain in all patients

23. Six months after enucleation, a patient returns to the office reporting mucoid discharge from the anophthalmic side. There is no pain. She states the prosthesis fits well. What is the most likely cause of the mucus discharge?
    a. papillary conjunctivitis
    b. implant extrusion
    c. implant infection
    d. lower eyelid entropion

24. What is one advantage of enucleation compared to evisceration?
    a. It is a technically easier procedure to perform.
    b. It results in better implant motility.
    c. It will not expose an occult intraocular malignancy.
    d. It has a lower rate of implant extrusion.

330 • Study Questions

25. Injury to the facial nerve can occur during what surgical maneuver?
    a. dissection superficial to the superficial musculoaponeurotic system (SMAS) inferior to the zygoma
    b. eyelid crease incision
    c. dissection deep to the temporoparietal fascia above the zygoma
    d. dissection superficial to the periosteum over the zygoma bone

26. What is the best way to minimize the incidence of brow ptosis after superficial temporal artery biopsy?
    a. Perform the biopsy close to the zygomatic arch.
    b. Make the incision 2.5 cm lateral to the lateral canthus.
    c. Biopsy the parietal branch of the artery.
    d. Perform the biopsy below the level of the brow.

27. What anatomic structure's function results in lower eyelid retraction in downgaze?
    a. The capsulopalpebral fascia is linked to the fascia of the inferior rectus muscle.
    b. The orbital septum retracts the eyelid as the suborbicularis fat contracts during infraduction.
    c. The inferior oblique muscle sends muscle fibers (the inferior tarsal muscle) to the inferior tarsus.
    d. The inferior tarsal muscle is a direct extension of the inferior rectus muscle.

28. During upper eyelid blepharoplasty, an ophthalmologist identifies the peripheral arterial arcade. This finding means that the ophthalmologist has dissected down to what structure?
    a. orbital septum
    b. Müller muscle
    c. levator aponeurosis
    d. conjunctiva

29. The suborbicularis oculi fat layer is anatomically equivalent to what other facial fat layer?
    a. orbital fat
    b. subcutaneous fat
    c. retro-orbicularis oculi fat
    d. temporal fat pad

Answer Sheet for Section 7 Study Questions

Question	Answer	Question	Answer
1	a b c d	16	a b c d
2	a b c d	17	a b c d
3	a b c d	18	a b c d
4	a b c d	19	a b c d
5	a b c d	20	a b c d
6	a b c d	21	a b c d
7	a b c d	22	a b c d
8	a b c d	23	a b c d
9	a b c d	24	a b c d
10	a b c d	25	a b c d
11	a b c d	26	a b c d
12	a b c d	27	a b c d
13	a b c d	28	a b c d
14	a b c d	29	a b c d
15	a b c d		

Answers

1. **d.** The clinical scenario presented is a right orbital floor fracture. The infraorbital groove and infraorbital canal, which transmit the infraorbital artery and the maxillary division of the trigeminal nerve, travel along the orbital floor and can be injured. Clinically, patients are likely to present with cranial nerve (CN) V_2 hypoesthesia that is typically transient. Epistaxis is more likely to occur after medial wall fracture or trauma. Cerebrospinal fluid rhinorrhea is likely to occur after an orbital roof fracture. Diplopia following a floor fracture is more likely to occur in vertical gaze rather than horizontal gaze.

2. **b.** Checkpoint inhibitors have been approved for use in the treatment of recurrent melanoma. They work by "unleashing" T cells that are normally kept in check by signaling proteins. This allows for an immune response against the melanoma. Checkpoint inhibitors target the PD-1 protein, not CTLA-4, to boost the immune response against melanoma cells. They are not used for the treatment of either basal cell carcinoma or recurrent multiple myeloma. The sonic hedgehog signaling pathway of basal cell carcinoma is treated by a variety of sonic hedgehog inhibitors (eg, vismodegib), not checkpoint inhibitors.

3. **a.** A perineural spread of a cutaneous squamous cell carcinoma (SCC) along the facial sensory nerves into the skull base (orbital apex and cavernous sinus) should be suspected in any patient with actinic changes or a history of facial cutaneous malignancies who presents with progressive periocular sensory and motor changes. SCC has a propensity for sensory nerves, and it occurs much more frequently in individuals with chronic immunosuppression (eg, those who have undergone renal transplantation). Bacterial sinusitis typically occurs in a fulminant fashion, and orbital involvement usually manifests with external eyelid changes (eg, erythema, edema) and proptosis. However, more indolent fungal sinusitis, especially aspergillosis, may occur in a slowly progressive manner. Tolosa-Hunt syndrome is an ill-defined cavernous sinus inflammation that presents with explosive pain and responds to systemic corticosteroids. It is a diagnosis of exclusion, because other pathologies may mimic its symptoms. Microvascular cranial neuropathy typically affects only 1 cranial nerve and typically resolves within 100 days. It does not usually affect sensory nerves.

4. **c.** Dog bites are polymicrobial; they include anaerobes and aerobes (both gram-positive and gram-negative), as well as specific species such as *Pasteurella canis*. Therefore, bites should be treated with broad-spectrum coverage.

5. **a.** Although observing the contour of the eyelids and the position of the puncta, reviewing the medical history and the mechanism of the trauma, and probing and irrigating the lacrimal outflow may all provide some information about the status of the canthal tendons and their possible need for repair, the only definitive (and therefore mandatory) way to determine whether there is an avulsion involves pulling directly on the eyelid, against the vector of the tendon. Probing and irrigation assess tear outflow, which could be affected by a medial canthal injury.

6. **b.** Eyelid retraction in downgaze that causes an increase in the margin–reflex distance 1 (MRD_1) is typical of congenital ptosis, in which the muscle is maldeveloped and is thus unable to relax and stretch in downgaze. However, this may also be true for infiltrative and compressive lesions involving the levator muscle, and in congenital ptosis, there should be normal retropulsion of the globes. The presence of a superior orbital mass may result

in decreased retropulsion of the globe with associated ptosis. Ocular myasthenia is associated with fluctuating ptosis, and this is not discussed in this scenario. Finally, dehiscence of the aponeurosis is not associated with lid lag as noted in downgaze.

7. **b.** Considering the constellation of ptosis, breathing difficulties, and trouble swallowing, myasthenia gravis is a reasonable and somewhat urgent concern, and the patient should undergo electromyography and erdrophonium (Tensilon) testing to confirm the diagnosis. Although antibody testing is useful, it will take time to get the results. Surgery is typically considered only after a diagnosis has been made and, if possible, the condition has been medically managed.

8. **d.** Disorders of eyelid closure associated with ocular surface and tear film irregularities would be the most likely cause, particularly in a patient who has undergone an overly aggressive brow-lift and/or upper eyelid blepharoplasty. Central retinal artery occlusion (CRAO) and soft tissue necrosis are certainly potential complications from injection of fillers; however, the former would present with frank and complete or partial vision loss without discomfort, and the latter would cause fairly immediate redness and swelling as well as facial (but not necessarily eye) discomfort. Facial palsy is a less likely complication from skin-tightening procedures than are paresis or lagophthalmos.

9. **a.** Because herpes virus reactivation can lead to severe facial skin infection and permanent scarring, most surgeons prophylactically treat patients with antiviral medication against outbreaks of herpes simplex virus prior to laser skin resurfacing. Eyelid malposition can occur with excessive tightening of skin and may require additional surgeries to treat lagophthalmos or ectropion (not entropion). Fat removal is not treated with laser resurfacing, but rather with blepharoplasty. Pigmentary skin changes, particularly with darker-pigmented patients, may be a relative contraindication for the procedure. In many cases, skin resurfacing serves as an adjunct procedure with blepharoplasty in order to better correct tissue laxity.

10. **c.** The lacrimal gland is not fully developed and functional until the infant is about 6 weeks old. Thus, newborn infants do not produce tears when crying.

11. **d.** Canalicular obstruction resulting from chemotherapeutic agents such as docetaxel (or 5-fluorouracil) is treated with conjunctivodacryocystorhinostomy, because a dacryocystorhinostomy procedure requires intact canaliculi through which the intubation tubes are placed. Intermittent irrigation is usually not sufficient to treat the tearing, and prophylactic intubation is best done prior to the onset of chronic tearing and structural canalicular stenosis. Punctal plugs are used to treat aqueous tear deficiency and are not appropriate in the setting of a canalicular obstruction.

12. **c.** Enophthalmos may occur as a result of volume expansion of the orbit (fracture), in association with orbital varix or secondary to sclerosing orbital tumors (eg, metastatic breast carcinoma). Metastatic prostate carcinoma is most likely to displace the globe anteriorly, especially if it has metastasized intraconally. Similarly, meningiomas typically displace the globe anteriorly. A maxillary sinus tumor is most likely to invade the orbit from the floor, displacing the globe superiorly.

13. **c.** Computed tomography (CT) and magnetic resonance imaging (MRI) are both important imaging modalities in the detection and characterization of orbital and ocular diseases. For evaluating a trauma, however, CT is currently the primary and single most–useful orbital imaging technique. It is often readily available and rapidly provides the

information necessary for decision-making. Although contrast agents can be used, they are not necessary for orbital evaluation following trauma. MRI generally provides better tissue contrast than CT; however, in most orbital conditions, the orbital fat provides sufficient natural tissue contrast to allow ready visualization of orbital tumors on CT.

14. **a.** During resection of a dermolipoma, the overlying conjunctiva should be preserved. Care must be taken to avoid damage to the lacrimal gland ducts, the extraocular muscles, and the levator aponeurosis. Although the glands of Wolfring are salivary excretory glands, these are fewer in quantity and distribution along the conjunctiva. The meibomian glands and the glands of Zeis are sebaceous glands that contribute to the tear film on the eyelid margin and on the lash cilia, respectively, and neither would likely be involved during the excision of a dermolipoma.

15. **c.** The clinical scenario presented is new-onset thyroid eye disease. Although the symptoms are moderate, the next appropriate step is to complete the workup to establish the diagnosis and the stage of the disease process. The surface disease should be managed nonsurgically for now and response to treatment reevaluated prior to proceeding with surgical intervention. Surgery may be required, but the typical pattern of management is orbital decompression, followed by strabismus surgery, and then eyelid retraction.

16. **d.** Immunoglobulin G4–related disease (IgG4-RD) is a fibroinflammatory disorder that may affect 1 or more organs. The disease most commonly affects the lacrimal gland within the orbit. Histologic examination shows lymphoplasmacytic infiltrates with large numbers of IgG4-positive plasma cells, storiform fibrosis, obliterative phlebitis, and eosinophil infiltration. In most cases, the ratio of IgG4/IgG plasma cells is greater than 40%. Serologic testing may show peripheral eosinophilia and elevated IgG4, but IgE is not typical. Interleukin-2 (IL-2), a lymphokine produced by activated T cells, has a wide variety of actions and plays a central role in immune regulation; however, IL-2 histology is not necessary for IgG4-related diseases. TNF-α levels are not diagnostic for IgG4-RD.

17. **d.** Silent sinus syndrome results from chronic subclinical sinusitis, which causes thinning of the bone of the involved sinus, leading to enophthalmos due to collapse of the orbital floor. The spontaneous collapse often occurs in association with a recent significant change in atmospheric pressure, for example in airplane travel or scuba diving. Osteoma is a nonepithelial tumor that can invade the orbit from the sinuses, nose, and facial bones. It is not typically spontaneous nor rapid in progression; thus, time to diagnosis may be slow. At the time of diagnosis, there may be extensive orbital involvement, a palpable orbital mass, and ocular muscle restriction. Plexiform neurofibromas are tumors formed by diffuse proliferation of Schwann cells within nerve sheaths. They are often associated with von Recklinghausen disease (neurofibromatosis 1), in which hamartomas may develop in the skin, eyes, central nervous system, and viscera. The most common orbital finding associated with plexiform neurofibromatosis is infiltration of the lateral upper eyelid, which causes an S-shaped contour to the eyelid margin and possible proptosis. Pseudotumor cerebri (also known as idiopathic intracranial hypertension) can cause cranial nerve VI palsy, which causes horizontal deviations, not vertical deviations.

18. **b.** Orbital compartment syndrome (OCS) may occur in a variety of settings (eg, posttraumatic or postsurgical hemorrhage, abscess formation, noninfectious inflammation). Posttraumatic OCS usually results from hemorrhage. Large orbital fractures expand the orbital compartment into the adjacent paranasal sinuses, and this may be relatively protective against the development of OCS. However, if bleeding continues, blood will fill

this larger compartment, resulting in OCS. Therefore, it is important not to discount the possibility of OCS in patients with orbital fractures. Prompt lateral canthotomy and cantholysis should be performed by the emergency department physician, particularly if the ophthalmologist is not able to perform the procedure in a timely fashion. Inadequate cantholysis will not relieve the OCS, and complete release should be verified once the ophthalmologist has arrived. Conservative management with IV fluids and pain management will only mask the pain noted in OCS. OCS is a clinical entity that can result in permanent visual loss if diagnosis is delayed. Therefore, definitive management should not be delayed by waiting for CT. OCS rarely manifests as a discrete hematoma on CT, but rather appears as an increased reticular signal in the intraconal fat. Posterior globe tenting may be seen on axial and parasagittal images, because the posterior sclera is distorted by proptosis and a stretched optic nerve. Bony orbital decompression is rarely needed in a patient with OCS. Use of intravenous mannitol may temporarily stabilize the OCS. If the OCS has not resolved, orbital surgery may be required.

19. **b.** Wooden orbital foreign bodies are the most common vegetal matter to enter the orbit. They often splinter upon orbital entry, and this may make them difficult to identify and remove during orbitotomy. It is not unusual for the patient to need several surgeries for removal, because each individual retained splinter causes orbital infection over time. In most cases, wooden orbital foreign bodies appear radiolucent on CT, although treated or painted lumber may appear radiopaque. The CT signal of wood is often misinterpreted as air. However, careful measurement of the specific Hounsfield units of the suspected wood and comparison to known air (eg, in the paranasal sinuses) by the radiologist often clinches the diagnosis and is a tool that should be used by the clinician. Wooden foreign bodies are notorious for causing severe orbital infections with atypical organisms, and these infections can result in permanent visual loss or spread along the skull base. However, the majority of these organisms are bacterial, not fungal. Concomitant intracranial involvement may occur with orbital wooden foreign bodies, but this is an exception rather than the rule. That said, any break in the orbital roof on CT should raise this possibility.

20. **c.** Orbital roof fractures occur much more commonly in young children than adults for 2 main reasons. First, pneumatized frontal sinuses, the structures that absorb much of the force of a frontal blow in adults, are not yet developed in children. This absence of pneumatized frontal sinuses allows force to be transferred directly to the orbital roof, resulting in fracture. Second, an infant or toddler has a much higher cranial vault-to-face ratio than an adult (8:1 vs 2:1, respectively) along with a flatter face, lacking the midfacial and nasal projection of adults. This results in a larger and more prominent forehead that is more susceptible to injury. The frontal lobe is not underdeveloped in young children.

21. **b.** A transnasal endoscopic approach to the orbit is useful in managing disease in the medial orbit. One of the most common uses of the transnasal approach is for removal of the lamina papyracea during medial orbital wall decompression for thyroid eye disease. The technique provides an excellent view of the medial orbital wall, optic canal, and skull base. Additionally, it has the theoretical advantage of minimizing iatrogenic compression of orbital soft tissue in an already congested orbit, since bone is removed from "outside in," as opposed to the transcaruncular approach. This technique should not be used in accessing lesions lateral to the optic nerve (lateral orbital apex ciliary ganglion). A superomedial dermoid cyst is usually located relatively anteriorly within the orbit and requires wide dissection for complete excision to avoid rupture; this is best achieved using standard anterior orbitotomy techniques.

22. **b.** Following an orbitotomy, patients can be observed for several hours postoperatively and then discharged to their homes, especially if the surgery was limited to the anterior orbit. Intravenous or oral corticosteroids are often prescribed in the immediate postoperative period to reduce edema in the hope of minimizing optic neuropathy. However, there is no definitive evidence that corticosteroids or antibiotics are effective or essential in all orbitotomies. More complex or deeper orbitotomies with a higher risk of postoperative orbital hemorrhages may be observed overnight and may require a drain, but a drain is usually not essential in anterior orbitotomies. Pressure patching is useful during extubation, but the patch should be removed once the patient is awake enough to cooperate with a clinical examination, both to ensure that there is no iatrogenic optic neuropathy and to allow the patient to monitor visual function postoperatively.

23. **a.** Chronic mucus discharge from an anophthalmic socket is usually due to a papillary conjunctivitis. This is thought to occur from protein buildup on the surface of the prosthesis, which then induces a conjunctival reaction. Prosthesis polishing and a course of topical corticosteroid drops often improve the symptoms. Implant extrusion can present in a similar fashion, but it is less common than papillary conjunctivitis. Implant infection is usually painful, and examination reveals purulent discharge. The weight of the prosthesis can stretch the lower eyelid over time, but this typically manifests as lower eyelid laxity with or without ectropion rather than entropion.

24. **c.** It is likely that the biggest advantage of enucleation over evisceration is that it will not expose an occult intraocular malignancy or disseminate it into the orbit. Evisceration should never be performed without a preoperative B-scan ultrasound to effectively rule out an intraocular mass. Neither CT nor MRI is as sensitive as B-scan in this regard. The possible increase in sympathetic ophthalmia (SO) rates following evisceration is controversial. Because of the rarity of SO, there is no large study proving the association between evisceration and SO. Evisceration is technically simpler to perform than enucleation, often requiring less intraoperative time and anesthesia. Implant motility is as good or better for evisceration compared with enucleation. Implant extrusion rates are likely equivalent between enucleation and evisceration; when performing evisceration on a phthisical eye, posterior sclerotomies are often necessary to accommodate the implant.

25. **d.** The facial nerve moves from a location deep to the superficial musculoaponeurotic system (SMAS) below the zygoma to superficial to the SMAS above the zygoma (the temporoparietal or superficial temporalis fascia); therefore, dissection in these locations requires caution. The innervation of the orbicularis is broad across the eyelid, so an eyelid crease incision does not paralyze the muscle.

26. **c.** The safest area to perform a temporal artery biopsy (TAB) of the frontal branch of the superficial temporal artery (STA) is either above the brow or more than 3.5 cm lateral to the lateral canthus. Brow ptosis is not an issue at all if the parietal branch of the STA is biopsied, but this usually requires shaving back the hairline. Although this adds a step to the procedure, it also hides the incision once the hair has grown back. The frontal branch of the facial nerve runs very superficially along the zygomatic arch and is vulnerable to injury if a TAB is performed in this location. Similarly, studies have shown that incisions within 3.5 cm of the lateral canthus or lateral eyebrow and below the brow have a higher incidence of brow ptosis. The area that lies between the zygomatic arch and the brow vertically and the lateral canthus to 3.5 cm lateral to it horizontally has therefore been dubbed the "danger zone" and should be avoided.

27. **a.** The anatomy of the lower eyelid is more primitive than that of the upper eyelid, but does allow for lower eyelid retraction during infraduction to clear the visual axis. This occurs because of a linkage between the inferior rectus and the inferior tarsus via the capsulopalpebral fascia (CPF). The outer fascia of the inferior rectus extends anteriorly to split around the inferior oblique muscle (IOM, which runs roughly perpendicular to the inferior rectus muscle) and then fuses at the anterior edge of the IOM to form the Lockwood suspensory ligament. The CPF arises from this area to attach to the inferior tarsus. Thus, as the inferior rectus muscle contracts to infraduct the eye, the CPF is pulled posteriorly and the tarsus (and lower eyelid) retracts inferiorly. The orbital septum is a static structure best described as an extension of periosteum arising at the arcus marginalis (orbital rim). The inferior tarsal muscle is a rudimentary smooth muscle akin to the superior tarsal muscle (Müller muscle) of the upper eyelid and is difficult to identify as a separate layer during surgery. From a practical standpoint, surgeons simply refer to the fused inferior tarsal muscle and CPF as one surgical layer (the "lower eyelid retractors"). Note that the inferior tarsal muscle is sympathetically innervated and can become paretic in Horner syndrome, resulting in a "reverse ptosis" of the lower eyelid; in other words, in Horner syndrome, the affected lower eyelid would be higher than the normal side.

28. **b.** The peripheral arterial arcade is an important anatomic landmark in upper eyelid surgery. It is located between the levator aponeurosis and Müller muscle just above the superior border of tarsus. Identification of the arcade during upper eyelid surgery means that the levator aponeurosis has dehisced. If this occurs during upper eyelid blepharoplasty, it may result in postoperative ptosis due to levator dehiscence. If the arcade is noted during blepharoplasty, the levator may need to be reattached to tarsus. Also, it is important to remember that both the upper and lower eyelid contain a marginal arterial arcade, but usually only the upper eyelid harbors a peripheral arcade.

29. **c.** Both the suborbicularis oculi fat (SOOF) and retro-orbicularis oculi fat (ROOF) separate facial mimetic muscles (orbicularis) from underlying periosteum. Orbital fat is behind the septum, a completely separate anatomic space, although the prolapse of orbital fat, SOOF, and ROOF contributes to aging effects. The temporal fat pad is sandwiched in as the deep temporalis fascia splits going over the zygomatic arch.

Index

(*f* = figure; *t* = table)